Management Practices for Controlling Nematode Parasites of Small Ruminants

_____

Management Practices for Controlling Nematode Parasites of Small Ruminants

Edited by

James E. Miller

Joan M. Burke

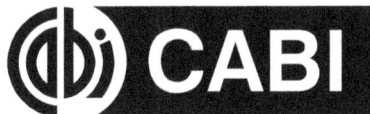

CABI is a trading name of CAB International

CABI
Nosworthy Way
Wallingford
Oxfordshire OX10 8DE
UK

CABI
200 Portland Street
Boston
MA 02114
USA

Tel: +44 (0)1491 832111
E-mail: info@cabi.org
Website: www.cabi.org

T: +1 (617)682-9015
E-mail: cabi-nao@cabi.org

The views expressed in this publication are those of the author(s) and do not necessarily represent those of, and should not be attributed to, CAB International (CABI). Any images, figures and tables not otherwise attributed are the author(s)' own. References to internet websites (URLs) were accu-rate at the time of writing.

CAB International and, where different, the copyright owner shall not be liable for technical or other errors or omissions contained herein. The information is supplied without obligation and on the understanding that any person who acts upon it, or otherwise changes their position in reliance thereon, does so entirely at their own risk. Information supplied is neither intended nor implied to be a substitute for professional advice. The reader/user accepts all risks and responsibility for losses, damages, costs and other consequences resulting directly or indirectly from using this information.

CABI's Terms and Conditions, including its full disclaimer, may be found at https://www.cabidigital-library.org/terms-and-conditions.

A catalogue record for this book is available from the British Library, London, UK.

ISBN-13: 9781800623743 (hardback)
          9781800623750 (ePDF)
          9781800623767 (ePub)

DOI: 10.1079/9781800623767.0000

Commissioning Editor: Alex Lainsbury
Editorial Assistant: Theresa Regueira
Production Editor: James Bishop

Typeset by Exeter Premedia Services Pvt Ltd, Chennai, India
Printed in the USA

Contents

Contributors

_____

Scott A. Bowdridge, School of Food and Agriculture, West Virginia University, Morgantown, West Virginia, USA. Email: scott.bowdridge@mail.wvu.edu.

Joan M. Burke, USDA, ARS, Dale Bumpers Small Farms Research Center, Booneville, Arkansas, USA. Email: joan.burke@usda.gov.

Ken Coffey, University of Arkansas System Division of Agriculture, Fayetteville, Arkansas, USA.

Richard A. Ehrhardt, Department of Animal Science, College of Agriculture and Natural Resources, Michigan State University, East Lansing, Michigan, USA, and Department of Large Animal Clinical Sciences, College of Veterinary Medicine, Michigan State University, East Lansing, Michigan, USA. Email: ehrhard5@msu.edu.

Heather Glennon, Agricultural Sciences Department, University of Mount Olive, Mount Olive, North Carolina, USA.

Hervé Hoste, Université de Toulouse, UMR 1225 IHAP INRAE/ENVT (retired), Toulouse, France.

Ray M. Kaplan, Department of Infectious Diseases, College of Veterinary Medicine, University of Georgia, Athens, Georgia, USA.

Kwame Matthews, Department of Agriculture & Natural Resources, Delaware State University, Dover, Delaware, USA.

James E. Miller, Department of Pathobiological Sciences (Emeritus), School of Veterinary Medicine, Louisiana State University, Baton Rouge, Louisiana, USA. Email: Jembrla@gmail.com.

James L.M. Morgan, Round Mountain Consulting, Fayetteville, Arkansas, USA.

Michael Pesato, Four State Veterinary Services, Newark, Delaware, USA. Email: mpasatodvm@gmail.com.

Dan Quadros, University of Arkansas System Division of Agriculture, Little Rock, Arkansas, USA. Email: dquardos@uark.edu.

Susan Schoenian, University of Maryland Extension (retired), Western Maryland Research & Education Center, Keedysville, Maryland, USA.

Leonor Sicalo Gianechini, Department of Infectious Diseases, College of Veterinary Medicine, University of Georgia Athens, Georgia, USA. Email: sicalo.leonor@uga.edu.

Thomas H. Terrill, Department of Agricultural Sciences Agricultural Research Station, Fort Valley State University, Fort Valley, Georgia, USA. Email: terrillt@fvsu.edu.

Juan Felipe de J. Torres-Acosta, Facultad de Medicina Veterinaria y Zootecnia, Universidad Autónoma de Yucatán, Mérida, Yucatán, México.

Adriano F. Vatta, Department of Pathobiological Sciences, Louisiana State University School of Veterinary Medicine, Baton Rouge, Louisiana, USA. Email: avatta2@lsu.edu.

Andrew R. Weaver, Department of Animal Science, North Carolina State University, Raleigh, North Carolina, USA.

Niki C. Whitley, Department of Agricultural Sciences Cooperative Extension, Fort Valley State University, Fort Valley, Georgia, USA. Email: whitleyn@fvsu.edu.

Anne Zajac, Department of Biomedical Sciences and Pathobiology (Emeritus), Virginia-Maryland College of Veterinary Medicine, Virginia Tech University, Blacksburg, Virginia, USA.

Introduction

How does one cope with the dangerous effects of small ruminant gastrointestinal nematode parasitism? Gastrointestinal nematodes are a continual major constraint to small ruminant production worldwide. Problems are often classified as a chronic subclinical/clinical production disease with losses that include reduced weight gain, weight loss, reproductive inefficiency, poor health, and death. The cost of treatment and prevention also needs to be considered. Loss estimates are difficult to measure because production diseases and disorders may result from interaction with other factors such as nutritional and environmental stresses, management methods, concurrent diseases, genetic predispositions, etc.

The age of modern anthelmintic control prevailed through the last half of the 20th century with the introduction of a series of effective anthelmintics. Anthelmintics became the accepted method for control as they are relatively easy to administer, and productivity thrived. Control programs based on frequent deworming of all animals in a flock or herd reduced the ability of gastrointestinal nematodes to affect animal health and production. However, it became apparent in the 1980s and 1990s that the efficacy of those anthelmintics was waning. To complicate matters, introduction of new anthelmintics was slow.

This book is a compilation of the research and extension efforts of members and colleagues that comprise the American Consortium for Small Ruminant Parasite Control (ACSRPC, www.wormx.info). The Consortium was formed in 2003 to address the need to investigate various alternatives, in addition to anthelmintic therapy, for controlling gastrointestinal nematode parasites of small ruminants due to the increased presence of reduced efficacy (i.e., resistance). If small ruminant production is to survive the continuous threat of infection and losses, a more integrated approach to control needs to be considered. Thus, the Consortium has worked over the past two decades to research and provide information on using anthelmintics smartly and providing alternatives that can be integrated for maintaining effective control. The bottom line is to be able to choose from all available methods to achieve an acceptable level of productivity.

James Miller is a retired Emeritus Professor, Louisiana State University School of Veterinary Medicine, Baton Rouge, Louisiana. USA. He taught ruminant parasitology to professional, graduate, and undergraduate students and conducted small ruminant nematode parasite research for 33 years. He received a BS degree (Biology) from the University of New Mexico, and DVM, MPVM (Preventive Medicine) and PhD (Parasitology) degrees from the University of California, Davis. He is board certified in parasitology in the American College of Veterinary Microbiology. After retirement, he elected to remain an active participant on several projects. He is a founding member of the ACSRPC. He is author and/or coauthor of numerous refereed journal articles, technical/report papers, proceedings papers, abstracts, and book chapters. He has been a research collaborator with national and international colleagues/organizations. He is a member of several professional organizations and participates as a consultant on two United States Department of Agriculture national projects: Increased Efficiency of Sheep Production and Sustainable Small Ruminant Production in the Southeastern US. His research interests have been epidemiology, control, and genetics of ruminant nematode parasitism and during his active career his research program focused on improving small ruminant production using an integrated approach to controlling parasites, specifically gastrointestinal nematodes of small ruminants.

Joan Burke is a research animal scientist with the United States Department of Agriculture-Agricultural Research Station, Booneville, Arkansas, USA. She received a BS degree (Animal Science) from Cornell University and PhD degree (Animal Science) from Oregon State University. She is a founding member of the ACSRPC. She conducts research on small ruminants with a focus on holistic gastrointestinal nematode parasite control. She has published research articles and factsheets and contributed to outreach events on management of gastrointestinal nematode parasites including use of FAMACHA©, copper oxide wire particles, sericea lespedeza, rotational grazing, genetic and genomic selection for parasite resistance, resilience and tolerance, and *Duddingtonia flagrans* (nematode-trapping fungus) as alternatives for traditional anthelmintic use. The genetic resistance of Katahdin sheep to nematode parasites along with selection for economically important traits led to collection of genotypes that were developed into genomic-enhanced estimated breeding values in the US National Sheep Improvement Program.

Chapters of the book include (1) Small Ruminant Gastrointestinal Nematode Biology and Epizootiology—life cycles and host/parasite/environment interactions are key to understanding, developing and using appropriate control methods; (2) Role of Nutrition in Small Ruminant Production and Gastrointestinal Nematode Management—nutrition is a key component in various management systems to keep animals healthy and productive; (3) Anthelmintics, Resistance, and Guidelines for Use in Controlling Gastrointestinal Nematodes of Small Ruminants—evolution of anthelmintics, mechanism of action, how resistance developed and how to use those that may still work; (4) Alternative Methods for the Control of Gastrointestinal Nematodes in Small Ruminants—alternatives to traditional drugs have been evaluated by the ACSRPC and others. Methods include copper oxide wire particles, nematode-trapping fungus, herbal remedies, diatomaceous earth, etc.; (5) Genetics of Gastrointestinal Nematode Resistance in Small Ruminants—differences exist within and between breeds and species and the role of genetic and genomic selection as a longer-term impact on developing parasite-resistant/resilient lines; (6) Benefits of Grazing Management and Pasture Species Rotation Systems for Integrated Gastrointestinal Nematode Parasite Management in Small Ruminant Production—role of pasture, animal grazing behavior, and herd/flock management so as to reduce exposure to gastrointestinal nematode parasites; (7) Bioactive Forages for the Control of Gastrointestinal Nematodes of Small Ruminants—role of forages that have been shown to have antiparasitic activity, including sericea lespedeza, birdsfoot trefoil, sanfoin, tropical species, etc.; (8) Diagnostics for the Management of Gastrointestinal Nematode Infections in Small Ruminants—various techniques are used for diagnosing gastrointestinal nematode infection, including fecal egg count, worm recovery/identification, FAMACHA/blood work, Drench-Rite™, etc.; (9) Improving the Effectiveness and Sustainability of Gastrointestinal Nematode Control in Cattle: Applying Lessons Learned from Small Ruminants to Forge a Brighter Future—gastrointestinal nematode control used in small ruminant production that might benefit cattle production, and vice versa; and (10) The Role of Extension in Gastrointestinal Nematode Control and Management—the importance of extending current control information/technologies from scientific discovery to applied application.

The information provided is intended to expand the "toolbox" for effective control. Information derived from current and future research will continuously evolve. For example, considering use of plants or secondary plant compounds, extracts, or combinations; the search for the perfect parasite-resistant genetics combined with optimal production traits; and knowledge of immune responses of responses that might be commercialized. There will always be a wish for a magic bullet—an effective anthelmintic that evades development of resistance by gastrointestinal nematodes without harm to the animal or environment. However, until then, we should consider what we know about the biology of the parasites and the animals, good management and nutrition, an awareness of risk factors that predispose animals to gastrointestinal nematode infection and using methods of control that readily apply to each individual farm. Funding for research on small ruminants, particularly in the US, is quite limited and relies on piecing together various opportunities and collaborations, or borrowing what is learned from other economically important farm species.

1 Small Ruminant Gastrointestinal Nematode Biology and Epizootiology

James E. Miller[1]* and Anne Zajac[2]

[1]*Department of Pathobiological Sciences (Emeritus), School of Veterinary Medicine, Louisiana State University, Baton Rouge, Louisiana, USA;* [2]*Department of Biomedical Sciences and Pathobiology (Emeritus), Virginia-Maryland College of Veterinary Medicine, Virginia Tech University, Blacksburg, Virginia, USA*

Abstract

Control of gastrointestinal nematode (GIN) parasites requires some nominal knowledge of the relevant parasites, the life cycles involved and the epizootiological/environmental aspects that affect transmission/infection. There are a multitude of complex interactions that are involved and it is impossible to cover them all here. Textbooks have been written that cover in-depth details for those who desire to gain such knowledge. The purpose of this chapter is to provide some basic information and concepts for the reader to better understand what the chapters in this book present.

Introduction

Ruminants (cattle, sheep, goats, and camelids) in the US and around the world are infected with a broad range of internal and external parasites. Infection with gastrointestinal nematode (GIN) parasites is probably the most serious constraint affecting production worldwide. Economic losses are caused by decreased production, cost of prevention, cost of treatment, and even death of infected animals. It is difficult by any form of major survey or other estimation to establish precise figures on losses incurred in production from infection and disease. Even minimal accuracy of loss estimates is difficult because production diseases or disorders may result from interaction with nutritional and environmental stresses, management methods, concurrent diseases, genetic predispositions, or other

factors. Periodic reports on such losses from governmental agencies and others always range into millions of dollars per year and include all phases of production. As such, problems with GIN are often classified as a production disease (i.e. chronic subclinical condition affecting productivity such as weight loss, reduced weight gain, reproductive inefficiency, etc.).

In the US, the Department of Agriculture, Animal Plant Health Inspection Service-Veterinary Service, National Animal Health Monitoring System (NAHMS) program periodically surveys sheep and goat producers to provide information on how they are managing their operations and what problems/issues they perceive as threatening the health and wellbeing of their animals. Sheep studies were conducted in 1996, 2001, and 2011. Those studies indicated that GIN continued to be a concern for producer

*Corresponding author: jembrla@gmail.com

© CAB International 2026. *Management Practices for Controlling Nematode Parasites of Small Ruminants* (eds James E. Miller and Joan M. Burke)
DOI: 10.1079/9781800623767.0001

losses and the 2025 study will describe management practices that producers use to control GIN and reduce resistance to anthelmintics. Knowing that goats have the same GIN as sheep, goat producers have similar concerns, especially when goats are allowed to graze. The 2009 and 2019 NAHMS goat studies provided information on practices that have been used to combat infections and addressed the issue of how to prevent anthelmintic resistance. However, it should be noted that when goats are managed as browsers, exposure to GIN is reduced and subsequently the effects would not be as severe.

All grazing small ruminants are infected with GIN and low infection level will usually have little impact on animal health. However, as infection level increases, signs of infection such as reduced appetite and reduced weight gain may begin to appear. With even heavier infection levels, clinical signs including weight loss, diarrhea, anemia, and bottle jaw may develop. Camelids (llamas and alpacas) can also be infected with these GIN and can suffer the same signs of disease, especially when numbers are high. Adult cattle and horses, however, usually do not become severely infected with sheep and goat GIN as they are considered dead-end hosts.

The community of GIN that infect grazing small ruminants contributes to disease and production losses. With the development of modern anthelmintics beginning in the 1960s, control programs based on frequent deworming of all animals in a flock or herd substantially reduced the ability of GIN to affect animal health and production. However, those programs were not sustainable because they led to the rapid development of anthelmintic resistance. Adequate control of GIN now requires integrated parasite management practices that are most effective when they are based on adequate knowledge of the GIN involved and their biology and epizootiology.

Gastrointestinal Nematodes

Descriptions for the GIN and other parasites included here reflect conditions found in the US. All are found throughout the world where similar conditions exist.

Abomasum

Haemonchus contortus (barber pole worm)

While all GIN can contribute to disease in small ruminants, the one that dominates in importance throughout the US is *Haemonchus contortus*, also known as the barber pole worm.

Adult worms are found in the abomasum, or fourth stomach compartment, which is the true stomach of small ruminants. In camelids, they are found in the third stomach compartment which lacks the separation of the omasum and abomasum and is the camelid equivalent of the abomasum. *Haemonchus contortus* is rather large compared to other abomasal and intestinal worms, measuring up to 2.5 cm in length, and is readily visible. When large numbers are present, *H. contortus* can be seen as thin red hair-like worms on the abomasal mucosal surface (Fig. 1.1).

Female worms are prolific egg-laying machines, 5000–10,000 eggs per day, and in large numbers with favorable conditions, they can contaminate the environment with a very large number of eggs. One of the reasons why *H. contortus* is such an important GIN is its mode of feeding. Unlike most GIN that feed on mucosal tissue or fluids, *H. contortus* feeds directly on host blood. It is a voracious blood feeder and gets its name due to the barber pole appearance of female worms consisting of the white ovaries that twist around the red blood-filled gut (Fig. 1.2). The head of the worm has a lancet (small "tooth") that is used to lacerate the abomasal mucosal wall which initiates capillary blood flow (Fig. 1.3). Blood is then ingested via a small opening behind the tip of the lancet.

Animals infected with large numbers of *H. contortus* show signs associated with loss of red blood cells and blood proteins that result in anemia and bottle jaw. Anemia is best visualized as pale mucous membranes (most visible by viewing inside the lower eyelid using the FAMACHA© technique). Bottle jaw is seen as pendulant edema, best seen as an accumulation of fluid under the chin (Fig. 1.4). The greater the infection level, the more blood is lost and eventually the animal becomes depressed, lethargic, anorexic, and may die. Severe infections are most likely to occur in young animals less than 6 months before immunity has developed. Long-term infection

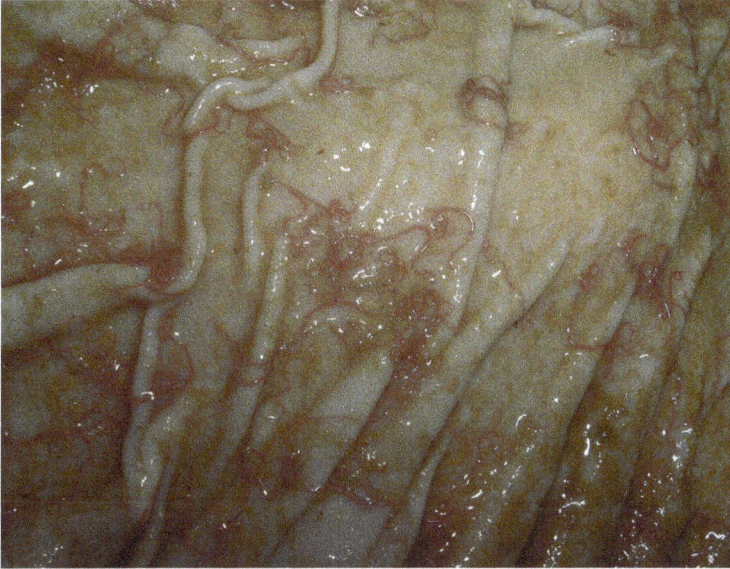

Fig. 1.1. Adult *Haemonchus contortus* on the abomasal mucosa. Courtesy of R. Kaplan, used with permission.

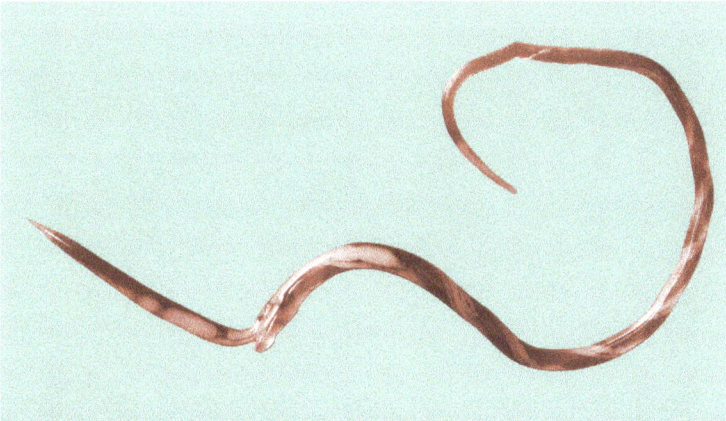

Fig. 1.2. Female *Haemonchus contortus* showing barber pole appearance with white ovaries twisted around the red blood-filled gut. Courtesy of J. Gilleard, used with permission.

with moderate numbers of *H. contortus* may lead to reduced growth and less severe anemia. This is especially likely to occur in animals on a nutritionally inadequate diet or with other chronic disease conditions.

Haemonchus contortus is found predominantly in tropical and subtropical regions of the world where environmental conditions are more conducive (i.e. hotter and wetter) for survival and development of the free-living larval stages on pasture. These conditions prevail in the south-eastern region of the US. However, in the rest of the US where similar environmental conditions are encountered during the summer, *H. contortus* transmission also frequently occurs. Transmission and infection are at the lowest level during the winter when environmental conditions are not conducive (i.e. colder and

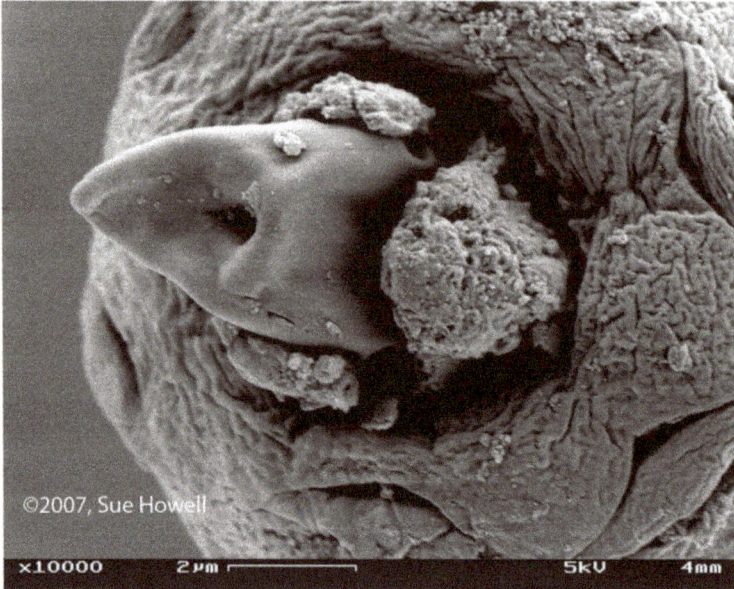

Fig. 1.3. Electron micrograph of *Haemonchus contortus* head end showing the lancet. Courtesy of S. Howell, used with permission.

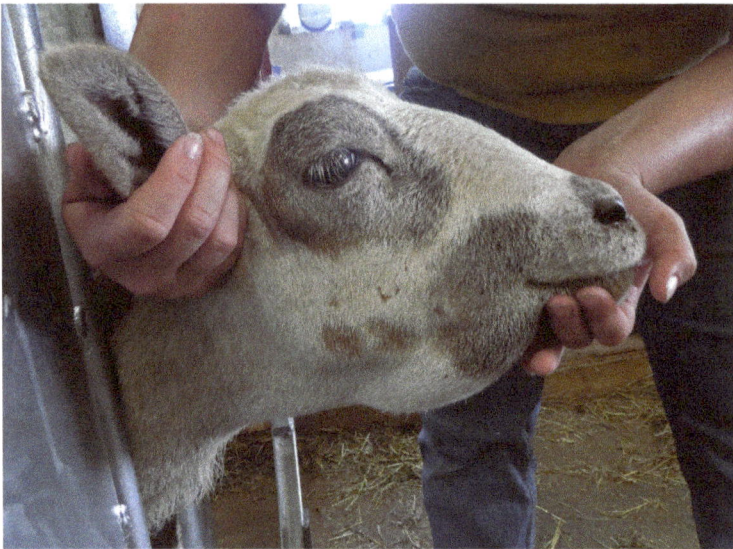

Fig. 1.4. Lamb with intermandibular edema (bottle jaw). Courtesy of S. Schoenian, used with permission.

dryer) to survival and development of the free-living larval stages. Transmission and infection increase with warmer temperatures and increasing moisture during the spring and peak during the summer. As temperatures dissipate during the fall, transmission and infection decrease. Hypobiosis (see below) occurs over winter in more northern/western temperate (cold/dry) regions of the US. It has not been observed to occur to any great extent in the south-eastern US because the life cycle can be maintained year around.

Teladorsagia circumcincta (brown stomach worm)

Another abomasal worm of major importance is *Teladorsagia circumcincta* which is smaller than *H. contortus* and not readily visible. This worm thrives in cooler wet environmental conditions which are encountered in the more temperate northern regions of the US (excludes most of the south-east). These worms feed mostly by consuming nutrients in mucus and do not feed on blood *per se*, but can ingest some blood if present. Female worms do not produce as many eggs as *H. contortus*, so contamination of the environment is not as high. Infection causes direct damage to the abomasal mucosa as they mature from larvae to adult worms, thereby interfering with digestion and appetite. Entwined masses of worms are found on the mucosa of the abomasum, which is inflamed, thickened, red, and covered with whitish nodules. Hypobiosis occurs when environmental conditions are too cold (northern/winter) or too dry (western/summer) with lesions on the mucosal wall of the abomasum which give it a leathery appearance.

Infection is usually considered a production disease as animals do not grow very well and death is not that common. Affected animals have reduced appetite and protein loss into the gut, resulting in a drop in weight gain. In sheep, wool growth and milk production can both be reduced before clinical signs become apparent. When infection reaches levels that cause clinical disease, the primary signs are diarrhea and emaciation. However, under very high infection conditions, death can result.

Trichostrongylus axei (stomach hair worm)

Trichostrongylus axei occurs commonly, often in association with *T. circumcincta*, but appears to be relatively harmless as the numbers are few. Adult worms are very small (smaller than *T. circumcincta*), slender, hair-like, and reddish-brown. Heavy infections may exacerbate inflammation of the abomasal mucosa caused by *T. circumcincta*.

Small intestine

Trichostrongylus colubriformis (bankrupt worm)

Trichostrongylus colubriformis is the most predominant small intestinal GIN. It is a very small hair-like worm and is found throughout the US where it seems to thrive better under northern temperate cooler and wetter conditions, like *T. circumcincta*. Together with *H. contortus*, these two worms account for the majority of problems on most farms. As with *T. circumcincta*, this worm feeds along the mucosa and interferes with nutrient absorption and diarrhea may ensue. It is called the bankrupt worm because death is seldom the result and animals become poor doers (lethargy and collapse, weight loss, damage and inflammation of the mucosa), leading to loss of production and income.

Nematodirus spp. (thin-necked intestinal worm)

Nematodirus spp. are relatively large worms which are easy to see. They are found in a small number of animals in the US except in cooler temperate areas where worms may accumulate in greater numbers. Problems are rare in the south-eastern region of the US. Damage to the mucosa is usually rare but mild inflammation may occur. Serious problems can occur in young animals, especially after grazing new short green forage subsequent to rain after dry periods. Such heavy infection results in lethargy and collapse, weight loss, severe inflammation, and diarrhea. Production and income losses are similar to those of *T. colubriformis*. While infection can cause disease in adult sheep, it is not very common as sheep develop a strong immunity. In contrast, adult goats do not develop such a strong immunity and disease is possible. It should be noted that *N. battus* is very pathogenic in areas of the world where it is present, but it is not present in most of the US except sporadically in parts of the north-west.

Cooperia curticei

Cooperia curticei is found mostly in small numbers in animals in the northern cooler temperate regions of the US. They are considered relatively nonpathogenic and are found coiled close along the mucosal wall of the small intestine. Infection does not usually cause disease or any characteristic signs but may contribute to the severity of disease in mixed infections especially with *T. circumcincta* and *T. colubriformis*.

Strongyloides papillosus (threadworm)

Strongyloides papillosus is a small thread-like worm often seen in animals throughout the US. Infection can result in mucosal inflammation and diarrhea typified by weight loss. The life cycle is not typical as for other GIN (see below) as it is more complex. Only parthenogenetic females are found in the animal. Eggs containing first-stage larvae (L1) are passed in the feces and development to the second- and third-stage larvae (L2 and L3, respectively) occurs on pasture. Infection may be direct by oral ingestion of L3 from forage or by L3 skin penetration, usually through the foot. Under moist conditions on pasture, some L3 continue development to mature adult worms and a sexual reproductive cycle may take place. Subsequently, L3 from that mating can continue the sexual reproductive cycle or be consumed during grazing where only parthenogenetic females survive to maturity. Heavy infection is associated with moist unhygienic conditions and high stocking rates.

Bunostomum phlebotomum (hookworm)

Bunostomum phlebotomum is rarely found in the US. It is a stout, readily visible worm with a large mouth and a body that may appear to be hook shaped. They prefer warmer, higher rainfall regions. They are usually not a problem but they are blood feeders and can contribute to anemia, being caused by *H. contortus*, and diarrhea, caused by other worms. Infection can be by oral ingestion of L3 during grazing or by skin penetration, usually around the feet which can lead to sore feet.

Large Intestine

Oesophagostomum spp. (nodular worm)

Oesophagostomum spp. is another large and clearly visible worm. They are found throughout the US, usually in rather small numbers. They feed on blood, contributing to the overall anemia being caused by *H. contortus* and other blood-feeding worms. Adult worms are found only in the large intestine and developing larvae are found in the mucosa of both the small and large intestine where they form nodules that are clearly visible, thus the name nodular worm. As larvae develop, they leave these nodules and migrate to the large intestine where they reside and mature to adults. Large numbers of these worms can cause severe disease resulting in lethargy, weight loss, and damage and inflammation of the mucosa (redness, thickening, and edema). A persistent green mucoid diarrhea may then occur. Young animals stressed by weaning typically show ill-thrift, lose condition, and become lethargic.

Trichuris spp. (whipworm)

Trichuris spp. is found throughout the US, usually in small numbers. They do not have a typical worm shape. The posterior end of the worm is rather large and can be easily seen. The anterior end of the worm is thin and thread-like (hard to see), thus the name whipworm. The head end of these worms imbeds in the mucosa and causes damage to capillary beds which can result in hemorrhage. They feed on fluids and blood and can contribute to the overall anemia being caused by *H. contortus* and other blood-feeding worms.

Other Internal Parasites

The following are not GIN parasites but deserve mention as they can be involved with overall mixed infections that commonly affect grazing animals and contribute to pathogenicity. In addition, their life cycles are different and involve some unique aspects.

Moniezia expansa (tapeworm)

Moniezia expansa is found throughout the US under all environmental conditions. They are flatworms composed of many segments and adults reside in the small intestine where they attach to the mucosa and feed by absorbing nutrients through the integument from surrounding digested materials. They grow longer (few feet) by adding new segments. Eventually, the most posterior egg-containing gravid segments break off and are expelled with the feces. Producers may become concerned about tapeworms when they can see the white grain-like gravid segments moving in freshly deposited feces. Eventually the segments deteriorate, and eggs are ingested by field mites and develop to the infective cysticercoid. Grazing animals ingest these mites and are infected when the cysticercoids develop to adult worms. Usually only one or two adult worms survive and become established in the animal. They do not cause much physical damage but infected young animals may not grow well, and intestinal blockage may rarely occur due to the worm mass. Fortunately, they do not live that long and are expelled due to a strong host immune response. Adult animals are rarely affected as immunity is considered lifelong.

Fasciola hepatica, Fascioloides magna (liver fluke)

Fasciola hepatica is found in low-lying perennial wet areas where the intermediate snail host is present. Adult flukes are flat and leaf-shaped and reside in the liver bile ducts where they deposit eggs which are passed in the feces. If the feces are deposited in water, the eggs will hatch and release a free-swimming miracidium which finds and infects a snail. Asexual reproduction occurs in the snail and several cercaria develop that then leave the snail and encyst on forage as metacercaria. Metacercaria are ingested by grazing animals and develop into immature flukes that find and migrate through the liver. Eventually immature flukes end up in the bile ducts and mature to adults. Damage from migrating immature flukes can be extensive and result in unthriftiness, weight loss, reduced gains, and sometimes death.

Infection with another liver fluke, the deer fluke (*Fascioloides magna*), is rare but should be considered where deer have access to pastures grazed by small ruminants. This fluke can kill animals by destroying the liver.

Dictyocaulus filaria, Muellerius capillaris, Protostrongylus spp. (lungworm)

Problems with lungworm infection are usually sporadic. Adult *Dictyocaulus filaria* (most pathogenic) live in the bronchi of the lungs and deposit eggs that are coughed up and hatch during transit through the gastrointestinal tract. The released L1 are then passed in the feces. The now free-living L1 develop to the infective L3 on pasture and are consumed by grazing animals. Infection results in respiratory distress (chronic coughing), unthriftiness, and sometimes death.

There are two other minor lungworms (*Muellerius capillaris* and *Protostrongylus* spp.) that require land snails/slugs as intermediate hosts to complete the life cycle. These worms reside in the lung parenchyma and are relatively isolated from the bronchi, thus not allowing very many eggs to reach the gastrointestinal tract to continue the life cycle. Fortunately, infection and pathogenesis are rare.

Parelaphostrongylus tenuis (meningeal worm)

Parelaphostrongylus tenuis frequently infects llamas, alpacas, and sometimes small ruminants, primarily goats. White-tailed deer are the natural host for this worm, so infection occurs where small ruminants interact with white-tailed deer. Adult worms reside in meningeal tissue of white-tailed deer and lay eggs which hatch into L1 that then migrate to the lungs via the blood. The L1 are shed in the feces where they are consumed by slug/snail intermediate hosts where they develop into L2 and L3. Small ruminants, which are not normal hosts, can ingest the slugs/snails harboring the L3 during grazing. The L3 migrate to locations where they do not normally reside in the deer. They migrate up the spinal nerves to the spinal cord and then they seem to 'wander' throughout the spinal cord and the brain (not in but around the spinal cord and brain). The central nervous system is damaged, and death may result. Often, only one animal is infected at a time on a single farm. Infected animals will display signs such as rear leg weakness/incoordination, paralysis, circling, abnormal head position, blindness, and gradual weight loss. Other than signs of infection, diagnosis is difficult in the live animal and usually made when the animal dies and larvae are found on examining the spinal cord and brain microscopically.

Eimeria spp. (coccidia)

Coccidia are protozoan parasites found throughout the US. They infect mucosal cells in the small and large intestine. Unsporulated oocysts are released from intestinal mucosal cells and pass out in the feces. The oocyst then sporulates (develops) to produce many infective sporozoites (within the oocyst). Upon ingestion by grazing animals, infective sporozoites are released and invade intestinal mucosal cells and undergo asexual reproduction, producing many infective merozoites. There are usually 2–4 asexual generations depending on the species, and this reinfection exacerbates the disease process. Eventually sexual reproduction occurs, which results in the formation of next-generation oocysts to complete the cycle. Devastating losses can occur quickly because the asexual reproductive process results in destruction of intestinal muscosal cells, leading to scours, unthriftiness, weight loss/reduced weight gains, and sometimes death.

Coccidiosis is primarily a problem in young animals and is associated with filth, moisture, and times of stress (depressed immunity) such as weaning or during transportation. Fortunately, a solid immunity develops subsequent to infection. However, if infection was severe, stunting of growth usually results.

Gastrointestinal Nematode General Life Cycle

It is important to understand the life cycle of these GIN before control measures can be considered which will be addressed in the other chapters of this book. The life cycle consists of part being spent inside the animal and part outside the animal on the pasture (Fig. 1.5).

An important concept to remember here is that the greatest proportion of the worm population (eggs and developing larvae) is on pasture and the worm population in the animal is much

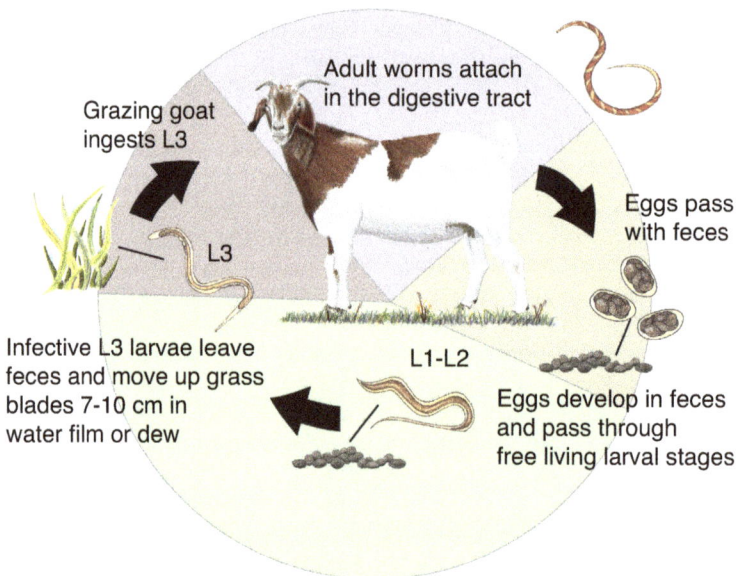

Fig. 1.5. Gastrointestinal nematode general life cycle. Courtesy of R. Merkel; illustrated by K. Williams, used with permission.

less. So, most of the population is present outside the host.

All GIN follow a relatively similar life cycle in which infection starts when L3 are consumed and infect a host during grazing. The L3 migrate to their respective parts of the gastrointestinal tract where they penetrate the mucosa and migrate through tissue, becoming fourth-stage larvae (L4). The L4 returns to the lumen and becomes the fifth-stage larvae (L5, immature adult) which then mature into adults. Once male and female worms are mature, they mate and females begin to produce eggs. This process from L3 ingestion to egg-laying females is called the prepatent period, which usually takes about 3 weeks. *Haemonchus contortus*, for example, are remarkably prolific and each female worm can produce 5000–10,000 eggs/day whereas the other worms produce fewer eggs. There is always a mixed infection of worms, and it is not unusual for young animals to be infected with hundreds or thousands of these worms. With *H. contortus* present, millions of eggs could be produced daily. Individual adult worms have a limited life span and usually survive for a few months. Unembryonated eggs are passed out in the feces and development to L1 occurs within the eggs in the feces which provides some protection from adverse environmental conditions. The eggs hatch and release the L1 which then feeds on bacteria and other organic material. Development to L2 and then to L3 occurs while remaining in the feces. When environmental conditions provide a moisture medium (dew, rain, flooding, etc.), the L3 migrates out of the feces onto the surrounding forage where they are available to be consumed during grazing, thus completing the cycle.

The time for development from egg to L3 can be about 7–10 days (especially during the summer months); therefore, transmission (reinfection) and continual pasture contamination can be quite rapid. However, during the colder months, larval development on pasture is delayed and may take up to a month or two to reach the L3 stage. Also, many of the developing larvae will die off due to cold/freezing conditions, thus pasture contamination and reinfection is minimized.

The L1 and L2 are not protected and can die off when conditions are too hot, too cold or too dry. The L3 are enclosed in a protective sheath, making them relatively resistant to adverse environmental conditions and can survive for months, thus extending transmission potential. As long as the temperature and moisture conditions remain warm and wet (especially following periods of substantial rainfall), development and survival continue, resulting in further accumulation of pasture contamination. As with L1 and L2, if conditions get too hot/cold/dry, L3 can die off and pasture contamination dissipates. Depending on the worm species, the time of the year that is most favorable for transmission varies. Transmission of GIN can be reduced by implementing control measures to eliminate the worms from the animal (deworming) and/or reducing the chances that L3 reinfect the animal (management).

The success of GIN egg and larval development and survival in the environment has an enormous influence on the number of worms that will eventually infect animals. In general, development of eggs and larvae occurs in a temperature range of approximately 10–35°C. *Haemonchus contortus* is so important in small ruminants in the US in large part because the climate in much of the country is favorable for development to and survival of L3. *H. contortus* develops most successfully in warm, wet climates; eggs and larvae do not tolerate cold temperatures well. The south-eastern US, with its hot, humid summers and long grazing season, is very well suited for *H. contortus*. Outside the south-east, the northern regions of the US and even further north into Canada, shorter summer grazing season conditions still provide an appropriate environment for *H. contortus* development and transmission, leading to disease in vulnerable animals. Thus, *H. contortus* is very important in these areas as well, although the period of active transmission is shorter than in the south-eastern region.

In south-western areas with colder winters and hot/dry summers, *H. contortus* becomes less important. However, they can become more of an issue if summer irrigation is practiced. Irrigation provides conditions for forage growth that are suitable for transmission of *H. contortus* and other GIN. In contrast, conditions are not suitable for transmission on nonirrigated pasture.

The length of time required for development of the egg to L3 has an impact on the design of pasture rotation systems. If grazing starts in cool spring weather, it may take a couple of weeks or more for development to L3. Once hotter humid summer weather comes on, the minimum length of time required for the development to L3 is about 7–10 days and numbers of L3 can build up quickly. Larval numbers on pastures in more northern colder areas may not substantially increase until well into the summer. Then, as cooler conditions return in the fall, development again is curtailed.

The activity of dung beetles and earthworms can break up fecal material. This activity can help to reduce the number of L3 by exposing developing L1 and L2 stages to desiccation and ultraviolet light which prevent further development.

Because larvae develop within the fecal pellets, frequent removal of feces should provide some control of GIN. Unfortunately, fecal removal is seldom practical with small ruminants, because of the small size and random distribution of fecal pellets on pasture. With camelids, however, manure removal is a very useful strategy for control. Camelids typically use communal fecal piles that can be easily removed to extensively limit contamination of pasture with L3 that are in close proximity to the piles. If the time for development of eggs to the L3 is considered (7–10 days), then removal of manure piles at least twice a week should be effective.

The L3 must leave the fecal pellet and migrate onto the forage. Rain, irrigation, flooding, and heavy dew provide the moisture necessary for migration of L3 from feces. During dry weather, L3 will be retained in the pellets. With rain, there can be a burst of L3 release. There may be an outbreak of GIN disease a few weeks after rain, especially if it follows a period of drought. Animals will then be exposed to large numbers of newly available L3.

Larvae of *H. contortus* and most other GIN do not develop or survive well on other than grass pasture and little transmission occurs in housing or on drylots. However, even the smallest tufts of grass can support larval development and survival where infection can occur in animals kept on dirt paddocks with small grass areas or where animals can access grass through fences.

The L3 can migrate laterally and vertically in films of moisture on grass and other plants as provided by rainfall and morning dew (Fig. 1.6). The ability of L3 to migrate is affected by air

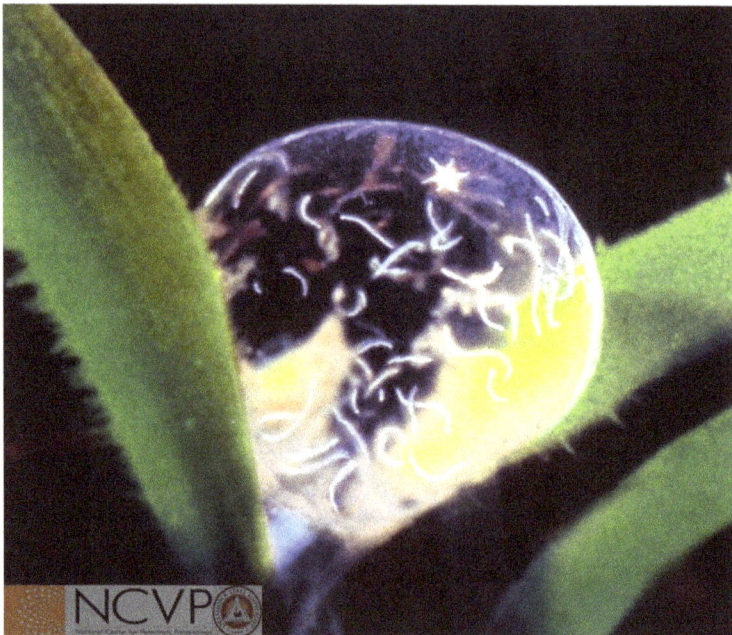

Fig. 1.6. Nematode larvae in water droplet. Courtesy of National Center for Veterinary Parasitology.

temperature, soil moisture, and relative humidity. Vertical migration of most L3 is limited to about 7–10 cm from the ground. Most L3 stay within a 30–45 cm radius after migrating out of feces, although some can move out up to 90 cm. If pastures can be maintained to preserve a forage height above 15 cm, exposure to L3 can be reduced. Additionally, when animals are allowed to browse on bushes and other taller plants, infection will be reduced. Goats are browsers by nature and provision of browse plants is strongly recommended in GIN control programs.

The length of time that L3 can survive on the pasture is also important for pasture management programs that aim to control GIN. Larvae are covered by a tough semi-permeable outer layer called the cuticle. The cuticle is replaced with each molt, but the L3 retains the cuticle of the L2 as a sheath. While the sheath gives the L3 greater resistance to environmental conditions, it also prevents them from feeding. Once an L3 utilizes its stored metabolic reserves, it will die. Consequently, hot/dry conditions cause quicker demise of L3 and cool/moist conditions best support survival because metabolic reserves will deplete slowly. In the hot summer grazing season, numbers of L3 are usually significantly reduced (e.g. safe pasture) after a rest period of 2–3 months. In cooler temperate regions, a grazed pasture should be rested for 6 months (maybe longer) to be considered relatively safe.

If pasture regrowth is used for hay or the pasture is plowed and reseeded, L3 will die more quickly. When utilizing pasture rest or rotation as a method of GIN control, these time periods need to be considered.

the year when environmental conditions are least favorable for development and survival of eggs and larvae outside the host. In areas with cold winters, most GIN survive primarily by hypobiosis.

Even without anthelmintic treatment, in regions with cold winters, *H. contortus* problems usually resolve at the end of the grazing season. This is because most newly ingested L3 will become arrested in the host and eggs that are shed at the end of the grazing season are unlikely to develop or develop very slowly, preventing further build-up of L3 on pasture. Where winters are very mild, hypobiosis appears to be less important in the epizootiology of transmission. In the south-eastern US, for example, levels of hypobiotic larvae are not substantial throughout the year, although the highest proportion of hypobiotic larvae tend to be in the fall/winter.

In areas where winter hypobiosis occurs, emergence and development of adult worms in late winter and spring are followed by an increase in fecal egg output. This rise in egg output is magnified in ewes and does in late pregnancy and early lactation by a relaxation of immunity that increases survival and egg production of existing GIN, which also increases susceptibility to further infection. This relaxation in immunity typically begins 2–4 weeks prior to and peaks around 2–4 weeks post kidding/lambing. This phenomenon is called the periparturient rise (PPR) in fecal egg count which can make an important contribution to the L3 population on pasture as young, susceptible animals begin grazing.

Hypobiosis

The epizootiology of important species of GIN is also strongly influenced by aspects of host/parasite biology after infection occurs. Larvae (L3 or L4 depending on species) of important GIN can undergo a period of arrested development (hypobiosis) in the host. Following infection, larvae may become metabolically inactive for a period that may last several months before resuming development. The greatest proportion of incoming L3 will become arrested at the L4 stage (some species at the L3 stage) at a time of

Epizootiology

Another way to look at the life cycle is in four phases. Phase 1 is the parasitic phase which is the interaction between the animal and the worm. Phase 2 is the contamination phase which is the result of eggs that are passed in the feces during defecation. Phase 3 is the free-living phase when larval stages develop and survive. Phase 4 is the infection phase when available L3 are consumed during grazing. There are many factors that affect what happens and influence

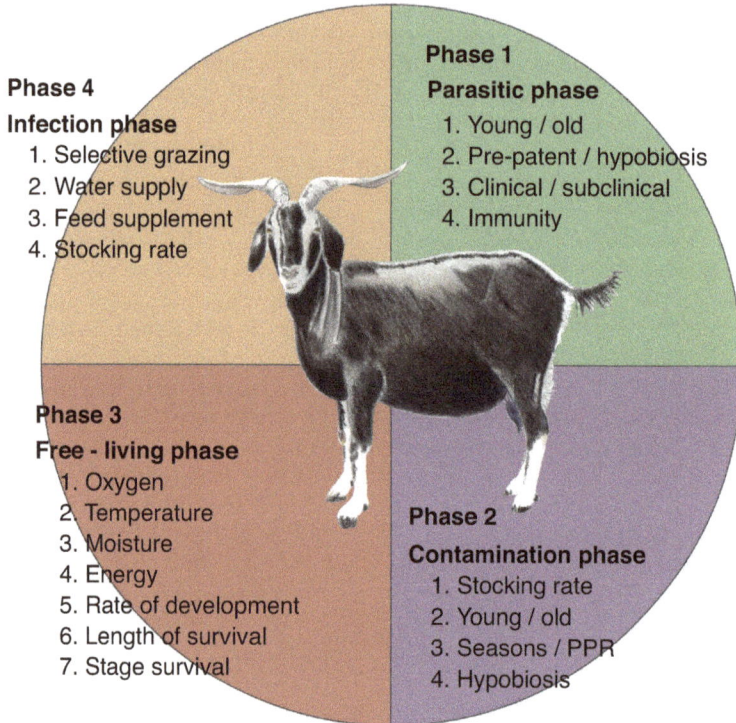

Fig. 1.7. Epizootiology cycle of small ruminant gastrointestinal nematodes. Courtesy of R. Merkel; illustrated by K. Williams, used with permission.

control strategies during each of these phases (Fig. 1.7).

Phase 1 – Parasitic phase

During Phase 1, worms develop and survive in the host. After ingestion, L3 lose their protective sheath and invade the mucosa of the abomasum, small intestine or large intestine depending on which worm is involved. While in the mucosa, larvae develop to L4 and then return to the surface of the gut mucosa where they develop to immature adults (L5) and then mature adult worms.

The animal's major defense mechanism against GIN is the immune system. When infectious agents enter the body, the immune system reacts through a series of pathways that mobilize various components (antibodies, macrophages, killer cells, etc.) that then attack and kill the invaders. These components act on the larval stages in the mucosa and the adults. How strongly the immune response persists depends on several factors. The immune system matures with age. When born, the young are somewhat protected by the dam's colostrum which provides antibodies to help prevent infection. After the effect of colostrum wanes, young animals (3–8 months of age) are relatively susceptible to infection, harbor the heaviest worm loads and suffer the most severe consequences. Animals over 8 months of age have developed stronger immunity and harbor lower infection levels.

One way in which infection level is measured is by quantifying the number of eggs being passed in the feces. So, relatively high and low egg counts are usually seen in young and adult animals, respectively. Young animals are more subject to clinical disease where signs of infection (diarrhea, rough hair coat, anemia, weight loss, bottle jaw, etc.) are seen. In older animals, infection usually becomes more subclinical where the only subtle sign may be weight loss. However, nutrition and/or stress can alter a host's immune competence. Under poor nutrition and/or stressful conditions, the immune system loses some effectiveness and cannot respond adequately. Therefore, no matter what the age of the animal, the effects of infection will become worse. As mentioned before, the prepatent period of most worms is about 3 weeks, but this period can be extended for worms that undergo hypobiosis (see above).

deposited in feces. However, when hypobiotic larvae resume development (especially in the spring coinciding with parturition/lactation), massive numbers can become mature adults over a short period of time. The resultant egg production (contributing to the PPR) and deposition in the feces can be very high which results in major pasture contamination and potential infection, especially for the young. An increased worm burden can also have severe adverse effects on the adult animal.

Phase 2 – Contamination phase

The magnitude of pasture contamination during Phase 2 is affected by stocking rate (number of animals per grazing area), age of the animals, season of the year, and hypobiosis. The higher/lower the stocking rate, the more/less feces are deposited on pasture, thus more/fewer eggs. More eggs are also passed from younger than older animals. Most worms have a definite seasonality so during their "season," more eggs are produced and passed. Of particular note in small ruminants, there is a phenomenon called the PPR in fecal egg output. This occurs at or around parturition (lambing/kidding) and extends through most of the lactation period. Because parturition and lactation are stressful conditions, the dam's immune system is compromised. Furthermore, nutrients are partitioned preferentially to support mammary and fetal development and then lactation, which also decreases the animal's ability to generate an effective immune response to worm infection. Providing a high-protein diet will help partitioning to support immune function. In addition, hormonal changes during lactation have been associated with the PPR. Thus, existing female worms increase the number of eggs produced and deposited in the feces.

Depending on location, some worm species undergo hypobiosis. In cold temperate climates, hypobiosis occurs over winter and all animals, male and female, pregnant and open, are affected. Thus, the development time to the adult stage is extended by several months. This will result in fewer adult worms during the hypobiosis period and fewer eggs

Phase 3 – Free-living phase

Development and survival of the free-living stages during Phase 3 depend on prevailing environmental (temperature and moisture) and nutritional (oxygen and energy) conditions. Initially, the L1 develop in the egg which then hatches. Development and survival to L2 and L3 occur within the fecal mass. The L1 and L2 are unprotected and need oxygen and energy as they feed on nutrients and microorganisms to grow. The L3 is enclosed in a protective sheath and does not feed. Temperatures conducive for normal development and survival are 10–35°C. The lower or higher the temperature gets, the more development and survival are reduced. Moisture is also crucial for development and survival. Because the initial development and survival occur within feces, moisture (greater than 75%) is usually adequate to complete development to the L3; however, if the feces dry out quickly, due to high temperatures and/or physical disruption, the L1 and L2 are susceptible to desiccation and will die. If feces remain intact, retain moisture, and do not get too hot or too cold, L3 may remain alive for months.

A moisture medium (rain/flooding/dew) is necessary for L3 to migrate out of feces. They are relatively resistant to environmental conditions due to their protective sheath. Temperature is usually the only factor that may adversely affect L3. Generally, L3 can survive very low temperatures but some may die off during hard freezes. Sustained temperatures above 35°C are usually lethal. The moisture conditions at ground level under forage cover usually are adequate for L3 to move around and survive. Since they do not feed, their length of survival depends on how fast they use up their energy reserves. So the hotter it is, the faster they move and use up energy stores and survival is shorter.

Eventually, L3 move up and down the forage when there is a moisture medium (i.e. advancing and receding dew). Rain and flooding also provide a moisture medium for larval movement on forage. For the most part, the majority of L3 do not migrate much past 7–10 cm up the forage or 30–45 cm from feces. So, the lower the animals graze forage and the closer to feces, consumption of L3 is increased and vice versa.

Phase 4 – Infection phase

Phase 4 is affected again by stocking rate in two ways. If the same animals are grazing, the stocking rate determines how many eggs initially contaminate the pasture (Phase 2) and, consequently, how many L3 will be available for consumption. If the initial contaminating animals are removed and replaced by new animals, the new stocking rate will determine the level of exposure each animal has to L3 during grazing, i.e. the higher the stocking rate, the more chance of exposure and vice versa. It is well known that animals usually do not graze close to feces so the further the distance between fecal deposits, the more exposure is reduced. Eventually feces disintegrate, forage grows well with fecal fertilization and animals will graze over the area where exposure can be high. Natural sources of water, such as streams, ponds or lakes, provide moisture along the banks where forage can grow readily. When animals congregate to drink and consume the attractive forage, defecation in these areas usually leads to increased contamination and eventually more L3. The same can be said for areas where supplements, especially hay, are fed on the ground where conditions might support development and survival of the free-living stages. Similarly, trees provide shade and an area for animal congregation. Under all these situations, essentially a high stocking

rate has been artificially created in a relatively small area where forage is kept closely grazed.

Conclusion

In summary, several elements of the biology, life cycle, and epizootiology of *H. contortus* and other GIN can be used in designing integrated parasite control programs that provide opportunities for decreasing or interrupting successful transmission, thereby reducing worm loads in animals. Examples include the following.

- Mixed or alternate grazing with horses or cattle helps reduce levels of L3 because each animal host has its own species of GIN (an exception is that young cattle can be infected with *H. contortus*).
- Because L3 usually do not migrate higher than 7–10 cm on forage, managing pastures to minimize grazing below that level can reduce exposure to L3. Similarly, allowing goats to utilize browse plants will reduce exposure.
- If using strip grazing for control, move animals every 1–3 days so no eggs have a chance to develop to L3 before the move.
- Significant numbers of L3 can be removed from pasture by allowing a period of pasture rest for at least 2–3 months in the grazing season, or by using the pasture regrowth of a grazed pasture for hay or plowing and reseeding pasture.
- Utilize knowledge of parasite biology in managing the PPR. Birthing in drylots or during times of year when larvae do not develop or survive well on pasture can substantially reduce initial infection of lambs and kids when they begin grazing.

Similarly, understanding important aspects of the response of small ruminants to GIN infection provides additional opportunities for successful control, including use of smart deworming principles, FAMACHA©, targeted selective treatment, nutritional management, breeding for parasite resistance, alternative treatments, etc. These essential strategies are the subjects of the other chapters in this book.

Further Reading

Dunn, A.M. (1978) *Veterinary Helminthology*, 2nd edn. Heinemann, Oxford.

Emery, D.L., Hunt, P.W. and LeJambre, L.F. (2016) *Haemonchus contortus*: The then and now, and where to from here? *International Journal for Parasitology* 46, 755–769. DOI: 10.1016/j.ijpara.2016.07.001.

Fleming, S., Craig, T., Kaplan, R.M., Miller, J., Navarre, C. *et al.* (2006) Anthelmintic resistance of gastro-intestinal parasites in small ruminants. *Journal of Veterinary Internal Medicine* 20, 435–444. DOI: 10.1111/j.1939-1676.2006.tb02881.x.

Kearney, P.E., Murray, P.J., Hoy, J.M., Hohenhaus, M. and Kotze, A. (2016) The 'Toolbox' of strategies for managing *Haemonchus contortus* in goats: What's in and what's out. *Veterinary Parasitology* 220, 93–107. DOI: 10.1016/j.vetpar.2016.02.028.

Kenyon, F., Sargison, N.D., Skuce, P.J. and Jackson, F. (2009) Sheep helminth parasitic disease in south-eastern Scotland arising as a possible consequence of climate change. *Veterinary Parasitology* 163, 293–297. DOI: 10.1016/j.vetpar.2009.03.027.

Levine, N.D. (1963) Weather, climate and the bionomics of ruminant nematode larvae. *Advances in Veterinary Science* 8, 215–261.

Miller, J.E. (2015) Internal parasites of goats. In: Merkel, R.C., Gipson, T.A. and Sahlu, T. (eds) *Meat Goat Production Handbook*, 2nd edn. American Institute for Goat Research, Langston, Oklahoma, pp. 143–156.

Miller, J.E., Bahirathan, M., Lemarie, S.L., Hembry, F., Kearney, M. *et al.* (1998) Epidemiology of gastro-intestinal nematode parasitism in Suffolk and Gulf Coast Native sheep with special emphasis on relative susceptibility to *Haemonchus contortus* infection. *Veterinary Parasitology* 74, 55–74. DOI: 10.1016/s0304-4017(97)00094-0.

Starkey, L.A. and Pugh, D.G. (2021) Internal parasites of sheep, goats and cervids. In: Pugh, D.G., Baird, A.N., Edmonson, M. and Passler, T. (eds) *Sheep, Goat and Cervid Medicine*, 3rd edn. Elsevier, London, UK, pp. 97–117.

Sutherland, I. and Scott, I. (2010) *Gastrointestinal Nematodes of Sheep and Cattle. Biology and Control.* Wiley-Blackwell. Ames, Iowa.

Waller, P.J., Rudby-Martin, L., Ljungstrom, B.L. and Rydzik, A. (2004) The epidemiology of abomasal nematodes of sheep in Sweden, with particular reference to over-winter survival strategies. *Veterinary Parasitology* 122, 207–220. DOI: 10.1016/j.vetpar.2004.04.007.

Westers, T., Jones-Britton, A., Menzies, P., Vanleeuwen, J., Poljak, Z. *et al.* (2017) Comparison of tar-geted selective and whole flock treatment of periparturient ewes for controlling *Haemonchus* sp. on sheep farms in Ontario, Canada. *Small Ruminant Research* 150, 102–110. DOI: 10.1016/j.smallrumres.2017.03.013.

Zajac, A.M. (2006) Gastrointestinal nematodes of small ruminants: Life cycle, anthelmintics and diagnosis. *Veterinary Clinics of North America: Food Animal Practice* 22, 539–541. DOI: 10.1016/j.cvfa.2006.07.006.

2 Role of Nutrition in Small Ruminant Production and Gastrointestinal Nematode Management

Dan Quadros[1]* and Ken Coffey[2]

[1]*University of Arkansas System Division of Agriculture, Little Rock, Arkansas, USA;*
[2]*University of Arkansas Dale Bumpers College of Agricultural, Food and Life Sciences, Fayetteville, Arkansas, USA*

Abstract

Small ruminants are adapted to a variety of environments and cultures as they are raised worldwide to convert forages into meat, milk, and fiber. Nutrition, which is the interrelated process of assimilating and using nutrients, is essential for the health and productivity of sheep and goats. Proper nutrition ensures adequate growth, reproduction, and immune system function. However, gastrointestinal nematodes (GIN) can be a significant threat to small ruminants, especially in warm, humid environments, causing production and economic losses. This chapter outlines the general aspects and role of nutrition in small ruminant health, production, and welfare, exploring the impacts of GIN parasitism on nutrition and metabolism, and how diet manipulation can be used as a tool to increase both resistance and resilience of small ruminants to GIN infections.

Introduction

Sheep and goat numbers are increasing worldwide (FAOSTAT, 2024) because of their adaptability and ability to thrive in harsh environmental conditions with minimal competition with humans for food. Their ruminant digestive system allows them to consume feedstuffs that are high in fiber and convert these feedstuffs into meat, milk, fiber, and other products that are readily consumed by the growing human population.

Nevertheless, gastrointestinal nematodes (GIN) constrain small ruminant production by decreasing productivity, negatively affecting welfare, and, eventually, causing death. With the failure of chemotherapy, researchers have studied other tools for an integrated approach to parasite management (Burke and Miller, 2020). In this context, nutrition can be an asset to improving animals' immunological response to GIN infections, overcoming the negative effects of parasitism and increasing animal performance.

The purpose of this chapter is to give an applied overview of the general aspects of small ruminant nutrition, the role of nutrition on health, production, and welfare, the impacts of GIN parasitism on nutrition and metabolism, and, finally, how nutrition can be used to lessen GIN losses and increase productivity.

Consumption of nutraceutical forages with antiparasitic bioactive components such as condensed tannins and the utilization of copper

*Corresponding author: dquadros@uark.edu

© CAB International 2026. *Management Practices for Controlling Nematode Parasites of Small Ruminants* (eds James E. Miller and Joan M. Burke)
DOI: 10.1079/9781800623767.0002

oxide wire particles (COWP) are nutritional tools associated with small ruminant integrated parasite management. However, COWP and antiparasitic bioactive forages will not be directly reviewed in this chapter and more information about them can be found in Chapters 4 and 7, respectively. More details about pasture management, forage legumes, and annual grasses, which can contribute to improving small ruminant nutrition, can be found in Chapter 6.

General Aspects of Small Ruminant Nutrition

Digestive system

The digestive system of small ruminants begins with their wide mouth and prehensile lips, that allow them to gather large quantities of forage when biomass is low, and their tongue which is used both in acquiring and selecting biomass when quantities are greater. Consumed feed is then swallowed and passes into the reticulum followed by the rumen, where it is exposed to fermentation by a diverse microbial population. Muscular movement within the rumen and reticulum keeps the contents mixed and in contact with the liquid fraction that contains the viable microorganisms for digestion (Van Soest, 1994).

Small ruminants are by nature prey, and thus they consume their diets rapidly with minimal chewing, then move to safer areas for rumination. Ruminants regurgitate and remasticate consumed forage to increase the surface area for greater microbial attachment and fermentation, and to reduce particle size so undigested particles can pass through the digestive system (Mertens and Grant, 2020). After particle size is reduced, the undigested particles and liquid flow into the omasum and then to the abomasum or true stomach, where they are acted on by hydrochloric acid and pepsin, a digestive enzyme. After that, they flow into the small intestine, where they are subjected to several enzymes (Merchen, 1988). Digested nutrients are absorbed in the small intestine before the digesta flows into the large intestine, where water is absorbed and additional microbial fermentation occurs, albeit somewhat limited. What remains is excreted through the feces (Van Soest, 1994).

Nutrients

Diets of small ruminants are generally based on forage that contains water, carbohydrates, protein, fats, minerals, and vitamins. Water is necessary for the microorganisms in the reticulorumen to grow and flourish and for vital metabolic processes. In situations where water is limited, feed intake and digestion typically decrease.

The majority of nutrients in most feedstuffs utilized by small ruminants is carbohydrates. Carbohydrates range from simple sugars to very complex molecules. Starch and sugars are non-structural carbohydrates used as plant reserves, which can be digested by microbes in the rumen and enzymes in the small intestine. Cellulose and hemicellulose are structural carbohydrates that need microbial enzymes to digest. Cellulose, hemicellulose, and lignin make up what is considered the fiber fraction of forages. Lignin is a complex polyphenolic compound that binds to the hemicellulose and cellulose fractions, reducing fiber degradability by rumen microorganisms. These structural components increase in concentration as forages mature.

Proteins are compounds composed of amino acids. The chain length and sequence of amino acids vary greatly in animal feedstuffs. Most of the protein found in typical feedstuffs for ruminants contains fractions that are degradable (rumen degradable protein, RDP) and some that are not degradable by the microorganisms (rumen undegradable protein, RUP). This is very important to the efficient functioning of the rumen and the ultimate feeding of the animal itself. A certain amount of RDP is necessary in the diet because this is what feeds certain strains of bacteria such as the cellulolytic bacteria as described below. However, excess RDP may be utilized inefficiently so a proper balance is necessary to enhance animal efficiency and reduce environmental issues. Ultimately, what actually meets the protein requirements of the animal is metabolizable protein (MP) which is the true protein (i.e. amino acids) actually absorbed by the small intestine from both microbial protein and protein that escapes degradation in the rumen.

Fats are high-energy compounds that, in their natural forms, range in saturation, or number of double-bonded carbons, from no double bonds to many double bonds. They are chemically altered in the rumen and metabolized in the small intestine of the animal.

Minerals are categorized as either macro (Ca, P, K, Mg, Na, S) or micro (Cu, Co, Mn, Mo, Fe, Se, Zn) depending on their relative concentrations in the diet. Minerals vary greatly in their function in the animal including growth and development, immune function, electrolyte balance, and catalysts of numerous chemical reactions in the body. There are also numerous chemical forms of minerals and these often vary greatly in their absorption and utilization by the animal. Minerals also vary greatly in their availability in different regions of the world. A much more thorough discussion of the different minerals and their nutritional role can be found in NRC (2007) and Stewart et al. (2021).

A number of vitamins or their precursors are available in actively growing forages (Ballet et al., 2000). These include the vitamin A precursor β-carotene and the vitamin E precursor α-tocopherol. Forage curing and storage conditions can have a dramatic impact on the actual concentrations of these precursors. Therefore, some recommend additional fat-soluble vitamins to prevent subclinical or clinical deficiencies. Several vitamins including the water-soluble vitamins (B complex and vitamin K) are synthesized by rumen microorganisms. However, factors that affect microbial growth and efficiency can impact production of these vitamins (Van Soest, 1994).

Digestion and metabolism

Animal performance results from a combination of intake and digestion and is basically a function of the quantity of digestible nutrients the animal consumes. Intake and digestion interact with each other as well as a number of other factors, such as palatability, nutrient composition, animal production status, animal and plant species, and animal genetics (Mertens and Grant, 2020). Chemostatic and distension signals feed back to the brain to control intake (Van Soest, 1994). Factors that negatively impact digestion, such as lignification of the forage, suppress the rate of digestion and subsequent passage of the forage out of the rumen. This results in distension signal feedback to the brain, causing the animal to consume less forage. As a general rule, the greater the fiber concentration of the forage, the lower the forage intake by small ruminants (Meyer et al., 2010). However, if the fiber contains low concentrations of lignin, the digestibility may still be high, resulting in greater intake than might be expected.

In the reticulorumen of small ruminants, a very diverse population of microorganisms digest nutrients, such as structural carbohydrates, to provide energy (i.e. volatile fatty acids, VFA) and protein (i.e. microbial protein) for the animal. These microorganisms consist of bacteria, protozoa, fungi, and archaea but the system is dominated by bacteria. Numerous strains of bacteria are very diverse in their function but more importantly, they are highly interdependent and vary in their specific function and requirements for growth. Because the diet of small ruminants is typically high in cellulose, the bacterial population in the rumen is dominated by cellulolytic bacteria. For the cellulolytic bacteria to grow, they actually require ammonia, which comes from the breakdown of RDP by proteolytic bacteria.

Microbial fermentation of carbohydrates results in the formation of short-chain VFA as well as lactic acid, carbon dioxide, and methane. The majority of the VFA produced (e.g. acetate, propionate, butyrate) is absorbed across the rumen wall and enters the bloodstream to be used for energy. The rate of degradation of different carbohydrates is dependent upon a number of factors. Simple sugars are digested very rapidly in the rumen, whereas the rate and extent of starch digestion are affected by proteins and other compounds in conjunction with the starch. Rate and extent of cellulose and hemicellulose digestion are limited primarily by the degree of lignification. When both starch and cellulose are present in the rumen, the more rapid fermentation of starch leads to greater production of lactic acid, which is a strong acid and reduces ruminal pH. If the pH drops below 6.0, growth of the cellulolytic bacteria is suppressed and cellulose and hemicellulose digestion will be compromised (Owens and Goetsch, 1988). When ruminating, a substantial amount of saliva is produced, buffering rumen pH to the normal range (6.4–6.8). Rumen pH values less than 5.5 or greater than 7.0 are considered abnormal (Jasmin et al., 2011).

Protein can be digested both by the animal itself in the abomasum and small intestine but, more importantly, by proteolytic microorganisms in the rumen and reticulum (Merchen, 1988). The RDP is critical to the overall function of the rumen. The proteolytic microorganisms deaminate the amino acids, resulting in free ammonia and the carbon backbone of the specific amino acids, which is required for microbial synthesis.

Protein in forages is generally highly degradable with only a small portion (generally 20–30%) of RUP. High RDP may lead to excessive ammonia in the rumen. Much of this excess is absorbed and transported to the liver, where it is converted to urea at the cost of energy. Urea is released into the bloodstream and some of it is captured by the salivary glands and recycled back into the rumen. This urea is rapidly converted to ammonia and carbon dioxide. The ammonia may be captured by the rumen microorganisms if sufficient carbon skeletons are present for the bacteria to use to build their own amino acids, but much of this ammonia is again absorbed across the gut wall and transported to the liver. Most of the urea produced in the liver is filtered out by the kidneys and excreted in the urine, thus representing a loss to the animal.

The degradation of proteins by rumen microorganisms varies substantially because of the protein structure, heat damage, or presence of compounds that suppress action of proteolytic microorganisms. Heat can denature protein and render it more slowly degraded or prevent degradation all together. In the instance of forages, heating that occurs when harvested forages are packaged improperly, such as hay baled at excessive moisture, can reduce the ability of microorganisms to degrade the protein. Certain chemical components in forages and feedstuffs may suppress digestion of protein in the rumen. For example, condensed tannins bind to both the rumen microbes and the actual feed protein to reduce ruminal protein digestion in a dose-dependent manner (Min et al., 2003).

Fats may be added to ruminant diets to increase energy density. Fat that leaves the rumen is vastly different chemically from the fat that was fed because of several modifications carried out by the ruminal microorganisms, including the addition of hydrogen to saturate the fat (Byers and Schelling, 1988). Binding of hydrogen by fat has the benefit of potentially reducing methane production in the rumen (Rasmussen and Harrison, 2011). Methane, although necessary to remove the metabolic hydrogen in the rumen, represents energy loss in the digestion process, and it is an environmental concern as the most important greenhouse gas related to ruminant production (Fox et al., 2018). However, excess of fat in ruminant diets lead to a reduction in fiber digestion.

Feeds and feeding

Livestock feedstuffs are classified by the American Association of Feed Control Officials (AAFCO) into several categories by collective terms. These terms include forage products, roughage products, grain products, plant protein products, animal protein products, and molasses products.

Small ruminants are able to survive solely on forage and roughage diets in many instances as long as protein is adequate to maintain bacterial growth. Otherwise, other feedstuffs must be included to maintain satisfactory growth and performance or to increase productivity.

Historically, cereal grains were used to correct energy deficiencies and enhance animal performance. Energy from cereal grains is derived primarily from ruminal degradation of starch to VFA. At lower levels of supplementation, few problems are noted. However, when excessive levels of cereal grains are offered, rumen pH may drop below the normal range and cause acidosis and laminitis, among other digestive and health problems.

Today, there are numerous by-product feeds that are available for use as feedstuffs for small ruminants (Fadel, 1999; Aregheore, 2000; Yang et al., 2021). These by-products are the residue of processing grains or other feedstuffs for human consumption. Examples are dried distillers' grains with solubles (DDGS), corn gluten feed, wheat middlings, and soybean hulls. The composition of these by-products is variable due to the processes used in different plants or simply due to variation related to their production. As they have considerable fiber and low lignin contents, these feedstuffs are attractive for use in ruminant diets. Published energy values of these feedstuffs are generally lower than corn (NRC, 2007). However, in actual feeding situations where the by-products are only a portion of the entire diet, animal performance may not differentiate between these feedstuffs and corn on an equal inclusion basis. This is likely because when corn is used at increasing concentrations in the diet, fermentation of the starch results in reduced ruminal pH, while by-product feedstuffs result in less ruminal pH suppression, which in turn results in less suppressive impacts on forage intake. There are also many by-product feedstuffs available on a more local basis and their inclusion in small ruminant diets may be interesting depending on the composition, digestibility, expected animal performance, and costs (Fadel, 1999).

Protein sources used as livestock feedstuffs are also by-products of other processes, generally. Soybean meal and cottonseed meal, by-products of the extraction of cooking oils, have been fed to livestock for many years. These meals have a fairly high rumen degradability depending on whether the oil is extracted via solvent (higher RDP) or mechanical (lower RDP) processes. In recent years, oil extraction from other plant products (corn, canola, peanuts, sunflowers, etc.) has provided other high-protein by-products as feedstuffs. As with soybean and cottonseed meal, the rumen degradability of these feedstuffs is highly dependent on the amount of heat used in the oil extraction and subsequent drying process. Solvent extraction involves much less heat compared with mechanical extraction (i.e. crushing out the oil), and therefore results in greater rumen degradability. Amino acid balance of the particular protein sources is generally not a consideration when the rumen degradability is high but should be considered when rumen degradability is lowered by heating since a greater proportion of the undegraded protein source reaches the intestine to be broken up into the individual amino acids.

Several animal by-products (e.g. fish meal, meat meal, poultry meal, hydrolyzed feather meal, blood and plasma meal, etc.) are available to feed ruminant animals. Generally, palatability and the rumen degradability of these by-products are low. Therefore, using these by-products to provide a major part of the dietary protein can not only reduce intake but also reduce animal performance through inadequate rumen ammonia for bacterial growth. Also, since the RDP content of these by-products is low, consideration should be given to the amino acid profile, as the protein that is digested and utilized from these by-products by the animal will occur in the small intestine. Individuals should verify the current laws and regulations in their country regarding the use of animal products in ruminant feeds.

Nonprotein nitrogen sources such as urea can be used to an extent in small ruminants because of the ability of rumen microorganisms to utilize ammonia. These nonprotein nitrogen sources are rapidly hydrolyzed to ammonia in the rumen to provide nitrogen to rumen microorganisms, and consequently increase the MP supply in sheep and goat diets. However, adequate carbon structures must be available in synchrony with the ammonia for adequate incorporation into microbial protein. Thus, nonprotein nitrogen sources work much more efficiently when used in conjunction with high starch- or molasses-based supplements. Overall feed costs can be reduced by feeding nonprotein nitrogen sources since proper safety measures are observed (Stanton and Whittier, 2006).

There are several feed additives that are available for small ruminants. Feed additives are substances, microorganisms, or formulated products added to animal diets intending to improve feed quality/digestibility or animal health/performance. These additives include but are not limited to ionophores (e.g. monensin and lasalocid, which also act as coccidiostats), coccidiostats (e.g. decoquinate), microbials (e.g. probiotics), yeasts cultures and fermentation products, enzymes, condensed tannins, and essential oils.

Role of Nutrition in Small Ruminant Production, Health, and Welfare

Undoubtedly, nutrition is one of the most important factors influencing the sustainability of small ruminant production. Deficiencies and malnutrition severely impact animal performance and can lead to irreversible health conditions, disorders, and fatalities. Proper nutritional management provides the animals with nutrients necessary to grow, develop, and reproduce, and sustain strong immunity to fight off infections (Makkar, 2016). Nutritionally

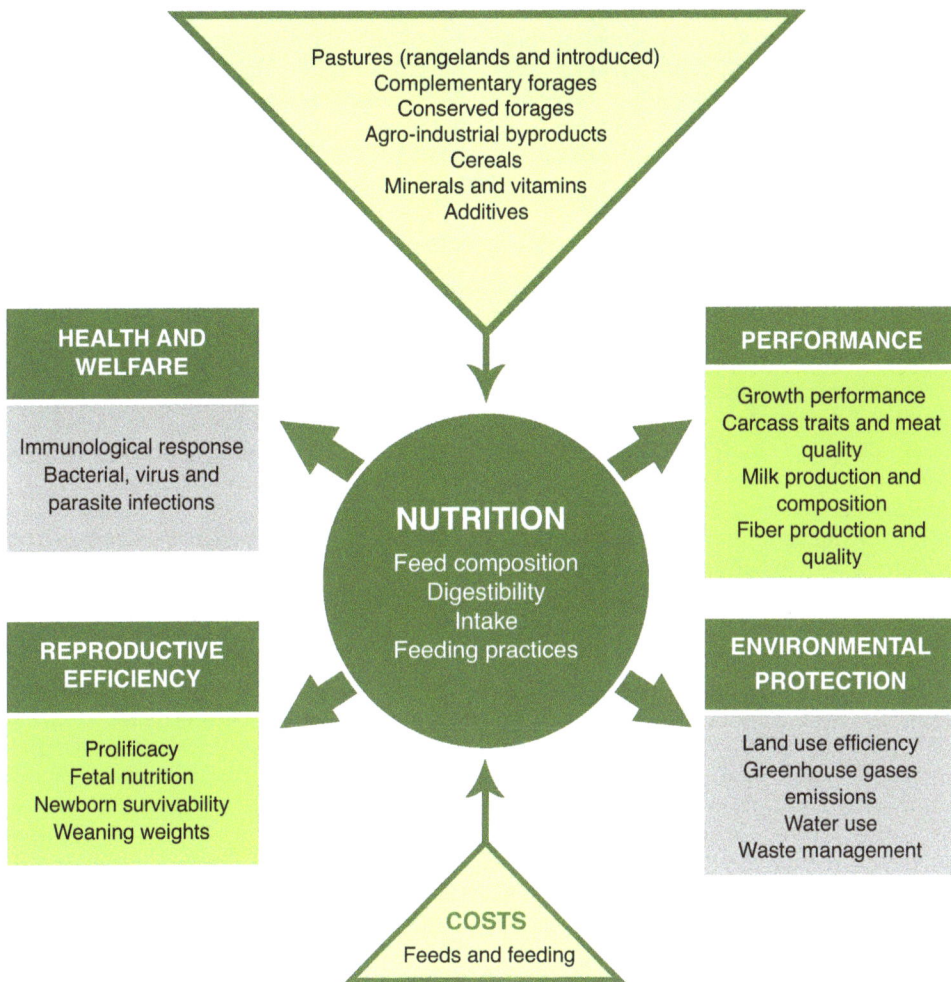

Fig. 2.1. Role of nutrition on health and welfare, reproductive efficiency, performance and sustainability of small ruminant production.

balanced diets increase reproductive efficiency, milk and fiber production, growth performance, and feed efficiency, reflected in the profitability and reduced environmental impact of small ruminant operations. From an economic standpoint, feeding represents the largest expense in the recurrent costs of a farm. Besides, improved feeding systems can mitigate environmental impacts, for instance by increasing land use efficiency and reducing waste and greenhouse gases emissions (Fig. 2.1).

Nutrition plays a key role in the reproductive performance of small ruminants. Implementing reproductive management with strategic feeding practices allows producers to control breeding and birth seasons, which can bring several benefits including marketing animals when prices are historically high, maximizing the number of animals born (e.g. maximizing ovulation rate and ensuring successful embryonic and fetal development), and ensuring the survival of the newborn and their ability to grow and mature into productive life efficiently (Martin *et al.*, 2004).

The proper nutrition during the final trimester of gestation of an ewe or doe, or the last 6–8 weeks before lambing/kidding, is critical. Dams in this phase have reduced dry matter intake (DMI) and it is likely that hay or pasture alone will not meet their nutritional requirements unless it is very high quality. Therefore, an increase in nutrient density is necessary, taking into consideration body condition score (BCS) and number of fetuses the ewe or doe is carrying (Gurung *et al.*, 2020). Nutritional requirements increase rapidly in the beginning of lactation, and an improper diet can result in a negative energy balance, accentuated loss in BCS, and occurrence of metabolic problems (Redden and Thorne, 2020). The peak in milk production is usually reached at around 4–6 weeks after birth. During this time, the diet must be able to supply enough energy and protein for the ewe/doe to produce the required milk and maintain her body condition. Thus, until around the age of 6–8 weeks, lambs/ kids receive much of their protein and energy for growth from the mother's milk. After that, their nutrition will depend on the forage and any concentrated feed they consume (Gurung *et al.*, 2020).

Animal growth is a function of genetic potential and the extent to which the environment allows this potential to be expressed. Among the main environmental variables that affect animal performance, nutrition is the most important. Therefore, the amount and composition of the feed consumed by the animal will dictate its growth pattern, within the constraints imposed by its genetic potential and climatic and pathogenic stresses (Oddy and Sainz, 2002). The plane of nutrition affects the growth of muscles, muscle fiber diameter, chemical composition (protein, fat, minerals, and vitamins), total energy deposited in the carcass, amount of fat and its distribution, and time to reach slaughter weight (Devendra, 1988; Goetsch *et al.*, 2011). Additionally, feeding systems affect multiple quality characteristics of meat products including attributes of quality related to commercial, sensorial, nutritional, technological, safety, and image aspects (e.g. meat color, tenderness, fatty acid profile, antioxidants, vitamins, muscle:fat ratio, flavor, and taste) (Zervas and Tsiplakou, 2011; Huang *et al.*, 2023).

Protein, energy, minerals, and vitamins influence wool, cashmere, and mohair production and quality because of their effects on fiber growth rate, fiber diameter, fiber length, staple strength, clean fiber yield, and color (Hynd and Masters, 2002; Di Trana and Sepe, 2007). Wool growth is dependent on energy intake. However, for the range of energy of most diets consumed by grazing sheep, wool growth rate will be limited by the supply of protein (i.e. amino acids) in the small intestine. A higher plane of nutrition increases both rate of fiber elongation and fiber diameter (Hynd and Masters, 2002). Angora goats respond to a dietary supplementation of good-quality protein with an increase in mohair yield but a decrease in its quality (Di Trana and Sepe, 2007).

Dairy systems vary dramatically from meat and fiber production systems in many regards, such as feeding practices, genetics, facilities, reproductive management, and health concerns. In order to increase sheep and goat milk production and ensure high feed efficiency, dairy farmers need to pay close attention to nutritional requirements of dairy animals which may differ during different stages of lactation (NRC, 2007). High nutrient requirements of dairy animals often necessitate the inclusion of concentrates in the diet. However, lack of fiber and inadequate feed particle length can alter rumen physiology and reduce milk fat content (Pulina *et al.*, 2007). Nutrition also affects both the yield and composition of the milk produced. As the majority of sheep and goat milk produced in the world is transformed into cheese, the effects of nutrition on the quality of milk influence cheese yield and quality (Never, 2015).

The relationship between nutrition and health is well known. Improper nutrition (i.e. under- or overfeeding, unbalanced diet) can impact health and welfare adversely by making animals more prone to diseases or metabolic disorders (Makkar, 2016). Providing the right amount of nutrients for maintenance, growth, and reproduction through balanced diets can directly affect the fitness of infectious pathogens, detrimentally alter the environment in which they reside, and improve host resistance to the pathogens (Bertoni *et al.*, 2016). Since host resistance to infection is mediated primarily through involvement of the immune system, the effects of nutrition on immune responses make an important contribution to animal health, welfare, and performance.

Effects of Nematode Parasitism on Nutrition and Metabolism

The magnitude of the deleterious effects of GIN on intake, digestibility, and nutrient utilization, and consequently on animal performance, depends on several factors related to both parasites (i.e. species and number, extent of larval challenge) and host (i.e. species, breed, age, physiological state, nutritional and immune status) (Coop and Sykes, 2002; Athanasiadou et al., 2008; Hoste et al., 2016). In a metaanalysis performed by Mavrot et al. (2015), the reduction of growth performance, wool growth, and milk yield in parasitized vs parasite-free sheep was observed in 77%, 90%, and 78% of the studies, respectively. However, GIN influenced milk yield and weight gain to a greater extent than wool production. The average daily gain (ADG) of sheep and especially goats decreases significantly when GIN infection increases. For each 1 unit increase in log FEC, ADG decreased by 1.55 and 4.55 g/kg $BW^{0.75}$ for sheep and goats, respectively (Ceï et al., 2018).

The primary pathophysiological effects of GIN on nutrition and metabolism that impair small ruminant production are: (i) a reduction of voluntary feed intake, (ii) decreased feed efficiency, and (iii) changes in nutrient utilization. Voluntary feed intake typically accounts for most of the variation in animal productivity since it determines the level of nutrients ingested and therefore the animal's response and function (Van Soest, 1994; Mertens and Grant, 2020). Intake may be reduced as much as 10–50% in subclinical infections (Sykes, 2000; Coop and Sykes, 2002; Méndez-Ortíz et al., 2019). Ceï et al. (2018) reported that DMI decreased 7.67 g/kg $BW^{0.75}$ for each 1 unit increase in log FEC in sheep and goats. Reduction in intake may be attributed to reduced gastric acid secretion and an increase in pepsinogen and gastrin levels with abomasal nematode infestation (Lawton et al., 1996; Fox, 1997). In intestinal nematode infection, the reduced DMI may be a consequence of an imbalance in the amino acids that reaches the liver and peripheral tissues (Coop and Sykes, 2002). Decreased DMI can be exaggerated by the reduction in GI motility and slower digesta flow, with longer transit time for subclinical infections of both intestinal (Trichostrongylus colubriformis,

bankrupt worm; Gregory et al., 1985) and abomasal (Haemonchus contortus, barber pole worm; Bueno et al., 1982) nematodes.

When grazing, sheep and goats parasitized with GIN are often presented with and forced to make foraging decisions involving trade-offs between the benefits of nutrient intake and the risks of parasitism. This is illustrated by avoiding grazing close to fecal contaminated forage, changing grazing behavior (e.g. reducing bite depth and increasing bite rate), and selecting more nutritive diets (Hutchings et al., 2000; Gunn and Irvine, 2003). However, the changes in strategies may not compensate for the negative effects of GIN, as parasitized sheep take briefer bites, have lower bite masses and depth, and move greater distances, resulting in reduced nutrient intake and increased nutrient expenditure (Hutchings et al., 2000; Yoshihara et al., 2023).

Larval and adult stages of GIN cause tissue damage by lancing abomasal tissue and sloughing epithelial cell layers, resulting in leakage of up to 10% of the circulating blood, plasma, and extracellular fluids because of H. contortus and 20–125 g protein per day in T. colubriformis infections (Coop and Kyriazakis, 1999; Sykes and Coop, 2001; Hoste et al., 2016). Haemonchus contortus is by far the most pathogenic GIN of small ruminants due to its blood-feeding activity and high fecundity. Blood losses can be much more significant than the blood consumption itself as H. contortus uses the lancet to cut the abomasal tissue and induce hemorrhages before ingesting the leaking blood (Rowe et al., 1988; Besier et al., 2016; Atiba et al., 2020). As a result, H. contortus infections in sheep and goats can induce hematological alterations (hypoproteinemia, hypoalbuminemia, and hypoglobulinemia) and depletion of serum macro- and microminerals (e.g. P, Ca, Fe, Zn, and Cu) (Coop and Sykes, 2002; Alam et al., 2020).

While most (i.e. 86%) of the endogenous loss of plasma protein from the digestive tract can be reabsorbed (Poppi et al., 1990), protein losses are large because of increased demand for amino acids during gastrointestinal (GI) repair processes and further limitation of overall nutrient availability by reductions in DMI (Coop and Kyriazakis, 2001). Diarrhea associated with large worm burdens, particularly Trichostrongylus and Teladorsagia species, enhances the loss of plasma protein, sodium, and chloride with an increase in potassium level, thereby altering acid–base balance (Sahoo and Karim, 2010; Jacobson *et al.*, 2020). Additionally, mixed infection of *H. contortus* with *T. colubriformis* may impair intestinal reabsorption of endogenous protein (Rowe *et al.*, 1988), and with *Teladorsagia circumcincta* (brown stomach worm, which is found in the abomasum) reduce N balance substantially, due to both reduction in DMI and increased urinary N excretion (Parkins and Holmes, 1989). Because of priority in the use of amino acids to repair the GI tissue, blood synthesis, mucus production and development of immunity, a parasitized sheep may need an additional daily supply of 50 g protein to cover these demands (Coop and Kyriazakis, 1999).

Although forage characteristics such as maturity determine potential digestibility, animal factors and other dietary components can dramatically affect forage digestion (Mertens and Grant, 2020). According to Ceï *et al.* (2018), organic matter digestibility (OMD) in sheep and goats decreased 1.21% for each 1 unit increase in log FEC. Intestinal GIN (e.g. *T. colubriformis*) can cause extensive villous atrophy, which significantly reduces the absorption of nutrients (Coop and Sykes, 2002). Parasitized animals not only have their digestion impaired due to the reduction of enzymatic functions and changes in HCl secretion but they also suffer from a decrease in nutrient absorption in the small intestine as a result of disrupted digestive processes, which finally culminate in a diversion of nutrients from tissues (e.g. muscle, udder, wool follicles) to compensate and replace losses caused by GIN (Roy *et al.*, 2003; Hoste *et al.*, 2016).

With scarce nutritive resources resulting from decreased DMI, OMD, and absorption, the allocation of remaining absorbed nutrients varies according to the order of priority, depending on physiological stages such as growth and reproduction (Coop and Kyriazakis, 1999). In all physiological stages, maintenance of body protein, including repair, replacement, and reaction to damaged or lost tissue, is the number one priority (Fig. 2.2). While the GI tract represents 3–6% of body mass, its metabolic requirements

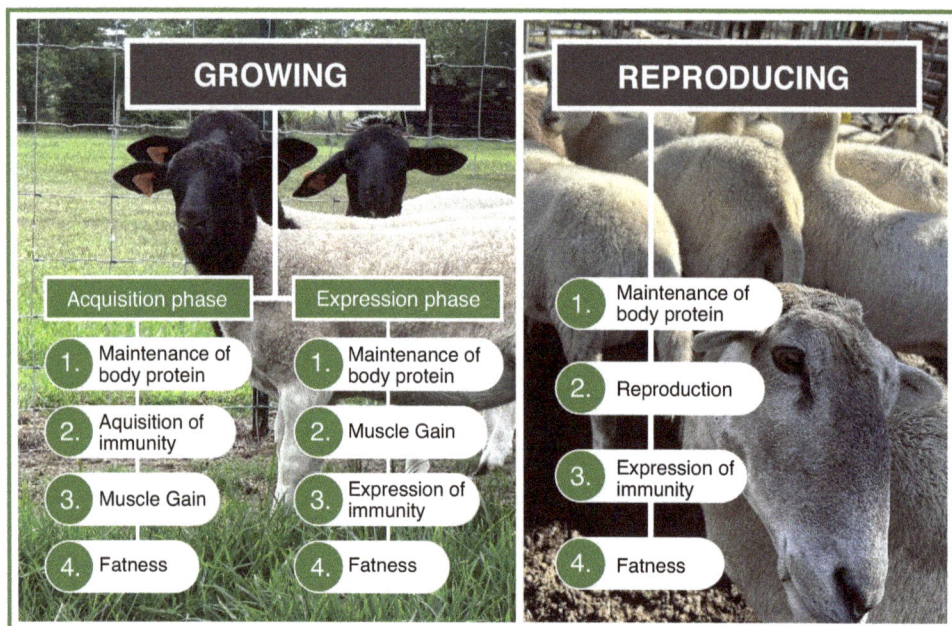

Fig. 2.2. Possible ordering of priorities (1 highest to 4 lowest) given by a growing or a reproducing animal to its various body functions when partitioning a scarce food resource. Source: Adapted from Coop and Kyriazakis (1999).

account for 20–50% of whole-body protein turnover and energy expenditure in sheep; therefore, any GI tract function and/or demand alteration (e.g. GIN infection) can have a dramatic impact on nutrient availability for other tissues (Roy et al., 2003).

For growing naive animals without prior exposure to a gastrointestinal nematode challenge, the phase of acquisition of immunity is separated from that of expression of immunity. Maintenance of body protein includes repair, replacement, and reaction to damaged or lost tissue.

Growth, reproduction, and other functions that ensure preservation of the species are given the second highest priority, depending on the physiological stage. For animals without prior exposure to a GIN challenge, the period of acquisition of immunity will be expected to be prioritized over growth, because otherwise the animal would succumb to the adverse consequences of parasitic burden before it reaches reproductive maturity (Coop and Kyriazakis, 1999). The acquisition of immunity to GIN is metabolically more expensive than the subsequent expression of immunity (Colditz, 2008). As the allocation of nutrients to reproduction (pregnancy/lactation) is prioritized before expression of acquired immunity, periparturient rise occurs, which is the rise in fecal parasitic output due to relaxation of acquired immunity to parasites around lambing/kidding (Hoste et al., 2008; Fthenakis et al., 2015). However, it should be noted that the supply of nutrients to the immune response in the gut comes from both feed and body reserves and the nutrient flow to attend the demands of other physiological processes is coordinated by hormones (Adams and Liu, 2003).

During an acute-phase response, which is the first line of defense against infections with acute-phase proteins as its agents, molecular resistance to the anabolic effects of insulin, growth hormone, and insulin-like growth factor 1 (IGF-1) reduces the capacity of muscle, skin, wool follicles, and mammary tissue to utilize nutrients for growth and production. Conversely, anabolic activity in liver and gut tissue is increased with production of acute-phase proteins (Colditz, 2008).

The immunity-associated response requires more protein than energy, particularly sulfur-containing amino acids such as cysteine and methionine (Liu et al., 2003), even though energy supply is essential for the synthesis of the increased mass of tissues associated with immunity and for immune cell functions (e.g. migration, cytokinesis, phagocytosis, antigen processing, antigen presentation, activation and effector; Méndez-Ortíz et al., 2019). Considerable demands for protein for immunity response create a strong competition for protein and decreases the animal's nutrient status. A GIN infection in sheep may result in a daily net protein loss equivalent to 0.57-, 0.71-, 0.14-, and 0.77-fold the protein requirements respectively for body growth, pregnancy, lactation, and wool production (Liu et al., 2003). Méndez-Ortíz et al. (2019) estimated protein and energy metabolic costs of 0.30 mg CP/kg BW$^{0.75}$ and 0.056 kJ/kg BW$^{0.75}$ per each adult parasite, respectively, considering a wide range of worm burden and diet quality.

Gastrointestinal parasitism has a major effect on energy metabolism of the host, largely through reductions in DMI (Coop and Sykes, 2002). Additionally, the efficiency of energy utilization is severely decreased. For instance, the efficiency of energy utilization in sheep infected with T. colubriformis and T. circumcincta is reduced by approximately 50% and 25%, respectively, which could be explained quantitatively by the anticipated additional protein synthesis in the gut (Van Houtert and Sykes, 1996). The extra energy requirement by T. colubriformis and T. circumcincta infections in sheep ranged from 0.170 to 0.421 Mcal/day, depending on the BW and ADG, and declined with increases in BW (Liu et al., 2005). Haemonchus contortus infections can reduce the efficiency of energy utilization due to, among other factors, an increase of 33% in methane production per kg of DMI (Fox et al., 2018). Not only can this decrease feed efficiency but it is also an environmental concern.

Goats seem to develop a lower immune response against GIN than sheep (Hoste et al., 2008) that can be related with their evolutionary circumstances, which resulted in distinct grazing behaviors (i.e. goats are intermediate browsers while sheep are grazers; Van Soest, 1994). In predominantly grass pastures, the exposition to GIN larval challenge provokes higher level of infections in goats than sheep, but the opposite response occurs when the animals have the opportunity to browse (Hoste *et al.*, 2008).

Effects of Nutrition on Nematode Parasitism

The role of nutrition in the ability of sheep and goats to cope with GIN has long been recognized (Poppi *et al.*, 1990; Van Houtert and Sykes, 1996). Manipulating diets is an important tool to increase resistance (i.e. ability to prevent or limit the establishment or development of infection) and resilience (i.e. ability to maintain a reasonable level of production when subjected to a parasitic challenge) of small ruminants to GIN (Tables 2.1 and 2.2). An increase in diet quality on pasture-based systems without supplementation can be achieved by planting forages with higher nutritive value than the existing ones and appropriate pasture management. Introducing forage legumes and overseeding annual grasses (e.g. summer annuals and small grains) on perennial grass pastures are practical examples that can result in more nutritious diets. Plants with nutraceutical properties, such as antiparasitic bioactive compounds (i.e. condensed tannins), can improve feed efficiency and decrease GIN infections, although their consumption may be low because of reduced palatability related to astringency. Nevertheless, the utilization of dietary supplements such as protein and energy feeds for small ruminants is an accessible, easy and fast way to increase the amount of nutrients in a given diet.

Nutrition provides nutrients to support the host's immune response and has a direct effect on GIN via modification of the digestive tract environment, which regulates their development (DeRosa *et al.*, 2005). Dietary interventions (e.g. roughage:concentrate ratio, probiotics, prebiotics, phytochemicals, dietary supplements) are associated with significant alterations of the gut environment and microbial composition that may contribute to the onset of parasitic gastroenteritis (Cortés *et al.*, 2020). In fact, many bodily functions including immune functions are penalized at times of nutrient scarcity (Houdijk, 2012); therefore, theoretically, the supplementation

of any limiting nutrient can improve the host's response to GIN infections (Athanasiadou *et al.*, 2008).

Protein

Protein has understandably been the most studied nutrient because of its importance in repairing damaged tissues, offsetting endogenous protein losses and its role in immunological responses of the host (Coop and Sykes, 2002). The expression of immunity depends on the levels of protein, and particularly RUP and certain amino acids (e.g. sulfur-containing amino acids), due to the proteinaceous nature of many components of the immune response (Coop and Kyriazakis, 2001; Houdijk, 2012). Protein supplementation can influence different effector mechanisms of the immune response towards GIN such as proliferation of inflammatory cells (i.e. mucosal mast cells, globule leukocytes, eosinophils, and goblet cells), associated release of effector molecules (e.g. mast cell proteases, leukotrienes and mucoprotein-containing mucus), and production of immunoglobulins (e.g. IgA and IgE; Athanasiadou *et al.*, 2008).

Sheep can acquire considerable resistance to GIN by 6–8 months of age, but the acquisition and expression of immunity seem to take longer to develop in goats (Hoste *et al.*, 2008). The development of immunity is impacted by the nutritional status of the animal which also interacts with animal age and infection rate (Coop and Holmes, 1996; Kahn *et al.*, 2000; Sykes, 2000). Protein intake does not appear to influence the initial parasite establishment in naive sheep, but animals with lower protein intake generally display more severe pathophysiological consequences of GIN. Lamb supplemented with a high protein (17% CP) diet developed apparent resistance to a continuing *H. contortus* infection, while those receiving a low protein (8.8% CP) diet showed no evidence of the development of any resistance (Abbott *et al.*, 1988).

As mentioned previously, an increase in the MP requirement in parasitized animals occurs because of digestion and absorption impairments as well as tissue damage and blood loss. Increasing dietary MP during the early period of

Table 2.1. Protein and energy supplementation on improving sheep resistance and resilience parameters in response to gastrointestinal nematode (GIN) infections.

Type/breed	Type of experiment	Diet[a]	Treatment[b]	Gastrointestinal nematodes (GIN)	Resistance[c]	Resilience[d]	Author(s)	Notes[e]
Protein								
Lambs Finn Dorset and Scottish Blackface	Pen	TMR containing soybean meal	8.8 vs 17% CP	H. contortus	Worm burden	PCV, growth performance	Abbott et al. (1985, 1988)	
Lambs Hampshire (H) and Scottish Blackface (SB)	Pen	TMR	9.8 vs 17.3% CP, testing the inclusion of soybean meal	H. contortus	FEC (H)	PCV, plasma protein and albumin (H), growth performance (SB), more muscle and less fat in the carcasses; leaner and more proteinaceous meat	Wallace et al. (1995, 1996)	Breed with low (H) or high (SB) GIN resistance
Lambs Hampshire	Pen	Sugar beet pulp, barley siftings	2.2% urea to increase MP in ~50%	H. contortus		PCV, plasma albumin, growth performance, feed efficiency	Wallace et al. (1998)	In infected animals. No difference in noninfected ones.
Lambs Crossbred	Pen	TMR containing cottonseed meal and urea	10–22% CP	H. contortus	FEC, antibody response	PCV, DMI, growth performance	Datta et al. (1998)	Long-term effects of diets (Datta et al., 1999)
Lambs Merino	Pen	Oat hay (oaten chaff)	3% of urea	H. contortus and T. colubriformis	FEC (mixed and H. contortus), worm burden (T. colubriformis)	DMI, growth performance and wool growth	Knox and Steel (1999)	Urea increased wool fiber diameter
Lambs Texel × Greyface	Pen	TMR containing Soypass®	9.6% vs 16.5% CP	T. colubriformis		Growth performance, feed efficiency	Kahn et al. (2000)	
Lambs Suffolk, Suffolk crossbred, Suffolk × Dorset	Grazing	Pasture +1% or 2% BW of supplement	19% CP, testing fish meal as RUP source	Mixed (73% Haemonchus spp., and 27% Teladorsagia spp. +Trichostrongylus spp.	FEC	PCV, growth performance	Crawford et al. (2020)	Advantages of fish meal inclusion and supplementation at the level of 2% BW

Continued

Table 2.1. Continued

Type/breed	Type of experiment	Diet[a]	Treatment[b]	Gastrointestinal nematodes (GIN)	Resistance[c]	Resilience[d]	Author(s)	Notes[5]
Ewes Coopworth	Pen	Hay + concentrate	0.8 to 1.25 times protein requirements with the inclusion of fish meal	Mixed (*T. circumcincta, T. colubriformis* and *T. colubriformis*)	FEC postpartum, worm burden	BW gain before parturition, lamb birth weight and growth performance	Donaldson *et al.* (1998)	Reduced periparturient rise
Ewes, Merino, GIN resistant (R) and randomly selected (S)	Grazing	Pasture + cottonseed meal	0 or 250g per day cottonseed meal before parturition or after parturition	Mixed (*Trichostrongylus* spp., *Haemonchus* spp., *Oesophagostomum* spp., *Teladorsagia* spp.)	FEC postpartum	BW pre- and postpartum, clean wool growth rate, lamb birth weight	Kahn *et al.* (2003a,b)	Reduced periparturient rise
Energy								
Lambs Pelibuey	Pen	TMR (sugarcane + concentrate)	Low and high energy (2.6 vs 3 Mcal/Kg ME, using sorghum + molasses)	*H. contortus*	FEC	PCV, TPP, growth performance	López-Leyva *et al.* (2020)	Better results with high-energy diets regardless of protein content (9% vs 12% CP)
Energy/protein								
Lambs Dorset × Hampshire	Grazing	Pasture + supplement	DDGS vs soybean hulls	Mixed		FAMACHA© score, PCV, growth performance	Felix *et al.* (2012)	Higher ADG of nondewormed fed DDGS
Lambs Corriedale crossbred	Grazing	Pastures + urea-molasses block	Urea-molasses block	Mixed (predominantly *H. contortus*)	FEC, worm burden	Growth performance	Waruiru *et al.* (2017)	
Lambs Crossbred (Dorset, Suffolk, Hampshire)	Grazing	Pasture + concentrate	1% BW concentrate (~48% CP)	Mixed (predominantly *H. contortus*)	FEC	FAMACHA© score, PCV, growth performance	Campbell *et al.* (2021)	Grazing established pastures

Lambs	Grazing	Pasture + concentrate	1.7% BW concentrate (~20% CP and 2.8 Mcal/kg ME)	Mixed	FEC	Growth performance, wool growth	Tafernaberry et al. (2022)	DDGS to partially replace sorghum and soybean meal did not affect the results
Lambs Crossbred (Ile de France, White Dorper, Texel)	Grazing/pen	Pasture + concentrate	15% of whole cottonseed replacing 50% of corn and 75% of soybean meal	Mixed (GIN and coccidia)	FEC	Thiol, TEAC AOPP, FOX	Kozlowski Neto et al. (2023)	

[a]TMR, total mixed ration.
[b]CP, crude protein; MP, metabolizable protein; RUP, rumen undegradable protein; ME, metabolizable energy; DDGS, distillers' grains with solubles.
[c]FEC, fecal egg counting.
[d]PCV, packed cell volume (hematocrit); DMI, dry matter intake; BW, body weight; TPP, total plasma protein; TEAC, trolox equivalent antioxidant capacity; AOPP, advanced oxidation protein products; FOX, ferric-xylenol orange.
[e]BW, body weight; CP, crude protein; ADG, average daily gain; DDGS, distillers' grains with solubles.

Table 2.2. Protein and energy supplementation on improving goat resistance and resilience parameters in response to gastrointestinal nematode (GIN) infections.

Type	Type of experiment	Diet	Treatment[a]	Gastrointestinal nematodes	Resistance[b]	Resilience[c]	Author(s)	Notes
Protein								
Kids Small East African	Grazing	Pastures + urea-molasses block	Urea-molasses block	Mixed (predominantly H. contortus)	FEC, worm burdens	Growth performance	Waruiru et al. (2004)	
Kids Creole	Pen	Hay + 2% protein supplement	Protein supplement (23.3% CP) with RUP	H. contortus	FEC, worm fecundity, IgA	PCV, growth performance	Cériac et al. (2019)	
Does Alpine, High (H) and low (L) milk production	Pen	Fibrous roughages and commercial concentrates	120% or 130% of protein requirements	T. colubriformis	FEC	Milk production and composition (H)	Etter et al. (2000)	
Does Alpine, high (H) and low (L) milk production	Pen	Hay, barley, and commercial concentrates	106% or 125% of protein requirements	Mixed (predominantly Trichostrongylus sp.)		Milk production, longer lactation	Chartier et al. (2000)	
Energy								
Kids Criollo	Grazing (browsing)	Pasture + corn	0%, 1%, and 1.5% BW of ground corn	H. contortus, T. colubriformis and O. colombianum	FEC, worm length, worm burden (T. columbriformis) and fecundity (H. contortus and T. columbriformis)	Growth performance	Gárate-Gallardo et al. (2015)	1.5% corn was the best treatment
Energy/protein								
Primiparous West African Dwarf × Sahelian does	Grazing (browsing)	Pasture + supplement	Whole cottonseed (200g before and 300g after parturition) + rice bran (200g before parturition)	Mixed	FEC (mid-dry season)	BW during lactation, milk production, kids' growth performance	Faye et al. (2003)	Periparturient rise control (trend)

[a]CP, crude protein; RUP, rumen undegradable protein; BW, body weight.
[b]FEC, fecal egg counting; IgA, immunoglobulin A.
[c]PCV, packed cell volume (haematocrit); BW, body weight.

infection can influence the later stages of development of sheep resistance and resilience to *H. contortus* (Datta *et al.*, 1999) and *T. colubriformis* (Kahn *et al.*, 2000). Interestingly, feeding sheep higher MP diets for a relatively short period (i.e. 9 weeks) can result in long-term benefits (i.e. over a year), probably due to enhanced immunoresponsiveness to GIN and consequently higher DMI, and absorption and utilization of nutrients (Datta *et al.*, 1999). The levels of MP in relation to maintenance requirements and the demand of other physiological functions influence the potential for MP to enhance resistance to GIN infections (Kahn *et al.*, 2000).

In order to increase supply of MP in small ruminant diets, utilization of protein feeds with a greater proportion of RUP, such as animal protein products, is the first rationale. For instance, fish meal (66% RUP and 46.2% MP) fed above the dietary protein requirement can be used to offset hypoproteinemia of predominantly *H. contortus*-parasitized sheep, which resulted in significant effects on immunological responses indicated by fecal egg count (FEC) reductions, increased packed cell volume (PCV), and growth performance (Crawford *et al.*, 2020).

Protein supplements are costly, so from a practical standpoint it is important that improvements in health and performance are sufficient to cover the investment. In this context, more emphasis on protein supplementation can be given specifically in more susceptible animals, such as young, late gestating, and lactating animals, as will be discussed in the section on supplementation practices.

It is useful to compare different protein sources considering their protein content, protein quality (e.g. RDP, RUP, MP), and prices. Several papers have reported increased sheep resilience (Abbott *et al.*, 1985; Wallace *et al.*, 1995, 1996), with fewer clinical signs of haemonchosis (i.e. anorexia, hypoproteinemia, hypoalbuminemia, weight loss, and edema), and resistance, with lower FEC (Wallace *et al.*, 1995) and worm burdens (Abbott *et al.*, 1988) as a result of supplementation with soybean meal (35% RUP and 34.3% MP). Furthermore, there are ways to treat soybean meal and other oil seed meals to increase RUP and intestinal amino acids supply. One is a nonenzymatically browned soybean meal (SoyPass®, LignoTech

USA, Rothschild, WI) that ensured greater MP supply and improved resilience of infected lambs as indicated by growth performance and feed efficiency after *T. colubriformis* infections (Kahn *et al.*, 2000). Other treatments include heating, enzyme (e.g. xylose) extrusion, alkalis, tannic acid, and formaldehyde treatment. Kid goats supplemented with rumen-protected protein enhanced their resistance to *H. contortus* (i.e. lower FEC, parasite prolificacy; Cériac *et al.*, 2019). However, rumen-protected methionine supplementation did not influence the level of *H. contortus* parasitism in kid goats despite an increase in PCV, hemoglobin, and serum IgA concentrations (Montout *et al.*, 2023).

Some plant protein products have a considerable RUP content, such as corn gluten meal (62%), cottonseed meal (43%), DDGS (53%), brewers' grains (60%), and other by-products that can be less expensive than animal protein products or soybean meal and still result in good outcomes in terms of increasing MP in small ruminant diets. For instance, supplementation of grazing lambs with DDGS allowed for increased growth and reduced anthelmintic treatment and the risk of becoming anemic because of GIN infections (Felix *et al.*, 2012). Supplementing grazing lambs with whole cottonseed (30% RUP and 3.42 Mcal/kg of energy) induced a decrease in oxidants such as ferric-xylenol orange and an increase in trolox equivalent antioxidant capacity that may benefit control of natural GIN and coccidia mixed infections (Kozlowski Neto *et al.*, 2023).

Nonprotein nitrogen such as urea can increase MP supply in sheep and goat diets and at the same time reduce the proportion of true protein supplements and supplementation costs. The addition of urea to increase by ~50% the dietary MP enhanced resilience (i.e. PCV, plasma albumin concentrations, and growth performance) of lambs infected with *H. contortus* (Wallace *et al.*, 1998), and feeding a supplement containing 3% of urea improved resilience (i.e. growth performance and wool production) and resistance mechanisms against infections of *H. contortus* (FEC), *T. colubriformis* (worm burden), and both (FEC), in young sheep fed low-quality roughage diets (Knox and Steel, 1999).

When testing supplements containing cottonseed meal and urea to achieve

10–22% CP in the diets of lambs infected with *H. contortus*, Datta *et al.* (1998, 1999) observed that groups fed with up to 16% CP lost weight and those fed over 19% CP gained weight. In these studies, FEC were significantly lower in infected lambs with higher protein diets, showing that a combination of NPN and RUP was effective. Wool production and quality improved quadratically, reaching a peak with 19% CP.

In an attempt to maximize microbial protein synthesis, urea and molasses have been used together because both present fast degradation in the rumen. Urea-molasses block enhanced resistance (i.e. FEC, worm burdens) and resilience (i.e. growth performance) in naturally infected grazing goats (Waruiru *et al.*, 2004) and sheep (Waruiru *et al.*, 2017), a strategy that can be especially relevant in extensive rangelands as feeding blocks can contain numerous agro-industrial by-products, urea, and minerals. Coating technologies have been used to develop slow-release urea products that could control urea degradation and release of ammonia into the rumen. Coated urea successfully replaced soybean meal in supplements for grazing lambs naturally infected with GIN, which might be economically advantageous as no differences in FEC, growth performance, body condition, and FAMACHA© scores were observed (Roberto *et al.*, 2023).

In small ruminant supplementation programs, the inclusion of alternative agro-industrial by-products and forage legumes containing antiparasitic plant secondary metabolites (e.g. condensed tannins) can contribute to integrated parasite management with their nutraceutical properties and cost-effectiveness (Torres-Acosta *et al.*, 2012; Hoste *et al.*, 2016). Condensed tannins in ruminant diets increase RUP and reduce methane emissions, which can affect feed efficiency positively but can restrict DMI depending on the level of inclusion (Kelln *et al.*, 2020).

There is an interaction between nutrition and genetics affecting the host's immune response, in which breeds or selected lines more resistant to GIN do not respond to protein supplements to overcome negative effects of parasitism to the same extent as less resistant ones. Dietary protein did not affect

the establishment of *H. contortus* in Scottish Blackface lambs, a breed considered highly resistant to GIN; however, in Finn Dorset lambs (more susceptible breed), high-protein diets decreased FEC and more severe clinical signs than those fed low protein (Abbott *et al.*, 1985). Protein supplementation helped Hampshire lambs (more susceptible to GIN) develop better immunity to overcome the pathogenic effects of haemonchosis, but in Scottish Blackface lambs, innate resistance masked the effects of protein supplementation (Wallace *et al.*, 1995, 1996). Merino ewes selected for *H. contortus* resistance had lower response to increased MP supply than unselected ewes, probably due to the partitioning of amino acids between the gut and other tissues that had been altered as a consequence of selection (Kahn *et al.*, 2003a, b).

The level of production is another factor that affects the response of protein supplementation on resistance and/or resilience to GIN infections. High-producing dairy goats have more severe consequences on milk production when facing *H. contortus* and *T. colubriformis* infections than low-producing ones (Hoste and Chartier, 1993). Chartier *et al.* (2000) observed partial improvements of resistance and resilience in naturally infected (primarily with *T. circumcincta* and *T. colubriformis*) high-producing does with additional protein, resulting in greater BCS and milk production, and suggested that the manipulation of protein level in their diets could reduce larval contamination of pastures. Low and high milk-producing goats infected with *T. colubriformis* had lower FEC and higher eosinophil counts when offered high-protein diets (130% of requirements), indicating that resistance was enhanced by protein supplementation; however, milk production and milk composition parameters were improved with high protein diet only in high-producing does (Etter *et al.*, 2000).

Energy

Energy supply is essential for the synthesis of tissues associated with immunity and immune cell functions such as migration, cytokinesis, phagocytosis, antigen processing, antigen presentation, activation and effector functions (Liu *et al.*, 2005). Thus, protein supplementation without a simultaneous provision of energy might not provide the expected effect for small ruminants (Torres-Acosta *et al.*, 2012), perhaps because the protein that is excess to requirements is catabolized by the animal for energy and the excess nitrogen excreted in the urine (Van Soest, 1994). Although CP × infection level is the best predictor of DMI in lambs, the association between ME intake and infection level is the best predictor of BW change, as infected animals must receive energy supplements to maintain similar BW to noninfected animals (Méndez-Ortíz *et al.*, 2019).

The consumption of carbohydrates influences the GI tract environment and, consequently, affects parasite survival in ruminants (Athanasiadou *et al.*, 2008). When energy feeds rich in starch or rapidly fermentable carbohydrates are consumed, ruminal pH drops (Mertens and Grant, 2020) and there is evidence that lower rumen fluid pH reduced the exsheathment efficiency of *Ostertagia ostertagi* in cattle (DeRosa *et al.*, 2005). Lambs parasitized with *H. contortus* receiving a high-energy (3 Mcal/Kg metabolizable energy, ME) diet had lower FEC regardless of whether they received a high (~12% CP) or low (~9%) level of protein, when compared to a low-energy (2.6 Mcal/Kg ME) diet (López-Leyva *et al.*, 2020). These authors found that the difference of high and low energy level on FEC increased over time, resulting in greater PCV, total plasma protein values, and growth performance. Supplementing browsing goat kids, naturally infected with GIN (*H. contortus*, *T. colubriformis*, and *Oesophagostomum columbianum*, which is known as nodular worm and found in the large intestine) with 1.5% of their BW in ground corn (covering 44.3% of ME and 34.7% of MP requirements) increased resistance (i.e. FEC, worm length, *T. colubriformis* worm burden and *H. contortus* and *T. colubriformis* fecundity) and resilience (i.e. growth performance) of the animals compared to unsupplemented ones, adding an additional US$5.8 per head in animal value (Gárate-Gallardo *et al.*, 2015).

Minerals and vitamins

It is known that deficiency of minerals can limit the ability of animal immune systems to deal with many diseases, including GIN parasitism (Atiba *et al.*, 2020), and that vitamins play important roles in animal health by inactivating harmful free radicals produced through normal cellular activity and from various stressors (MacGlaflin *et al.*, 2011). However, there is limited information about how each mineral and vitamin could affect small ruminant resistance and resilience to GIN. Hughes *et al.* (2023) showed that lambs receiving mineral and vitamin supplementation had lower FEC and greater energy utilization and ADG than unsupplemented ones.

Hypophosphatemia was reported because of intestinal nematode infection (Sykes and Coop, 2001). Disturbances in phosphorus (P) metabolism and, by association, calcium (Ca) can lead to severe osteomalacia and osteoporosis in parasitized sheep (Coop and Sykes, 2002). Phosphorus supply can influence resistance of sheep to *Trichostrongylus vitrinus*, which infects the small intestine, as parasitism combined with low P diets can reduce the level of P in the rumen below the threshold required for optimal microbial protein synthesis (Sykes, 2000).

Concentrations of microminerals required for healthy animals are often below what is required for animals experiencing an immunological challenge (Fekete and Kellems, 2007). Cobalt (Co) deficiency can induce higher FEC and increased pepsinogen levels in lambs infected with *T. circumcincta* (Coop and Holmes, 1996), likely because a deficiency in Co leads to vitamin B_{12} deficiency and a resultant reduction in parasite resistance (Sykes and Coop, 2001; McClure, 2003). Zinc (Zn) is directly involved in biochemical processes that affect the host's immune response, such as maturation and function of immune cells, among others, by protecting developing lymphocytes from apoptosis (Fekete and Kellems, 2007; Atiba *et al.*, 2020). Organic Zn supplementation enhanced the antioxidant status of lambs infected with *H. contortus*, which can help them to overcome the oxidative stress due to the formation of a large number of reactive molecules derived from oxygen (e.g. superoxide radicals, hydroxyl radicals, hydrogen peroxide) induced by the nematode (Čobanová *et al.*, 2020).

Copper (Cu) has been used as an anthelmintic and immunity boost in parasitized sheep and goats. COWP, initially used as mineral supplement, became an alternative to anthelmintic drugs since they possess anthelmintic activity against abomasal nematodes (Burke and Miller, 2020). COWP act on adult nematodes through the increased copper status of the host, or directly due to increased copper in the abomasum, which could potentially damage and penetrate the cuticle of *H. contortus* (Atiba *et al.*, 2020; Burke and Miller, 2020).

Addition of molybdenum (Mo, ~5 mg/kg DM) to lamb diets greatly increased host resistance to *H. contortus* (Suttle *et al.*, 1992a) and *T. vitrinus* (Suttle *et al.*, 1992b) by reducing FEC and worm burdens. Molybdenum is a well-known Cu antagonist in ruminant nutrition, but these effects could not be attributed to Cu depletion. Diets containing 6–10 mg Mo/kg DM increased lamb resistance to *T. colubriformis* indicated by lowering FEC and worm burdens compared with lambs fed diets containing Mo above or below this range (McClure, 2003). Correlated responses in intestinal antibody, jejunal mast cell, and blood eosinophil numbers suggest that Mo has an important enabling role in the cell-mediated immune response. It is possible that Mo is toxic to GIN or enhances the inflammatory response by increasing superoxide radical concentration in the mucosa, either directly or by reducing the effectiveness of local trace element-dependent antiinflammatory enzymes (Suttle *et al.*, 1992a, b). However, the Mo concentration of 6–10 mg/ kg DM reported by McClure (2003) to maximize host resistance is above the maximum tolerable level of Mo for sheep (5 mg/kg DM) according to the NRC (2007), but toxic levels depend on the chemical form of Mo, type of the diet, concentration of S, and Cu status of the animals. In grazing goats supplemented with mineral blocks, Mo reduced FEC and increased PCV, haemoglobin concentration, and growth performance, with no difference between blocks with 2 or 10 mg/ kg Mo (Mahusoon *et al.*, 2004).

Selenium (Se) has a vitamin E-independent immunostimulant effect in marginally supplied animals (Fekete and Kellems, 2007). Selenium is deficient in soils and forages in a considerable part of the US and many other countries, and small ruminant deficiency is an issue in some years as the mineral uptake into forage depends on multiple factors (e.g. type of forage, weather conditions, forage growth stage, soil mineral status; Hughes *et al.*, 2023). Selenium is an integral part of antioxidant enzymes and is important for adequate functioning of the immune system (Komáromyová *et al.*, 2021). However, according to Coop and Holmes (1996), apparent Se deficiency does not affect resistance to GIN infection. There is evidence that Se yeast reduced FEC in sheep infected with *H. contortus* after 90 days of infection but did not affect worm burden and growth performance (Komáromyová *et al.*, 2021). Parenteral administration of Se combined with Cu increased resistance (i.e. serum γ-globulin, FEC, worm burden) and resilience (i.e. growth performance) of lambs infected with *H. contortus* (Fausto *et al.*, 2014).

The most frequent cause of iron (Fe) deficiency in small ruminants is *H. contortus* infection, which is also implicated in anemia. Even though supplementation with Fe increased PCV and hemoglobin in lambs infected with *H. contortus*, it had no direct effect on GIN (Casanova *et al.*, 2018).

Although vitamins play an important role in animal health, more scientific work is necessary to elucidate the specific effects of vitamin supplementation on GIN as rumen microorganisms provide a constant supply of certain vitamins to the animal (Van Soest, 1994). Parasitized sheep had lower serum vitamin A, C, and E concentrations than uninfected sheep but the direct links between vitamin or vitamin precursor consumption and GIN loads were not made (Kozat *et al.*, 2007). Vitamin B_{12} is involved with a coenzyme form of the vitamin, adenosyl cobalamin, in glucose production from propionate, and methyl cobalamin, in methylation reactions to convert homocysteine to methionine, a precursor for synthesis of cysteine. As a result, the effects of vitamin B_{12} on amino acid availability to the host cannot be excluded (Sykes and Coop, 2001). The active form of vitamin D_3 regulates transcription at the cellular level, acts as an immunomodulator, and promotes phagocytosis (Fekete and Kellems, 2007), but its effects on GIN infections are still unknown.

NRC (2007) increased the recommended daily vitamin E requirement to boost immunocompetence in sheep based on virus challenge studies. However, biweekly parenteral vitamin E supplementation (15 or 30 IU d-α-tocopherol/kg BW) has no effect on FEC, PCV, and worm burden of lambs naturally infected with GIN (MacGlaflin *et al.*, 2011).

Supplementation practices

The main goal of a proper supplementation program is to balance all dietary nutrients and therefore, supplements based solely on protein or energy feeds would not yield an optimal response, especially under grazing/browsing conditions (Méndez-Ortíz *et al.*, 2019). The main influence of supplementation in an integrated parasite management program is on the degree of expression of immunity, indicated by reduced establishment or arrested development of incoming larvae as well as reduced survival and fecundity of the established worm population (Balic *et al.*, 2000).

Strategic supplementation, notably with increased protein supply, can be used to boost the immunological response in critical phases of small ruminant production, aiming, for instance, to reduce the periparturient rise (Donaldson *et al.*, 1998; Kahn *et al.*, 2003a; b) and lamb mortality around the time of weaning (Coop and Kyriazakis, 2001). *Teladorsagia circumcincta* and *T. colubriformis* burdens in periparturient sheep were reduced when fish meal was used to increase the amount of dietary protein above requirements; additionally, ewe BW gain before parturition, and lamb birth weight and growth performance were enhanced (Donaldson *et al.*, 2001). Grazing ewes receiving 250 g/day of cottonseed meal (corresponding to approximately 45 g/day MP and 2.6 MJ/day ME) for 5 weeks before or 6 weeks after parturition reduced FEC prepartum (Kahn *et al.*, 2003a) and postpartum (Kahn *et al.*, 2003b) compared to unsupplemented ewes. Variation in the temporal importance of supplementation was explained as a function of MP pressure, in which supplementation worked well during periods of high MP pressure as indicated from maternal BW loss. While maternal BW loss may be a practical indicator of the likely magnitude of the periparturient rise and subsequent immunoresponsiveness

to increased MP supply, it does not provide an indication as to the specific importance of body protein mass in the maintenance of immunity to GIN infection (Kahn, 2003). Lactating ewes fed a 15% CP diet had lower FEC and higher PCV than ewes receiving an 8% CP diet, regardless of the energy level (9.6 or 10.1 MJ/kg), while in pregnant and nonproductive (i.e. nonpregnant or lactating) ewes, no effect of dietary protein was observed (López-Leyva *et al.*, 2022).

Protein and/or energy supplementation trials with young sheep (Steel, 2003; Retama-Flores *et al.*, 2012; Chaudhary *et al.*, 2023) and goats (Torres-Acosta *et al.*, 2004) have shown enhanced resilience and/or resistance to GIN infections after weaning. According to Steel (2003), the increased supply of RUP enhances immune expression of young lambs in terms of reducing FEC and expelling adult worms but does not appear to limit the initial establishment of incoming larvae. Supplementary MP improves both development of immunity and resilience in lambs from sheep breeds susceptible to *H. contortus*; RUP enhances immune response to *T. circumcincta*; and the response to protein supplementation by lambs infected with *T. colubriformis* infections depends on MP content of the basal diet and period of exposure to incoming larvae (Steel, 2003). Supplementing 2-month-old kid goats with 100 g/day of sorghum and soybean meal (74%:26% respectively, fresh weight basis), when browsing native vegetation with naturally infected adult goats for 22 weeks, increased resistance (i.e. peripheral eosinophil counts) and resilience (i.e. growth performance, PCV, and hemoglobin) compared to unsupplemented ones (Torres-Acosta *et al.*, 2004). Four-month-old hair lambs grazing in silvopasture systems increased growth performance and reduced FEC at the end of 5 weeks when supplemented with 1.5% BW of corn, as a result of increased DMI, and ME and MP intakes (Retama-Flores *et al.*, 2012). Young Katahdin-St. Croix cross lambs along with their mothers raised in woodlands were more resilient to natural GIN infections (i.e. greater BW and BCS, and lower FAMACHA© scores) when supplemented with 0.5% BW of whole soybean compared to the same level of whole corn (Chaudhary *et al.*, 2023).

Lambs majorly infected with *H. contortus* (80%) offered a 48% CP supplement containing

DDGS, corn gluten meal, soybean meal and fat, at a level of 1% BW, increased growth performance and PCV, and decreased FEC and FAMACHA© scores, compared with unsupplemented lambs, when grazed predominantly on tall fescue (*Schedonorus arundinaceus*) established pastures (Campbell *et al.*, 2021). According to the data, the improvement in lamb growth by 9.4 kg in 112 days could pay off supplementation costs and resulted in US$1.27 per each US$1.00 invested in supplementation. However, when lambs grazed newly sown pasture converted from cropland, the same benefits of supplementation were not observed.

Energy-protein supplementation (i.e. whole cottonseed + rice bran) for primiparous does naturally infected with GIN, grazing semiarid rangelands, reduced FEC in mid-dry season and improved BW postpartum, milk production, and offspring growth performance. If not dewormed, supplemented does had significantly higher PCV than does offered the basal diet during the early and mid-dry season (Faye *et al.*, 2003).

High levels (1.7% BW) of energy-protein supplementation (~20% CP and 2.8 Mcal/kg ME) increased resistance (i.e. FEC, after the course of 69 days) and resilience (i.e. growth performance, wool growth) of grazing lambs naturally infected with GIN, compared with unsupplemented ones (Tafernaberry *et al.*, 2022). According to the data, using DDGS to replace approximately one-third of sorghum grain and half of the soybean meal did not change the results when the supplement energy and protein composition remained the same, which might be more economically advantageous.

A practical approach for supplementing sheep and goats in small operations is to use commercial formulations. *Haemonchus contortus*-infected goat kids fed low-quality hay (6.8% CP, 71% neutral detergent fiber, and 37.3% acid detergent fiber) and a commercial pelletized concentrate (150g/kg MP and 2.5 Mcal/kg ME) containing corn (68%), soybean meal (15%), wheat bran (11%), vitamin and mineral supplement (5%), and urea (1%), reduced FEC, regardless of the level (100–300 g/d), and increased growth performance (Bambou *et al.*, 2011). In that study, without supplementation, kid goats susceptible to GIN had 1.6 times higher FEC than resistant kids. However, FEC did not differ

among susceptible and resistant kids when supplementation was offered. In a subsequent study (Bambou *et al.*, 2021) using the same commercial concentrate at a rate of 20g/kg $BW^{0.75}$ per day for supplementing grazing goat kids naturally infected with GIN, the PCV, BCS, and growth performance increased with supplementation. Cograzing goats and cattle reduced FEC despite supplementation.

Supplementation practices for grazing small ruminants should consider complementary, substitution, and additive responses on forage DMI depending on the type and quantity of supplement offered. Complementary response is when supplement increases forage DMI (e.g. overcoming rumen degradable protein, mineral and/or vitamin deficiencies); substitution response is when the supplement consumption decreases forage DMI (e.g. high-energy/low-protein supplements); and additive response is when supplementation does not affect forage DMI (e.g. small quantities of grain) (Dove, 2002; Kawas *et al.*, 2012). The degree of substitution will be more accentuated with abundance of good-quality forage and large quantities of good-quality supplement, or when the animals do not have high demand for nutrients (Dove, 2002). The ingestion of infective larvae (L3) from contaminated pastures may be decreased when substitution response occurs, which could be advantageous from a GIN management perspective (Houdijk *et al.*, 2012; Hoste *et al.*, 2016). Substitution response could confound the interpretation of the effects of supplementation on resistance or resilience against GIN in grazing studies (Van Houtert and Sykes, 1996).

Small ruminant nutritional status can be assessed by appearance and by analyzing samples of blood and feces. Visual and palpation assessment of body condition (i.e. fat and muscle covering) can provide insight into an animal's current and future nutritional needs (Morand-Fehr, 2005; Kenyon *et al.*, 2014). A score of 1 indicates extreme thinness, while a score of 5 indicates extreme obesity. Blood serum metabolites (e.g. alanine aminotransferase, aspartate aminotransferase, alkaline phosphatase, total protein, albumin, creatine kinase, serum urea nitrogen, glucose, triglycerides), minerals (e.g. Ca, Mg, Se, Cu, Zn) and hormone (e.g. insulin-like growth factor, growth hormone, leptin) concentrations can provide a more accurate assessment of a sheep or goat's nutritional status (Hernández *et al.*, 2020; Stewart *et al.*, 2021). Additionally, fecal indices as predictors of nutrient intake have been widely used to assess the nutritional status in ruminants (Orellana *et al.*, 2019).

In recent years, metabolomic studies have identified serum biochemical markers associated with small ruminant nutrition, growth, and development (e.g. phosphatidylethanolamine, phosphatidylcholine, lysophosphatidylethanolamine, lysophosphatidylcholine, fatty acid esters of hydroxy fatty acids) (Zhang *et al.*, 2019; Goldansaz *et al.*, 2020; Li *et al.*, 2024).

Conclusion

Sheep and goat nutrition is one of the most important factors for sustainable small ruminant production, in which all nutrients necessary to grow, produce, reproduce, and boost immunity should be considered. Proper nutrition plays a key role in both resistance and resilience of small ruminants to GIN infections. Emphasis on providing nutrients that enhance immune function will help the animal resist GIN infection and improve performance, but other nutrients are required to replace and repair damaged tissues. Protein plays a key role in both of these functions since it is required to optimize immune status to help the animal resist GIN infection as well as replace lost blood components and repair damaged gut tissues. Extra energy is also required to carry out the processes of repair and replacement of damaged tissues as well as helping the animal to overcome GIN infections.

Certain trace elements are involved with immune function as well and therefore important to the animal's ability to fight off GIN infections. Therefore, care should be taken to meet not only the energy and protein requirements of the animal but also the mineral and vitamin requirements. Essential nutrient amounts will need to be increased in situations where animals carry greater GIN loads and when immune expression needs to be enhanced, such as during weaning, end of gestation and beginning of lactation periods.

Strategic supplementation is a practical technology to help sheep and goats raised in forage-based systems to cope with GIN infections and perform satisfactorily. For a successful GIN management program, an integrated approach should be adopted, which includes genetics, pasture management, utilization of nutraceutical plants, supplemental feeding, cograzing systems, biological control, and targeted selective treatment.

References

Abbott, E.M., Parkins, J.J. and Holmes, P.H. (1985) Influence of dietary protein on parasite establishment and pathogenesis in Finn Dorset and Scottish Blackface lambs given a single moderate infection of *Haemonchus contortus*. *Research in Veterinary Science* 38, 6–13.

Abbott, E.M., Parkins, J.J. and Holmes, P.H. (1988) Influence of dietary protein on the pathophysiology of haemonchosis in lambs given continuous infections. *Research in Veterinary Science* 45, 41–49.

Adams, N.R. and Liu, S.M. (2003) Principles of nutrient partitioning for wool, growth and reproduction: Implications for nematode parasitism. *Australian Journal of Experimental Agriculture* 43, 1399–1407.

Alam, R.T., Hassanen, E.A. and El-Mandrawy, S.A. (2020) *Haemonchus contortus* infection in sheep and goats: Alterations in haematological, biochemical, immunological, trace element and oxidative stress markers. *Journal of Applied Animal Research* 48, 357–364.

Aregheore, E.M. (2000) Chemical composition and nutritive value of some tropical by-product feedstuffs for small ruminants—*in vivo* and *in vitro* digestibility. *Animal Feed Science and Technology* 85, 99–109.

Athanasiadou, S., Houdijk, J. and Kyriazakis, I. (2008) Exploiting synergisms and interactions in the nutritional approaches to parasite control in sheep production systems. *Small Ruminant Research* 76, 2–11.

Atiba, E.M., Zewei, S. and Qingzhen, Z. (2020) Influence of metabolizable protein and minerals supple-
    mentation on detrimental effects of endoparasitic nematodes infection in small ruminants. *Tropical
    Animal Health and Production* 52, 2213–2219.
Balic, A., Bowles, V.M. and Meeusen, E.N. (2000) The immunobiology of gastrointestinal nematode infec-
    tions in ruminants. *Advances in Parasitology* 45, 181–241.
Ballet, N., Robert, J.C. and Williams, P.E.V. (2000) Vitamins in forages. In: Givens, D.I., Owen, E., Axford,
    R.F.E. and Omed, H.M. (eds) *Forage Evaluation in Ruminant Nutrition*. CAB International, Wallingford,
    UK, pp. 399–431.
Bambou, J.C., Archimède, H., Arquet, R., Mahieu, M., Alexandre, G. *et al*. (2011) Effect of dietary sup-
    plementation on resistance to experimental infection with *Haemonchus contortus* in Creole kids.
    Veterinary Parasitology 178, 279–285.
Bambou, J.C., Ceï, W., Arquet, R., Calif, V., Bocage, B. *et al*. (2021) Mixed grazing and dietary supplemen-
    tation improve the response to gastrointestinal nematode parasitism and production performances
    of goats. *Frontiers in Veterinary Science* 8, 628686.
Bertoni, G., Trevisi, E., Houdijk, J. and Calamari, L. (2016) Welfare is affected by nutrition through health,
    especially immune function and inflammation. In: Phillips, C.J.C. (ed.) *Nutrition and the Welfare of
    Farm Animals*. Springer, New York, USA, pp. 85–113.
Besier, R.B., Kahn, L.P., Sargison, N.D. and Wyk, J. (2016) The pathophysiology, ecology and epidemiol-
    ogy of *Haemonchus contortus* infection in small ruminants. *Advances in Parasitology* 93, 95–143.
Bueno, L., Dakkak, A. and Fioramonti, J. (1982) Gastro-duodenal motor and transit disturbances associ-
    ated with *Haemonchus contortus* infection in sheep. *Parasitology* 84, 367–374.
Burke, J.M. and Miller, J.E. (2020) Sustainable approaches to parasite control in ruminant livestock.
    Veterinary Clinics of North America: Food Animal Practice 36, 89–107.
Byers, F.M. and Schelling, G.T. (1988) Lipids in ruminant nutrition. In: Church, D.C. (ed.) *The Ruminant
    Animal: Digestive Physiology and Nutrition*. Prentice-Hall, Englewood Cliffs, USA, pp. 298–312.
Campbell, B.J., Marsh, A.E., Parker, E.M., McCutcheon, J., Fluharty, F. *et al*. (2021) The effects of protein
    supplementation and pasture maintenance on the growth, parasite burden, and economic return of
    pasture-raised lambs. *Translational Animal Science* 5, txab113.
Casanova, V.P., Aires, A.R., Collet, S.G. and Krause, A. (2018) Iron supplementation for lambs experimen-
    tally infected by *Haemonchus contortus*: Response to anemia and iron store in the bone marrow.
    Pesquisa Veterinária Brasileira 38, 1543–1548.
Cériac, S., Archimède, H., Feuillet, D., Felicite, Y., Giorgi, M. *et al*. (2019) Supplementation with rumen-
    protected proteins induces resistance to *Haemonchus contortus* in goats. *Scientific Reports* 9, 1237.
Ceï, W., Salah, N., Alexandre, G. and Archimede, H. (2018) Impact of energy and protein on the gastro-
    intestinal parasitism of small ruminants: A meta-analysis. *Livestock Science* 212, 34–44.
Chartier, C., Etter, E., Hoste, H., Pors, I., Mallereau, M. *et al*. (2000) Effects of the initial level of milk
    production and of the dietary protein intake on the course of natural nematode infection in dairy
    goats. *Veterinary Parasitology* 92, 1–13.
Chaudhary, S., Karki, U., Shrestha, B., Lamsal, S. and Karki, L. (2023) Supplement type influenced the
    performance and resiliency against gastrointestinal parasites of nursing lambs raised in woodlands.
    Professional Agricultural Workers Journal 9, 38–49.
Colditz, I.G. (2008) Six costs of immunity to gastrointestinal nematode infections. *Parasite Immunology*
    30, 63–70.
Coop, R.L. and Holmes, P.H. (1996) Nutrition and parasite interaction. *International Journal for Parasitology*
    26, 951–962.
Coop, R.L. and Kyriazakis, I. (1999) Nutrition–parasite interaction. *Veterinary Parasitology* 84, 187–204.
Coop, R.L. and Kyriazakis, I. (2001) Influence of host nutrition on the development and consequences of
    nematode parasitism in ruminants. *Trends in Parasitology* 17, 325–330.
Coop, R.L. and Sykes, A.R. (2002) Interactions between gastrointestinal parasites and nutrients. In: Freer,
    M. and Dove, H. (eds) *Sheep Nutrition*. CAB International, Wallingford, UK, pp. 313–331.
Cortés, A., Rooney, J., Bartley, D.J., Nisbet, A. and Cantacessi, C. (2020) Helminths, hosts, and their
    microbiota: New avenues for managing gastrointestinal helminthiases in ruminants. *Expert Review
    of Anti-Infective Therapy* 18, 977–985.
Crawford, C.D., Mata-Padrino, D.J., Belesky, D.P. and Bowdridge, S. (2020) Effects of supplementation
    containing rumen by-pass protein on parasitism in grazing lambs. *Small Ruminant Research* 190,
    106161.

Datta, F.U., Nolan, J.V., Rowe, J.B. and Gray, G. (1998) Protein supplementation improves the performance of parasitised sheep fed a straw-based diet. *International Journal for Parasitology* 28, 1269–1278.

Datta, F.U., Nolan, J.V., Rowe, J.B., Gray, G. and Crook, B. (1999) Long-term effects of short-term provision of protein-enriched diets on resistance to nematode infection, and live-weight gain and wool growth in sheep. *International Journal for Parasitology* 29, 479–488.

DeRosa, A.A., Chirgwin, S.R., Fletcher, J., Williams, J. and Klei, T. (2005) Exsheathment of *Ostertagia ostertagi* infective larvae following exposure to bovine rumen contents derived from low and high roughage diets. *Veterinary Parasitology* 129, 77–81.

Devendra, C. (1988) Nutrition and meat production. In: Devendra, C. (ed.) *Proceedings of the Workshop Goat Meat Production in Asia. Tando Jam*, Tando Jam, Pakistan. Available at: https://idl-bnc-idrc .dspacedirect.org/server/api/core/bitstreams/dcc39309-b40d-46a2-8c13-6ff3b8d911e2/content (accessed 9 July 2025).

Di Trana, A. and Sepe, L. (2007) Goat nutrition for fibre production. In: Cannas, A. and Pulina, G. (eds) *Dairy Goats: Feeding and Nutrition*. CAB International, Wallingford, UK, pp. 238–262.

Donaldson, J., Van Houtert, M.F.J. and Sykes, A.R. (1998) The effect of nutrition on the periparturient parasite status of mature ewes. *Animal Science* 67, 523–533.

Donaldson, J., Van Houtert, M.F.J. and Sykes, A.R. (2001) The effect of dietary fish-meal supplementation on parasite burdens of periparturient sheep. *Animal Science* 72, 149–158.

Dove, H. (2002) Principles of supplementary feeding in sheep-grazing systems. In: Freer, M. and Dove, H. (eds) *Sheep Nutrition*. CAB International, Wallingford, UK, pp. 119–142.

Etter, E., Hoste, H., Chartier, C., Pors, I., Koch, C. *et al.* (2000) The effect of two levels of dietary protein on resistance and resilience of dairy goats experimentally infected with *Trichostrongylus colubriformis*: Comparison between high and low producers. *Veterinary Research* 31, 247–258.

Fadel, J.G. (1999) Quantitative analyses of selected plant by-product feedstuffs, a global perspective. *Animal Feed Science and Technology* 79, 255–268.

FAOSTAT (2024) Food and Agriculture Organization of the United Nation. UNdata. Sheep, Goat. Available at: https://data.un.org/Data.aspx?d=FAO&f=itemCode%3A976 (accessed 9 July 2025).

Fausto, G.C., Pivoto, F.L., Costa, M.M., Lopes, S., Franca, R. *et al.* (2014) Protein profile of lambs experimentally infected with *Haemonchus contortus* and supplemented with selenium and copper. *Parasites & Vectors* 7, 1–6.

Faye, D., Leak, S., Nouala, S., Fall, A., Losson, B. *et al.* (2003) Effects of gastrointestinal helminth infections and plane of nutrition on the health and productivity of F1 (West African Dwarf × Sahelian) goat crosses in The Gambia. *Small Ruminant Research* 50, 153–161.

Fekete, S.G. and Kellems, R.O. (2007) Interrelationship of feeding with immunity and parasitic infection: A review. *Veterinarni Medicina-PRAHA* 52, 131.

Felix, T.L., Susin, I. and Shoup, L.M. (2012) Effects of supplemental dried distillers grains or soybean hulls on growth and internal parasite status of grazing lambs. *Sheep & Goat Research Journal* 27, 1–8.

Fox, M.T. (1997) Pathophysiology of infection with gastrointestinal nematodes in domestic ruminants: Recent developments. *Veterinary Parasitology* 72, 285–308.

Fox, N.J., Smith, L.A., Houdijk, J.G.M., Athanasiadou, S. and Hutchings, M. (2018) Ubiquitous parasites drive a 33% increase in methane yield from livestock. *International Journal for Parasitology* 48, 1017–1021.

Fthenakis, G.C., Mavrogianni, V.S., Gallidis, E. and Papadopoulos, E. (2015) Interactions between parasitic infections and reproductive efficiency in sheep. *Veterinary Parasitology* 208, 56–66.

Gárate-Gallardo, L., de Jesús Torres-Acosta, J.F., Aguilar-Caballero, A.J., Sandoval-Castro, C., Camara-Sarmiento, R. *et al.* (2015) Comparing different maize supplementation strategies to improve resilience and resistance against gastrointestinal nematode infections in browsing goats. *Parasite* 22, 19.

Goetsch, A.L., Merkel, R.C. and Gipson, T.A. (2011) Factors affecting goat meat production and quality. *Small Ruminant Research* 101, 173–181.

Goldansaz, S.A., Markus, S., Berjanskii, M., Rout, M., Guo, A. *et al.* (2020) Candidate serum metabolite biomarkers of residual feed intake and carcass merit in sheep. *Journal of Animal Science* 98, skaa298.

Gregory, P.C., Wenham, G., Poppi, D., Coop, R., MacRae, J. *et al.* (1985) The influence of a chronic subclinical infection of *Trichostrongylus colubriformis* on gastrointestinal motility and digesta flow in sheep. *Parasitology* 91, 381–396.

Gunn, A. and Irvine, R.J. (2003) Subclinical parasitism and ruminant foraging strategies: A review. *Wildlife Society Bulletin* 31, 117–126.

Gurung, N.K., Rush, J. and Pugh, D.G. (2020) Feeding and nutrition. In: Pugh, D.G., Baird, A.N., Edmondson, M.A. and Passler, T. (eds) *Sheep Goat and Cervid Medicine*. Elsevier, Amsterdam, The Netherlands, pp. 15–44.

Hernández, J., Benedito, J.L. and Castillo, C. (2020) Relevance of the study of metabolic profiles in sheep and goat flock. Present and future: A review. *Spanish Journal of Agricultural Research* 18, e06R01.

Hoste, H. and Chartier, C. (1993) Comparison of the effects on milk production of concurrent infection with *Haemonchus contortus* and *Trichostrongylus colubriformis* in high-and low-producing dairy goats. *American Journal of Veterinary Research* 54, 1881–1885.

Hoste, H., Torres-Acosta, J.F.J. and Aguilar-Caballero, A.J. (2008) Nutrition–parasite interactions in goats: Is immunoregulation involved in the control of gastrointestinal nematodes? *Parasite Immunology* 30, 79–88.

Hoste, H., Torres-Acosta, J.F.J., Quijada, J., Chan-Perez, I., Dakheel, M. *et al.* (2016) Interactions between nutrition and infections with *Haemonchus contortus* and related gastrointestinal nematodes in small ruminants. *Advances in Parasitology* 93, 239–351.

Houdijk, J.G. (2012) Differential effects of protein and energy scarcity on resistance to nematode parasites. *Small Ruminant Research* 103, 41–49.

Houdijk, J.G., Kyriazakis, I., Kidane, A. and Athanasiadou, S. (2012) Manipulating small ruminant parasite epidemiology through the combination of nutritional strategies. *Veterinary Parasitology* 186, 38–50.

Huang, Y., Liu, L., Zhao, M., Zhang, X., Chen, J. *et al.* (2023) Feeding regimens affecting carcass and quality attributes of sheep and goat meat — a comprehensive review. *Animal Bioscience* 36, 1314.

Hughes, M., Phillips, E.J. and Jones, R.A. (2023) Supplementation of minerals and vitamins influences optimal targeted selective treatment thresholds for the control of gastro-intestinal nematodes in lambs. *Veterinary Parasitology* 322, 110026.

Hutchings, M.R., Kyriazakis, I., Papachristou, T.G., Gordon, I. and Jackson, F. (2000) The herbivores' dilemma: Trade-offs between nutrition and parasitism in foraging decisions. *Oecologia* 124, 242–251.

Hynd, P.I. and Masters, D.G. (2002) Nutrition and wool growth. In: Freer, M. and Dove, H. (eds) *Sheep Nutrition*. CAB International, Wallingford, UK, pp. 165–187.

Jacobson, C., Larsen, J.W., Besier, R.B., Lloyd, J. and Kahn, L. (2020) Diarrhoea associated with gastrointestinal parasites in grazing sheep. *Veterinary Parasitology* 282, 109139. DOI: 10.1016/j.vetpar.2020.109139.

Jasmin, B.H., Boston, R.C., Modesto, R.B. and Schaer, T. (2011) Perioperative ruminal pH changes in domestic sheep (*Ovis aries*) housed in a biomedical research setting. *Journal of the American Association for Laboratory Animal Science* 50, 27–32.

Kahn, L.P. (2003) Regulation of the resistance and resilience of periparturient ewes to infection with gastrointestinal nematode parasites by dietary supplementation. *Australian Journal of Experimental Agriculture* 43, 1477–1485.

Kahn, L.P., Kyriazakis, I., Jackson, F. and Coop, R. (2000) Temporal effects of protein nutrition on the growth and immunity of lambs infected with *Trichostrongylus colubriformis*. *International Journal for Parasitology* 30, 193–205.

Kahn, L.P., Knox, M.R., Walkden-Brown, S.W. and Lea, J. (2003a) Regulation of the resistance to nematode parasites of single-and twin-bearing Merino ewes through nutrition and genetic selection. *Veterinary Parasitology* 114, 15–31.

Kahn, L.P., Knox, M.R., Gray, G.D., Lea, J. and Walkden-Brown, S. (2003b) Enhancing immunity to nematode parasites in single-bearing merino ewes through nutrition and genetic selection. *Veterinary Parasitology* 112, 211–225.

Kawas, J.R., Mahgoub, O. and Lu, C.D. (2012) Nutrition of the meat goat. In: Mahgoub, O., Kadim, I. and Webb, E. (eds) *Goat Meat Production and Quality*. CAB International, Wallingford, UK, pp. 161–195.

Kelln, B.M., Penner, G.B., Acharya, S.N., McAllister, T. and Lardner, H. (2020) Impact of condensed tannin-containing legumes on ruminal fermentation, nutrition, and performance in ruminants: A review. *Canadian Journal of Animal Science* 101, 210–223.

Kenyon, P.R., Maloney, S.K. and Blache, D. (2014) Review of sheep body condition score in relation to production characteristics. *New Zealand Journal of Agricultural Research* 57, 38–64.

Knox, M.R. and Steel, J.W. (1999) The effects of urea supplementation on production and parasito-logical responses of sheep infected with *Haemonchus contortus* and *Trichostrongylus colubriformis*. *Veterinary Parasitology* 83, 123–135.

Komáromyová, M., Mravčáková, D., Petrič, D., Kucková, K., Babják, M. *et al.* (2021) Effects of medicinal plants and organic selenium against ovine haemonchosis. *Animals* 11, 1319.

Kozat, S., Göz, Y. and Yörük, B.H. (2007) Some trace elements and vitamins A, C, and E levels in ewes infected with gastrointestinal parasites. *Yyü Vet Fak Derg* 18, 9–12.

Kozlowski Neto, V.A., Schmidt, E.M.D.S., Rubio, C.P., Silva, N., Tardivo, R. *et al.* (2023) Effect of sup-plementation of lambs with whole cottonseed: Impact on serum biomarkers and infection by gastro-intestinal parasites under field conditions. *Metabolites* 13, 398.

Lawton, D.E.B., Reynolds, G.W., Hodgkinson, S.M., Pomroy, W. and Simpson, H. (1996) Infection of sheep with adult and larval *Ostertagia circumcincta*: Effects on abomasal pH and serum gastrin and pepsinogen. *International Journal for Parasitology* 26, 1063–1074.

Li, Q., Chao, T., Wang, Y., Xuan, R., Guo, Y. *et al.* (2024) Comparative metabolomics reveals serum metabolites changes in goats during different developmental stages. *Scientific Reports* 14, 7291.

Liu, S.M., Masters, D.G. and Adams, N.R. (2003) Potential impact of nematode parasitism on nutrient par-titioning for wool production, growth and reproduction in sheep. *Australian Journal of Experimental Agriculture* 43, 1409–1417.

Liu, S.M., Smith, T.L., Karlsson, L.J.E., Palmer, D. and Besier, R. (2005) The costs for protein and energy requirements by nematode infection and resistance in Merino sheep. *Livestock Production Science* 97, 131–139.

López-Leyva, Y., González-Garduño, R., Huerta-Bravo, M., Ramírez-Valverde, R., Torres-Hernández, G. *et al.* (2020) High energy levels in the diet reduce the parasitic effect of *Haemonchus contortus* in Pelibuey sheep. *Heliyon* 6, e05870.

López-Leyva, Y., González-Garduño, R., Cruz-Tamayo, A.A., Arece-Garcia, J., Huerta-Bravo, M. *et al.* (2022) Protein supplementation as a nutritional strategy to reduce gastrointestinal nematodiasis in periparturient and lactating Pelibuey ewes in a tropical environment. *Pathogens* 11, 941.

MacGlaflin, C.E., Zajac, A.M., Rego, K.A. and Petersson, K. (2011) Effect of vitamin E supplementation on naturally acquired parasitic infection in lambs. *Veterinary Parasitology* 175, 300–305.

Mahusoon, M.M., Perera, A.N.F., Perera, E.R.K. and Perera, K. (2004) Effect of molybdenum supplemen-tation on circulating mineral levels, nematode infection and body weight gain in goats as related to season. *Tropical Agriculture Research* 16, 128–136.

Makkar, H.P. (2016) Animal nutrition in a 360-degree view and a framework for future R&D work: Towards sustainable livestock production. *Animal Production Science* 56, 1561–1568.

Martin, G.B., Milton, J.T.B., Davidson, R.H., Hunzicker, G., Lindsay, G. *et al.* (2004) Natural methods for increasing reproductive efficiency in small ruminants. *Animal Reproduction Science* 82, 231–245.

Mavrot, F., Hertzberg, H. and Torgerson, P. (2015) Effect of gastro-intestinal nematode infection on sheep performance: A systematic review and meta-analysis. *Parasites & Vectors* 8, 1–11.

McClure, S.J. (2003) Mineral nutrition and its effects on gastrointestinal immune function of sheep. *Australian Journal of Experimental Agriculture* 43, 1455–1461.

Méndez-Ortíz, F.A., Sandoval-Castro, C.A., Vargas-Magaña, J.J., Sarmiento-Franco, L., Torres-Acosta, J. *et al.* (2019) Impact of gastrointestinal parasitism on dry matter intake and live weight gain of lambs: A meta-analysis to estimate the metabolic cost of gastrointestinal nematodes. *Veterinary Parasitology* 265, 1–6.

Merchen, N.R. (1988) Digestion, absorption and excretion in ruminants. In: Church, D.C. (ed.) *The Ruminant Animal: Digestive Physiology and Nutrition*. Prentice-Hall. Englewood Cliffs, USA, pp. 172–201.

Mertens, D.R. and Grant, R.J. (2020) Digestibility and intake. In: Collins, M., Nelson, C.J., Moore, K.J. and Barnes, R.F. (eds) *Forages: The Science of Grassland Agriculture*, 7th edn. Wiley-Blackwell, Hoboken, USA, pp. 609–631.

Meyer, K., Hummel, J. and Clauss, M. (2010) The relationship between forage cell wall content and volun-tary food intake in mammalian herbivores. *Mammal Review* 40, 221–245.

Min, B.R., Barry, T.N., Attwood, G.T. and McNabb, W. (2003) The effect of condensed tannins on the nutrition and health of ruminants fed fresh temperate forages: A review. *Animal Feed Science and Technology* 106, 3–19.

Montout, L., Bahloul, L., Feuillet, D., Jean-Bart, M., Archimede, H. *et al.* (2023) Supplementation with rumen-protected methionine reduced the parasitic effect of *Haemonchus contortus* in goats. *Veterinary Sciences* 10, 559.

Morand-Fehr, P. (2005) Recent developments in goat nutrition and application: A review. *Small Ruminant Research* 60, 25–43.

Never, A. (2015) Effects of nutrition on yield and milk composition in sheep and goats. *Scientific Journal of Animal Science* 4, 1–10.

NRC - National Research Council, Committee on Nutrient Requirements of Small Ruminant (2007) *National Research Council, Committee on Nutrient Requirements of Small Ruminants*. National Academies Press, Washington, DC, USA.

Oddy, V.H. and Sainz, R.D. (2002) Nutrition and wool growth. In: Freer, M. and Dove, H. (eds) *Sheep Nutrition*. CAB International, Wallingford, UK, pp. 237–262.

Orellana, C., Parraguez, V.H., Arana, W., Escanilla, J., Zavaleta, C. *et al.* (2019) Use of fecal indices as a non-invasive tool for nutritional evaluation in extensive-grazing sheep. *Animals* 10, 46.

Owens, F.N. and Goetsch, A.L. (1988) Ruminal fermentation. In: Church, D.C. (ed.) *The Ruminant Animal: Digestive Physiology and Nutrition*. Prentice-Hall, Englewood Cliffs, USA, pp. 145–171.

Parkins, J.J. and Holmes, P.H. (1989) Effects of gastrointestinal helminth parasites on ruminant nutrition. *Nutrition Research Reviews* 2, 227–246.

Poppi, D.P., Sykes, A.R. and Dynes, R.A. (1990) The effect of endoparasitism on host nutrition – the implications for nutrient manipulation. In: *Proceedings of the New Zealand Society of Animal Production*, pp. 237–244 (Vol. 50).

Pulina, G., Nudda, A., Battacone, G., Fancellu, S. and Francesconi, A. (2007) Nutrition and quality of goat's milk. In: Pulina, G. and Bencini, R. (eds) *Dairy Goats Feeding and Nutrition*. CAB International, Wallingford, UK, pp. 1–30.

Rasmussen, J. and Harrison, A. (2011) The benefits of supplementary fat in feed rations for ruminants with particular focus on reducing levels of methane production. *International Scholarly Research Notices* 2011, 613172.

Redden, R. and Thorne, J.W. (2020) Reproductive management of sheep and goats. In: Blazer, F.W., Lamb, C. and Wu, G. (eds) *Animal Agriculture: Sustainability Challenges and Innovations*. Academic Press, Cambridge, USA, pp. 211–230.

Retama-Flores, C., Torres-Acosta, J.F.J., Sandoval-Castro, C.A., Aguilar-Caballero, A., Camara-Sarmiento, R. *et al.* (2012) Maize supplementation of Pelibuey sheep in a silvopastoral system: Fodder selection, nutrient intake and resilience against gastrointestinal nematodes. *Animal* 6, 145–153.

Roberto, F.F.D.S., Difante, G.D.S., Costa, R.G., Borges, F., Itavo, L. *et al.* (2023) Extruded urea levels in lamb supplementation in rainy tropical savanna conditions: The triad host-gastrointestinal nematodes-environment. *Tropical Animal Health and Production* 55, 193.

Rowe, J.B., Nolan, J.V., Chaneet, G.D., Teleni, E. and Holmes, P. (1988) The effect of haemonchosis and blood loss into the abomasum on digestion in sheep. *British Journal of Nutrition* 59, 125–139.

Roy, N.C., Bermingham, E.N., Sutherland, I.A. and McNabb, W. (2003) Nematodes and nutrient partitioning. *Australian Journal of Experimental Agriculture* 43, 1419–1426.

Sahoo, A. and Karim, S.A. (2010) Sheep and goat nutrition: Newer concepts and emerging challenges. *Indian Journal of Small Ruminants* 16, 18–28.

Stanton, T.L. and Whittier, J. (2006). Urea and NPN for Cattle and Sheep. Colorado State University Extension. Fact sheet 1.608. Available at: https://extension.colostate.edu/docs/pubs/livestk/01608 .pdf (accessed 9 July 2025).

Steel, J.W. (2003) Effects of protein supplementation of young sheep on resistance development and resilience to parasitic nematodes. *Australian Journal of Experimental Agriculture* 43, 1469–1476.

Stewart, W.C., Scasta, J.D., Taylor, J.B., Murphy, T. and Julian, A. (2021) Mineral nutrition considerations for extensive sheep production systems. *Applied Animal Science* 37, 256–272.

Suttle, N.F., Knox, D.P., Angus, K.W., Jackson, F. and Coop, R. (1992a) Effects of dietary molybdenum on nematode and host during *Haemonchus contortus* infection in lambs. *Research in Veterinary Science* 52, 230–235.

Suttle, N.F., Knox, D.P., Jackson, F., Coop, R. and Angus, K. (1992b) Effects of dietary molybdenum on nematode and host during *Trichostrongylus vitrinus* infection in lambs. *Research in Veterinary Science* 52, 224–229.

Sykes, A.R. (2000) Environmental effects on animal production: The nutritional demands of nematode parasite exposure in sheep. *Asian-Australasian Journal of Animal Sciences* 13, 343–350.

Sykes, A.R. and Coop, R.L. (2001) Interaction between nutrition and gastrointestinal parasitism in sheep. *New Zealand Veterinary Journal* 49, 222–226.

Tafernaberry, A., Romaniuk, E., Lier, E.V. and Reyno, R. (2022) High performance of growing lambs grazing *Paspalum notatum* INIA sepé with energy-protein supplement including sorghum-DDGS. *Agrociencia Uruguay* 26, 549.

Torres-Acosta, J.F.J., Jacobs, D.E., Aguilar-Caballero, A., Sandoval-Castro, C., May-Martinez, M. *et al.* (2004) The effect of supplementary feeding on the resilience and resistance of browsing criollo kids against natural gastrointestinal nematode infections during the rainy season in tropical Mexico. *Veterinary Parasitology* 124, 217–238.

Torres-Acosta, J.F.J., Sandoval-Castro, C.A., Hoste, H., Aguilar-Caballero, A., Camara-Sarmiento, R. *et al.* (2012) Nutritional manipulation of sheep and goats for the control of gastrointestinal nematodes under hot humid and subhumid tropical conditions. *Small Ruminant Research* 103, 28–40.

Van Houtert, M.F. and Sykes, A.R. (1996) Implications of nutrition for the ability of ruminants to withstand gastrointestinal nematode infections. *International Journal for Parasitology* 26, 1151–1167.

Van Soest, P.J. (1994) *Nutritional Ecology of the Ruminant*. Cornell University Press, New York, USA.

Wallace, D.S., Bairden, K., Duncan, J.L., Fishwick, G., Gill, M. *et al.* (1995) Influence of supplementation with dietary soyabean meal on resistance to haemonchosis in Hampshire Down lambs. *Research in Veterinary Science* 58, 232–237.

Wallace, D.S., Bairden, K., Duncan, J.L., Fishwick, G., Gill, M. *et al.* (1996) Influence of soyabean meal supplementation on the resistance of Scottish Blackface lambs to haemonchosis. *Research in Veterinary Science* 60, 138–143.

Wallace, D.S., Bairden, K., Duncan, J.L., Eckersall, P., Fishwick, G. *et al.* (1998) The influence of dietary supplementation with urea on resilience and resistance to infection with *Haemonchus contortus*. *Parasitology* 116, 67–72.

Waruiru, R.M., Ngotho, J.W. and Mutune, M.N. (2004) Effect of urea-molasses block supplementation on grazing weaner goats naturally infected with gastrointestinal nematodes. *Onderstepoort Journal of Veterinary Research* 71, 285–289.

Waruiru, R.M., Munyua, W.K., Mavuti, S.K., Otieno, R., Mutune, M. *et al.* (2017) Effects of medicated urea-molasses block supplementation on productivity and gastrointestinal nematode infestation of sheep in central Kenya. *Livestock Research for Rural Development* 29, 161.

Yang, K., Qing, Y., Yu, Q. and Tang, X. (2021) By-product feeds: Current understanding and future perspectives. *Agriculture* 11, 207.

Yoshihara, Y., Saiga, C., Tamura, T. and Kinugasa, T. (2023) Relationships between sheep nematode infection, nutrition, and grazing behavior on improved and semi-natural pastures. *Veterinary and Animal Science* 19, 100278.

Zervas, G. and Tsiplakou, E. (2011) The effect of feeding systems on the characteristics of products from small ruminants. *Small Ruminant Research* 101, 140–149.

Zhang, J., Gao, Y., Guo, H., Ding, Y. and Ren, W. (2019) Comparative metabolome analysis of serum changes in sheep under overgrazing or light grazing conditions. *BMC Veterinary Research* 15, 1–10.

Čobanová, K., Váradyová, Z., Grešáková, Ľ., Kucková, K., Mravčáková, D. *et al.* (2020) Does herbal and/or zinc dietary supplementation improve the antioxidant and mineral status of lambs with parasite infection? *Antioxidants* 9, 1172.

3 Anthelmintics, Resistance, and Guidelines for Use in Controlling Gastrointestinal Nematodes of Small Ruminants

Michael Pesato[1]* and Susan Schoenian[2]

[1]*Four State Veterinary Services, Newark, Delaware, USA;* [2]*University of Maryland Extension (retired), Western Maryland Research & Education Center, Keedysville, Maryland, USA*

Abstract

Deworming sheep and goats is a practice that has evolved over the decades. The three major classes of dewormers are benzimidazoles, macrocyclic lactones, and cholinergic agonists which were discovered in the 1960s, 1970s, and 1980s respectively. Each class has a unique function and affects the parasite in different ways. Although it was previously recommended to deworm animals often and aggressively, it is now recommended that a targeted deworming approach is followed. This approach includes both animal assessment using modalities like FAMACHA© scoring and the Five-Point Check and fecal assessment using fecal egg-counting techniques. Targeted deworming strategies aim to decrease anthelmintic resistance development amongst parasites.

Introduction

Parasites in small ruminants present a unique challenge for both producers and veterinarians alike. The ability of the parasite population within sheep and goats to develop resistance to current commercial therapies continues to complicate treatment. Multiple anthelmintics are commercially available for use in sheep and goats that range in efficacy depending on many factors. Use of these anthelmintics relies on judicious medicinal use practices which include a targeted deworming approach. This chapter will discuss currently available anthelmintic options as well as how to implement targeted deworming strategies.

History and Traditional Use of Anthelmintics

History of available anthelmintic compounds

There are three main classes of anthelmintics that are commonly used in small ruminant parasite control: the benzimidazoles, macrocyclic lactones, and cholinergic agonists (Fissiha and Kinde, 2021). Cholinergic agonists can be further subdivided into two classes: the imidazothiazole class and the tetrahydropyrimidine class. Each class has one or more compounds that are used for parasite control in the small ruminant. From the

*Corresponding author: mpasatodvm@gmail.com

© CAB International 2026. *Management Practices for Controlling Nematode Parasites of Small Ruminants* (eds James E. Miller and Joan M. Burke)
DOI: 10.1079/9781800623767.0003

benzimidazole class, fenbendazole and albendazole are the two most common compounds used in sheep and goats. Ivermectin and moxidectin are the two most common compounds from the macrocyclic lactone class while there are two main cholinergic agonists: levamisole and morantel tartrate. Levamisole belongs to the imidazothiazole class of anthelmintics while morantel tartrate is a tetrahydropyrimidine. These compounds have been the backbone of small ruminant parasite control for decades and their history, properties, and uses will be discussed throughout this chapter.

The first class of anthelmintics to be discovered was the benzimidazoles. The first veterinary benzimidazole, thiabendazole, was discovered in 1961 (Cantón et al., 2022). Following this discovery, many more benzimidazole variations were discovered including the benzimidazole methylcarbamates (Cantón et al., 2022). This classification of benzimidazole includes fenbendazole and albendazole. These sulfur-containing methylcarbamate derivatives were used extensively in small ruminants due to their exhibited high efficacy against both lungworms and gastrointestinal nematodes (Cantón et al., 2022). The mechanism of action of benzimidazoles is to bind to nematode tubulin and inhibit the formation of microtubules. The inhibition of these tubules leads to a build-up of secretory granules and/or enzymes in the cell cytoplasm, eventually leading to cell lysis and death of the parasite (Cantón et al., 2022).

In the 1970s, cholinergic agonists were discovered (Kaplan, 2009). Under this classification, there are two unrelated classes of anthelmintics that have similar mechanisms of action: imidazothiazole, represented by the compound levamisole, and tetrahydropyrimidine, represented by the compound morantel tartrate (Kaplan, 2009). Both compounds act on the nicotinic receptors at the neuromuscular junction, leading to spastic muscle paralysis of the parasite (Cantón et al., 2022). This spastic paralysis is a result of prolonged activation of the excitatory nicotinic acetylcholine receptors on muscle of the nematode body wall and will eventually lead to parasite death (Cantón et al., 2022).

Two groups exist within the macrocyclic lactone class: avermectins and milbemycins (Merola and Eubig, 2012). Both groups are derivatives of naturally occurring compounds that are secreted by soil-dwelling bacteria of the genus *Streptomyces* (Kaplan, 2009). There are 16 total members of the class within these two major groups (Cantón et al., 2022) but only two main compounds are used in small ruminants: ivermectin and moxidectin. Both discovered in the early 1980's, ivermectin is considered an avermectin while moxidectin is a milbemycin (Prichard et al., 2012). The difference between these two groups is related to the biochemical structure of the compounds (Cantón et al., 2022). Both compounds, however, perform the same task—they bind to γ-aminobutyric (GABA) and glutamate-gated chloride channels. Chloride enters the muscle of the nematode, causing paralysis and eventual death (Cobb and Boeckh, 2009). Morantel tartrate may also interfere with glucose metabolism of the nematode although this is mostly achieved at high concentrations (Sharma and Anand, 1997).

The newest class of anthelmintics, amino-acetonitrile derivatives, were first marketed in 2008 (Dilrukshi Herath et al., 2021). The only compound in this class is monepantel. Monepantel targets specific nicotinic acetylcholine receptors of the nematode and binds to these receptors. The compound mimics the acetylcholine and signals for muscle contraction, leading to spastic paralysis and death of the parasite. This compound is not readily available for use in small ruminants in the United States.

Currently, there are four products legally labeled for use in sheep in the United States: albendazole (Valbazen®), ivermectin (Ivomec®), moxidectin (Cydectin®), and levamisole (Prohibit®). All labeled products are formulated for oral use. There are three products legally labeled for goats in the United States: albendazole (Valbazen), fenbendazole (Panacur®, Safeguard®), and morantel tartrate (Rumatel®). All labeled products are also formulated for oral use only. It is strongly recommended that only anthelmintics formulated to be given orally be used in small ruminants. It is not recommended that products made for injectable or topical use be given orally to small ruminants as absorption may be variable, leading to increasing incidence of subtherapeutic dosing. All available products in the United States are labeled for the treatment of *Haemonchus* spp., *Teladorsagia* spp., and *Trichostrongylus* spp., the primary gastrointestinal nematodes affecting small ruminants.

Traditional use of anthelmintics

Each anthelmintic class and the compounds within these classes were viewed as valuable tools against the ever-present threat of parasitic disease in small ruminants. As each compound was introduced, new treatment options could be incorporated to control parasitic infection, often with very little consideration for judicious use. For example, when ivermectin became available in the early 1980s, producers and veterinarians alike had access to a relatively safe and inexpensive anthelmintic (FDA, 2023). This, coupled with the ease of oral administration, lead to efficient treatment of entire herds and flocks of small ruminants with an effective anthelmintic (FDA, 2023). Utilizing a highly effective treatment coupled with the practice of treating all animals within the herd or flock resulted in 100% parasite kill-off (FDA, 2023). This process, known as "blanket deworming," quickly became the recommended treatment strategy for all new anthelmintics.

The basis for traditional use of anthelmintics was to eliminate all parasites in the small ruminant frequently (Burke and Morgan, 2015). This ideology led to "scheduled" treatments that often occurred during certain times of the year. For example, any animal being moved to a new (or "clean") pasture was given anthelmintic to remove all parasites prior to entering the new pasture (Burke and Morgan, 2015). Another traditional recommendation was to treat all ewes and/or does prior to breeding and following lambing/kidding. This practice would "eliminate" parasites that could lead to disease during times when the animal may have a compromised immune system due to additional stressors on the body. Traditionally, it was also recommended that lambs and kids be treated with an anthelmintic every few weeks during the summer months (Burke and Morgan, 2015). Loosely based on the lifecycle of the gastrointestinal nematodes, it was thought that this practice would eliminate adult parasites and decrease the number of clinically affected lambs and kids.

Traditional use of anthelmintics did not just involve use of one product given often to all animals. It was also traditional to utilize multiple products throughout the year. Prior to the year 2000, it was recommended that different products should be rotated to prevent resistance development (Burke and Morgan, 2015). Rotation of anthelmintics was a popular practice that involved treating all animals with one class or compound followed by additional treatment of all animals with a different class or compound at the next scheduled treatment time. Often, all three common classes of anthelmintics were used multiple times throughout the year, exposing the entire population to all available medications.

Scheduled treatment times were a staple of traditional anthelmintic use. Entire herds and flocks were often scheduled for treatment two or more times a year. Anthelmintics were treated as prophylaxis and given to all animals regardless of suspected parasite burden. These compounds were thought to prevent parasitic infection; however, anthelmintics are a treatment and will only treat parasites currently affecting the host. Although anthelmintics may decrease the parasitic burden in an animal with high parasite numbers, these compounds will have little to no effect on animals with low parasite numbers.

Recommendations for use of anthelmintics have evolved during the decades that chemical products have become available. The effectiveness of these anthelmintics has also evolved over time. Safety recommendations, however, have remained static and provided the only restraint when it came to the traditional use of anthelmintics. A compound's relative safety would affect how frequently it was used and how much of it was given. It is important to recognize the safety recommendations for each compound to better understand why some compounds may have been used more often than others.

The benzimidazole class is generally considered to be very safe, with the toxic dose being anywhere from 10 to 100 times the recommended dose, depending on the compound (Kaplan, 2009). While risk of overdose is rare, albendazole is not recommended for treatment of sheep within the first 30 days of pregnancy due to possible teratogenic effects (Kaplan, 2009). The relative safety and availability of this anthelmintic class make it a popular choice for producers, leading to more exposure of the animal and parasites to both fenbendazole and albendazole.

One of the cholinergic agonists has the narrowest margin of safety of all anthelmintics. Levamisole, an imidazothiazole, can cause toxicity at 3–5 times the therapeutic dose (Kaplan, 2009). Clinical signs associated with overdose of levamisole include ataxia, muscle fasciculations, seizure, and excessive salivation (Kaplan, 2009). Although levamisole can be used in pregnant animals, overdose may lead to compromise of the pregnancy (Kaplan, 2009). Levamisole overdose can be fatal, and it is best to avoid use in animals that are not healthy. This major safety concern may be a deterrent for some producers, leading to less exposure of their animals to levamisole. Morantel tartrate, a tetrahydropyrimidine and another cholinergic agonist, is very safe for use in pregnant or debilitated animals. It is only formulated to be added to feed, which makes accurate dosing difficult (Kaplan, 2009). The combination of formulation and wide margin of safety often leads to exposure of entire herds or flocks, and their parasites, to this anthelmintic.

Macrocyclic lactones can lead to signs of toxicity when excessively overdosed. Typically, the blood–brain barrier will block macrocyclic lactones from crossing and causing signs of toxicity. However, with gross overdose, the blood–brain barrier becomes more permeable and allows the macrocyclic lactones to cross (Merola and Eubig, 2012). At lower concentrations, the macrocyclic lactones will lead to tremors and excitatory behavior. At higher concentrations, the animal will develop ataxia and depression. Since gross overdose is required for clinical signs to manifest, macrocyclic lactones are still considered relatively safe and are often used by producers, which leads to more animal and parasite exposure.

The traditional approach to anthelmintic use involved two things: treat often and treat all. Scheduled, systematic use of anthelmintics predominated ideology from the 1960s to the 2000s. Small ruminants were often treated for parasites in a prophylactic way—anthelmintics were given to animals during times of physiological stress to prevent parasitism from causing clinical signs. Rotation of anthelmintics at regular intervals lead to widespread exposure to every anthelmintic class. This strategy of regular and indiscriminate anthelmintic use over the course of decades has led to rampant resistance development amongst multiple species of parasites. One of the deadliest parasites, *Haemonchus contortus*, is also the most likely to develop resistance to all available anthelmintics. Resistance development amongst parasites is a direct result of the traditional practices associated with anthelmintic use.

Resistance Development Amongst Parasite Species

Anthelmintic resistance development amongst parasites has become one of the most important concerns for both small ruminant producers and veterinarians. Resistance development depends on multiple factors including the host, parasite, anthelmintic use, management of the farm, and climate characteristics (Fissiha and Kinde, 2021). Overuse of anthelmintics coupled with poor farm management (improper nutrition and poor sanitation, for example) will lead to increased resistance amongst parasites, especially in geographical areas with temperatures and humidity indices conducive to parasite survival. Unfortunately, anthelmintic resistance has been reported in all three of the major gastrointestinal nematodes that affect small ruminants—*Haemonchus* spp., *Teladorsagia* spp., and *Trichostrongylus* spp. This resistance has been reported for every class of anthelmintic currently available and is occurring worldwide (Fissiha and Kinde, 2021).

The length of time it takes for resistance to develop can be variable. Initially, it is rare to find nematodes with anthelmintic resistance-inducing mutations in such a large and diverse population of parasites (Kaplan, 2015). Factors that will expedite the volume of resistant parasites include frequency of treatment, targeting and timing of mass treatment, and anthelmintic dose rates (Fissiha and Kinde, 2021). Treatment with anthelmintics does not necessarily affect the resistant parasites but instead targets the anthelmintic-susceptible parasites. When this occurs, resistant nematodes are left behind and allowed to reproduce with limited competition (Kaplan, 2015). Therefore, each treatment with anthelmintic allows for the numbers of resistant nematodes to increase incrementally (Kaplan, 2015). Treating all small ruminants in a herd or flock also incrementally increases the number of nematodes exposed to the anthelmintic. Finally, proper dosing is important to limit survival of nematodes exposed to subtherapeutic doses of anthelmintic. As more nematodes are exposed to the anthelmintic and survive exposure, there is an elevated risk of increased resistant populations.

Resistance to anthelmintics is a trait that can be passed down from generation to generation within the parasite population. This heritable resistance is defined as a loss of sensitivity to an anthelmintic in a parasite population that was in the past susceptible to that anthelmintic (Fissiha and Kinde, 2021). Nematodes have several biological qualities that allow them to develop and propagate anthelmintic resistance within the population, including short life cycles, high reproductive rates, rapid rates of evolution, and extremely large population size (Kaplan, 2015). These factors combine to give nematodes a high degree of genetic diversity and more incidence of gene mutations that would support resistance development (Kaplan, 2015).

The primary mechanism of resistance for the parasite differs for different classes of anthelmintics. However, resistance is typically due to gene mutations that directly affect the mechanism of action of the anthelmintic. Macrocyclic lactones, for example, affect the parasite by allowing chloride to enter the muscle of the nematode after binding GABA and glutamate-gated chloride channels, leading to paralysis and death. Several factors are linked to resistance of macrocyclic lactones. This includes mutations of the glutamate-gated chloride receptors with a specific mutation at an allele of a GluCla-subunit gene (Fissiha and Kinde, 2021). Mechanisms that prevent the anthelmintic from reaching its target have also been reported, including the protein transporter P-glycoprotein. Finally, enzymes such as CYP34/35 that impact drug metabolism have been reported in parasites resistant to macrocyclic lactones (Fissiha and Kinde, 2021).

Benzimidazole-resistant parasites typically have mutations associated with β-tubulin, the primary binding site of the anthelmintic. A single amino acid mutation in the parasite's tubulin protein can cause benzimidazole binding to be blocked, leading to survival of the parasite (Fissiha and Kinde, 2021). Cholinergic agonist anthelmintics require the presence of nicotinic acetylcholine receptors. Resistant parasites will have alterations of these receptors that block binding of the anthelmintic. Shortened forms of two receptor subunits have been reported as

causes of resistance in *Haemonchus contortus*, *Trichostrongylus colubriformis*, and *Teladorsagia circumcincta* (Fissiha and Kinde, 2021). Gene mutation has allowed parasites to adapt and survive therapeutic doses of every anthelmintic currently available.

Multiple variations of anthelmintic resistance have been noted in nematodes affecting livestock. Three distinct types of resistance that have been observed are cross-resistance, side-resistance, and multiple resistances (Nipane *et al.*, 2008). Cross-resistance is defined as the ability of parasites to survive therapeutic doses of chemically unrelated drugs or drug classes with different mechanisms of action (Nipane *et al.*, 2008). Side-resistance describes parasites developing resistance to members of the same class with the same or similar mechanism of action, for example a parasite with known resistance to fenbendazole also exhibiting resistance to albendazole. Multiple resistances refer to parasites developing resistances to multiple classes of anthelmintics (Nipane *et al.*, 2008). Unfortunately, all three classifications of resistance are widespread globally.

Due to the high prevalence of resistance recognized globally and across multiple species of parasites, it is paramount that the efficacy of anthelmintics be confirmed as well as possible. It is recommended that resistance testing be performed on every farm every 2–3 years as a management standard (Kaplan, 2009). Presently, there were two primary ways to evaluate anthelmintic efficacy against small ruminant parasites: the fecal egg count reduction test (FECRT) and the larval development assay (LDA or DrenchRite® Assay) (Howell and Storey, 2012). The FECRT can be performed by producers or veterinarians and does not require a parasite diagnostic laboratory, whereas the LDA does require a parasite diagnostic laboratory that offers that service.

The FECRT is a practical and inexpensive method to evaluate anthelmintic resistance. First, initial fecal samples are collected from animals that are going to receive treatment with an anthelmintic. Fecal egg counts are performed utilizing a method that allows for quantification of the parasite eggs per gram of feces (for example, a McMaster slide or mini-FLOTAC system). Then, another fecal sample is collected from the same treated animals 10–14 days following anthelmintic treatment. Fecal egg counts are also performed on these samples. The two counts from the pretreatment and posttreatment samples are then compared to determine a percentage reduction. The formula used to determine this percentage is FECR% = 100 (1-Xt/Xu) where Xt is the posttreatment sample and Xu is the pretreatment sample (Kaplan, 2009). In order to determine the effectiveness of a dewormer on the farm, it is recommended that at least 10–15 animals are sampled. These animals should have fecal egg counts of 250 eggs per gram or more prior to anthelmintic administration (O'Brien, 2018). To save time, pooled fecal samples have been used in FECRTs (Kenyon et al., 2016; George et al., 2017); however, none of the currently available methods for analyzing the FECRT has been validated for pooled samples (Kaplan et al., 2023). For additional information on the FECRT, see Chapter 8.

Resistance development amongst all species of gastrointestinal nematodes is a recognized and concerning problem worldwide. These parasites have developed resistance to all anthelmintic classes and compounds available for use in small ruminants. Resistance development has allowed parasites to alter their response to anthelmintics, often due to genetic mutation that allows the parasite to avoid the anthelmintic's primary mechanism of action. This resistance will only be countered with diligence in monitoring by performing assessments such as the fecal egg count reduction test. The other avenue for reducing anthelmintic resistance is the practice of strategic management and anthelmintic use. Utilizing a targeted approach to anthelmintic use coupled with management strategies to reduce parasite exposure may help to turn the tides of anthelmintic resistance.

Targeted Selective Treatment

Long-term use (and sometimes misuse) of anthelmintics (dewormers) has resulted in worm populations that have become increasingly resistant to treatment. In the United States, anthelmintic resistance tends to be highest among the benzimidazoles (fenbendazole, SafeGuard; and albendazole, Valbazen) and avermectins (ivermectin, Ivomec), but is also common with levamisole (Prohibit, Leva-Med®) and moxidectin (Cydectin), depending upon geographic location and individual farm.

Targeted selective treatment (TST) is considered to be a necessary strategy for combating anthelmintic resistance. TST involves deworming only those animals that require treatment (or would benefit most from treatment). It differs from previous deworming recommendations which advocated whole-flock and/or calendar-based treatments and resulted in increased selection for resistant worms.

Refugia

Targeted selective treatments slow down anthelmintic resistance by reducing the number of treatments, which increases refugia. Refugia are worms that have not been exposed to dewormers. The goal of refugia-based strategies is to dilute the resistant worms (on a farm) so that a sufficient proportion of the worm population remains susceptible to antiparasitic drugs. This maintains the high efficacy of treatments, even though some resistant worms are still present. Refugia is deemed necessary to slow down the further development of resistant worms. Strategies which increase refugia, such as TST, are recommended. TST can also help to identify animals which are more resistant and especially more resilient (and conversely more susceptible) to parasitic infection.

There are several tools which can be used to identify which animals require or would benefit from deworming. These include the FAMACHA© eye anemia system, body condition scoring (BCS), and the Five Point Check©. Performance indicators, such as the Happy Factor™, are other options for implementing TST strategies. Fecal egg count is incorporated into some TST strategies.

The FAMACHA© system

The FAMACHA© eye anemia system was developed almost 30 years ago by South African researchers in response to growing dewormer resistance on sheep farms in South Africa. FAMACHA© was introduced to the US (and other countries) in 2002, where it was validated (and modified) for sheep, goats, and camelids (llamas and alpacas) (Kaplan *et al.*, 2004; Storey *et al.*, 2017).

FAMACHA© is a color eye chart (card) with five categories that estimates the level of anemia (blood loss) in the animal (Table 3.1). Anemia is the primary symptom of barber pole worm infection. The barber pole worm (*Haemonchus contortus*) is a highly pathogenic roundworm that thrives in warm, moist climates and/or during periods of seasonal rainfall. It is the primary parasite of small ruminants in many parts of North America and regions with similar climates.

Anemia is measured by packed cell volume (PCV) or blood hematocrit: the proportion (percentage) of red blood cells in whole blood. While there can be other causes of anemia, the barber pole worm is usually the most common (Zajac, 2016; Kaplan and Miller, 2002).

Anemia is also a symptom of liver fluke disease (fascioliasis) (Olah *et al.*, 2015), and FAMACHA© holds promise as a tool for selective treatment against *Fasciola hepatica*. Other causes of anemia include undernourishment or other diseases, such as paratuberculosis (Johne's disease), caseous lymphadenitis (CL), and protozoan parasites, such as coccidia and trypanosome (Zajac, 2016; Kaplan and Miller, 2002).

If there is a question as to whether barber pole infection is the cause of anemia, the fecal egg counts (FEC) of animals with FAMACHA© scores of 4 or 5 can be examined. If most pale animals have high fecal egg counts, then FAMACHA© is suitable as a deworming criterion.

The FAMACHA© card displays five color and treatment categories. Each category (or score) corresponds to a PCV value or range. A FAMACHA© score of 1 (red) is indicative of an

animal with a healthy or "high" PCV (>28%). At the other end of the scale is a FAMACHA© score of 5 (white) which is indicative of a very low or "deadly" PCV (<12%).

Treatment recommendations

It is recommended that sheep, goats, and camelids with FAMACHA© scores of 4 or 5 always be dewormed with effective drugs, whereas those with FAMACHA© scores of 1 or 2 not be dewormed, unless other signs of parasitism are present (Kaplan and Miller, 2002). It may be advisable to treat periparturient females with FAMACHA© scores of ≥ 3, especially if they are thin, young, and/or nursing multiple offspring. Because they have comparatively small blood volumes and can progress rapidly from moderate to severe anemia, consideration should be given to deworming lambs and especially kids with FAMACHA© scores of ≥ 3.

Some additional recommendations for FAMACHA© scores of 3 are to treat 3s if FAMACHA© scores are trending higher since the last time the animals were checked or if more than 10% of the group has FAMACHA© scores of ≥4 (Kaplan and Miller, 2002). Some producers will treat 3s if they are not able to recheck their animals in a timely fashion or if nutrition is suboptimal and/or the risk of reinfection is high.

For all species, FAMACHA© scoring is most sensitive when categories 3, 4, and five are treated. However, based on research (Kaplan *et al.*, 2004), 3s are only rarely anaemic, and treating all 3s will greatly increase the total number of treatments. However, treating FAMACHA© category three reduces the probability of missing an anaemic (clinically parasitized) animal. In contrast, when only categories 4 and 5 are treated, the probability of deworming an animal that does not require treatment decreases. Some producers choose to err on the side of caution and deworm any animal that has a FAMACHA© score of 3 or higher.

Using the FAMACHA© system

Proper training is required before using a FAMACHA© card (Kaplan and Miller, 2002). Small ruminant producers must take an approved training (certification) course in order to get a FAMACHA© card. Veterinarians may

Table 3.1. FAMACHA© system.

Category	Color	Treatment recommendation
1	Red	No
2	Pinkish-red	No
3	Pink	Maybe
4	Pinkish-white	Yes
5	White	Yes

Source: Bath and Van Wyk (2009), used with permission from Elsevier.

purchase FAMACHA© cards without certification, though training is still recommended. Louisiana State University is the sole North American distributor of FAMACHA© cards (famacha@lsu.edu). FAMACHA© workshops are conducted throughout the United States and in other countries. Several US universities offer online FAMACHA© certification. Online certification is available in both English and Spanish. For information about FAMACHA© certification, visit the website of the American Consortium for Small Ruminant Parasite Control (ACSRPC; wormx.info).

Proper FAMACHA© technique is essential and the main reason why training is mandatory. The phrase "Cover, Push, Pull, Pop" has been adopted to teach proper technique: (1) cover the eye with the top eyelid; (2) push down on the eye (gently); (3) pull down the bottom eyelid; and (4) the mucous membranes will "pop" into view (Petersson, 2016). You should not try to expose the membranes simply by pulling down on the eyelid (Petersson, 2016). It is important not to score the inner surface of the lower eyelid, but rather to score the darkest portion of the bed of mucous membranes. Both eyes should be scored since they can be different. You should always use the higher score and err on the side of caution. Half scores are not used. Any time the color seems to be between two scores, the higher score should be used. A FAMACHA© card (not memory) should always be used to assign FAMACHA© scores and make deworming decisions.

A handling system with a head gate is convenient for doing FAMACHA© scoring. Scoring can also be done chute-side, by leaning over the raceway panel. Producers who do not have handling equipment can crowd their animals into a pen or have someone else hold the animal for inspection. Animals can also be scored when they are haltered or on a milking or fitting stand. It is a good practice to FAMACHA© score an animal any time it is being handled or you have your hands on it. Camelids can be more challenging to score than sheep and goats. Smaller and more docile camelids may be manually restrained, whereas larger and more spirited animals may require a chute for safety purposes. FAMACHA© scoring of camelids may require more than one person.

FAMACHA© scoring can be done at the same time as other activities, such as weighing, sorting, body condition scoring, or vaccinating. It should be done in full daylight, not indoors or in the shade. Care should also be taken not to shade the eye when scoring. The FAMACHA© card should be stored in a dark place when it is not being used (to prevent fading). It should be replaced after 1–2 years of use, but the length of time is dependent on the extent of use and how the card is stored.

A suggested approach is to have two cards: one that is used (stored when not being used) and one that is kept in a dark place. Every few months, the cards should be compared and when the in-use card looks faded compared to the storage card, it should be replaced. Replacement cards can be purchased (from Louisiana State University) with proof of training (usually a certificate of competence). Under no circumstances should someone try to make their own card by copying the colors of the FAMACHA© card.

One of the challenges of the FAMACHA© system is that it can be labor-intensive, especially for larger flocks/herds. Animals need to be checked frequently (every 1–3 weeks) during the peak *H. contortus* transmission season. Outside the months of peak transmission, animals can be checked with less frequency. Depending upon climate, it may not be necessary to check animals during the winter months when worms are hypobiotic (arrested). However, in some climates, it may be necessary to do year-round FAMACHA© scoring. Pregnant females, which suffer a temporary reduction in immunity around the time of parturition, should always be checked during late gestation and dewormed (or not) accordingly to targeted selective treatment criteria.

For producers with large flocks or herds, a random sample of animals can be selected for FAMACHA© scoring. If the combined percentage of 1 s and 2 s exceeds 80–90%, and there are no category 4 or 5 animals in the selected group, it is unlikely that there is danger in not checking the whole flock/herd. Another check could be done in a few weeks. However, if there are some 4 s or 5 s, then the entire group should be checked or even treated, leaving some animals untreated to maintain refugia (Kaplan and Miller, 2002). Another option is to sort off the animals that lag behind (thus, are more likely to be parasitized) and subject them to scoring (Kaplan and Miller, 2002). In large flocks and herds, FAMACHA© can be used to select male and female replacements.

Body condition scoring

Body condition score (BCS) is a measure of the relative fatness of an animal. Low body condition scores (≤ 2) are usually indicative of a nutrition issue, and these animals are more prone to parasitic infection. Moreover, animals with low BCS and/or on a poor plane of nutrition are less able to cope with the effects of a parasitic burden (reduced resilience).

Various studies have shown BCS to be a reliable indicator of internal parasitism in adult small ruminants. In the tropics, research showed that hair sheep ewes with a BCS of 3 or greater can be maintained without anthelmintic treatment during the production year (Soto-Barrientos et al., 2018). Leaving ewes with higher BCS untreated helps to maintain refugia. Research has shown that camelids in optimal to overweight categories harbor fewer parasites (Storey et al., 2017). Body condition scoring is less effective as a tool for young growing animals.

Sheep, goats, and camelids are typically assigned body condition scores using a scale from 1 to 5, with 1 representing emaciated, 2 being thin, 3 average, 4 fat, and 5 obese. Half scores are used. Visual assessment of body condition can be misleading because fleece or hair coat (and even pregnancy) can hide the true status of an animal. It is usually necessary to touch the animal to assess body condition, and it is recommended to use a body condition scoring card (or fact sheet or video) for reference.

Body condition scoring involves feeling for fat and muscle over the backbone, loin, and ribs. Prominent bones are an indication of less fat cover, whereas bones that are difficult to detect can be an indication of overconditioning. Better conditioned animals also feel fuller in the loin. To get the most accurate body condition score, animals should be handled in a natural state, not when their feet are off the ground, or they are pushing strongly forward.

Body condition scoring is somewhat different in goats (and some sheep), as they carry more fat in their abdomen and less on their backs. It is normal for goats to carry less condition than sheep, dairy goats to carry less condition than meat goats, and hair sheep to carry less condition than wooled sheep. Finn sheep and St Croix hair sheep also fatten similarly to goats and hair sheep and do not usually handle with as much condition.

The Five Point Check

The Five Point Check was developed by the same South African researchers to address the limitations of the FAMACHA© system, which only assesses damage caused by blood-feeding parasites, such as H. contortus (Bath and Van Wyk, 2009). The Five Point Check is a simple extension of the FAMACHA© system. It utilizes five checkpoints (on the animal's body) to make deworming decisions (Bath and Van Wyk, 2009) (Table 3.2). These five checkpoints provide the criteria necessary for evaluating the impact of other parasites that can affect small ruminants, including those that cause digestive disturbances and infect the nasal passages (nasal bots). The Five Point Check also exemplifies the importance of considering multiple criteria when making deworming decisions.

In addition to assessing the damage caused by worms other than blood feeders, the Five Point Check is useful for making deworming decisions for animals with FAMACHA© scores of 3. For example, a small ruminant with a FAMACHA© score of 3 should be dewormed if it has bottle jaw, poor body condition, and/or moderate to severe diarrhea (dag score ≥ 3). If all other scores are "good," an animal with a FAMACHA© of 3 may not need to be dewormed.

The five check points are eye, jaw, back, tail, and nose. (1) The eye is examined to assess anemia and determine FAMACHA© score. (2) The jaw is examined to check for the presence (or absence) of bottle jaw (submandibular edema). (3) The back is felt to determine body condition score. (4) The tail is observed to determine the extent of fecal soiling. (5) The nose is observed for signs of a nasal discharge.

Bottle jaw

Submandibular edema is an accumulation of fluid under the jaw of the animal, commonly called "bottle jaw." Edema is caused by disruption of the normal balance of pressure and/or proteins between the blood and the spaces between cells located outside the blood vessels. All animals with

Table 3.2. The Five Point Check.

Checkpoint (criteria)	Observation (score)	Possibilities — diagnosis
Eye	Anemia FAMACHA© score, 1–5	Barber pole worm (*Haemonchus contortus*) Liver fluke (*Fasciola hepatica*) Other diseases Undernourishment
Jaw	Soft swelling under jaw Submandibular edema, "bottle jaw"	Barber pole worm (*Haemonchus contortus*) Liver fluke (*Fasciola hepatica*) Other diseases
Back	Body condition score, 1–5	Brown stomach worm (*Teladorsagia circumcincta*) Bankrupt worm (*Trichostrongylus* spp.) Nodular worm (*Oesophagostomum*) Other worms Other diseases Undernourishment
Tail	Fecal soiling, 0–5 Dag score	Bankrupt worm (*Trichostrongylus* spp.) Brown stomach worm (*Teladorsagia circumcincta*) Nodular worm (*Oesophagostomum*) Other worms Other diseases
Nose	Nasal discharge	Nasal bots (*Oestrus ovis*) Lungworms Pneumonia Other diseases

Adapted from Bath and Van Wyk (2009), used with permission from Elsevier.

bottle jaw, whether they appear anemic or not, should be dewormed (Kaplan and Miller, 2002). On the other hand, bottle jaw does not develop in the majority of animals that are clinically parasitized. It is seen primarily when anemia is severe. It seems to be more common in sheep than goats.

While there can be other causes of bottle jaw in small ruminants, the barber pole worm is the most common cause. However, it is important not to confuse bottle jaw with other conditions. Milk goiter (or neck) is a (lower) throat swelling, common to well-nourished kids and hair sheep lambs. An enlarged thyroid is caused by an iodine deficiency, not parasites. Tooth abscesses, periodontal disease, and "lumpy" jaw (caused by bacteria) can also look like bottle jaw.

Fecal soiling (or dag score)

Parasites which cause mild to severe diarrhea (scours) are more significant than the barber pole worm in some locations and regions of the world. The accumulation of feces (dags) on

the backside of a sheep can predispose it to fly strike. The tail (or hindquarters) of the animal should be examined to determine if diarrhea is present. Fecal soiling is usually assessed using a scale of 0–5, with 0 representing no fecal soiling and 5 representing very severe diarrhea, usually extending to the hocks. Treatment (or action) is usually considered at dag score 3 (moderate soiling, dag formation).

If fecal samples are collected, the consistency of the feces can also be examined. There is a scoring system for fecal consistency as well, with 1 representing pelleted feces, 2 being wetter, less formed pellets, and 3 (or more) being liquid (diarrhea) (WormBoss, 2022). As with the other checkpoints, there can be other causes of diarrhea besides worms.

Nasal discharge and coat condition

A clear or even purulent nasal discharge can be indicative of nasal bots. Nasal bots are a parasite of sheep and goats. While usually only a minor annoyance, they can cause serious problems in some instances. Female flies (*Oestrus ovis*) deposit their larvae in and around the nostrils of their host, causing sneezing and a snotty nose.

In goats, the nose checkpoint is sometimes changed to coat condition. A poor or rough hair coat can be indicative of parasitic infection. In fact, researchers have found coat condition to be a reliable indicator of welfare in dairy goats (Battini *et al.*, 2015). Like other parameters, a poor hair coat can have other causes including poor nutrition and/or other disease conditions; thus, it is important to consider additional checkpoints or criteria when making deworming decisions.

Performance indicators

Weight gain is another refugia-based strategy, especially in climates where the barber pole worm is not the primary parasite. The Happy Factor is a model that predicts a target weight for a growing lamb (McBean *et al.*, 2016). If the lamb fails to achieve its predicted level of performance, it is dewormed; otherwise, it is left untreated. Like FAMACHA©, the Happy Factor results in fewer treatments being given, thereby increasing refugia while maintaining productivity.

Brazilian researchers determined that refugia-based strategies that combined weight gain with FAMACHA© scores produced the best performance in lambs. In fact, they recommend against using FAMACHA© scores as the sole criteria when making deworming decisions, even in situations where the barber pole worm is the primary parasite. Similar experience in tropical areas of Latin America has shown that properly nourished lambs can be maintained without anthelmintic treatment, so long as they meet a standard of level of gain, e.g. ≥100 g or 0.22 lb per day (Rizzon Cinta *et al.*, 2019).

In Europe, milk production has been used as a criterion for deworming dairy goats, with does in their first lactation and with the highest level of production being targeted for treatment. British researchers have applied different deworming protocol (and nutrition) to ewes carrying single, twin, and triplet fetuses.

In many parts of the world, FEC is used to make deworming decisions, primarily because flock sizes are too large to make individual assessments. In these situations, fecal samples are collected from random animals (usually about 10) or a mob sample is utilized. Whole-flock treatments are administered when FEC reaches a certain threshold. The FEC that triggers deworming varies. Leaving some animals untreated (at least 10%, preferably 15–20% or more) assures that refugia is maintained (Leathwick, 2017). However, as a deworming criterion, FEC is most effective when it is combined with the other criteria.

Other combined TSTs

Similar to the Five Point Check, other combined TST strategies have been implemented around the world. In tropical areas, many animals struggle with undernourishment. Sometimes, they have poor BCS and/or FAMACHA© but low worm burdens. In these situations, Mexican researchers have suggested fecal sampling animals with poor BCS (≤ 2.5) and/or FAMACHA© scores (4, 5). If FEC reaches certain thresholds, the animals are dewormed. Otherwise, treatment is withheld, but skinny, pale animals are given improved nutrition (Torres-Acosta *et al.*, 2014).

Researchers in Ontario, Canada, compared whole-flock treatments (prelambing) of periparturient ewes with a TST strategy that used four criteria to determine deworming need (Westers *et al.*, 2017). Ewes were only dewormed if they met at least one of the four criteria: (1) last grazing season was first grazing season; (2) BCS ≤ 2; (3) FAMACHA© score ≥ 4; and/or (4) nursing three or more lambs. Similar to other studies, their research demonstrated that TST can be effective, so long as accurate indicators are used to identify animals that need treatment (Westers *et al.*, 2017).

Combination treatments

It is now recommended that clinically parasitized small ruminants be given combination treatments (Kaplan, 2018). A combination treatment is when more than one medication is given to kill the same worm species. Combination treatments have an additive effect on the worm population. The purpose of combination treatments is to kill as many worms as possible; worms that survive one drug can be killed by the second (or third). Of course, combination treatments will not be effective if none of the drugs used in the combination has enough potency. To be beneficial, each drug in the combination should reduce fecal egg count by at least 60% (Schoenian, 2020).

In non-US countries, combination drenches may be commercially available. In the US, it is necessary to purchase and administer each drug separately (Kaplan, 2018). The most effective drug from each class should be given. In the US, this is usually albendazole (Valbazen) + moxidectin (Cydectin) + levamisole (Prohibit, Leva-Med). A full dose of each drug (based on an accurate weight) should be given. Drugs should not be mixed, as they have different chemistries. Optimally, a different dosing syringe should be used for each drug, with treatments being given sequentially. The withdrawal period for the drug with the longest withdrawal should be followed (Kaplan, 2018).

In the US, veterinary approval (valid veterinarian–client–patient relationship; VCPR) is required to administer combination treatments to goats and camelids, as non-FDA-approved drugs are usually recommended. For sheep, there is an FDA-approved drug in each dewormer class.

When administering combination treatments, it is essential to follow TST guidelines to prevent resistance from developing to all drugs and chemistries simultaneously (Kaplan, 2018). When combination treatments are used in conjunction with other "best management practices," the susceptibility of the worms to individual drugs may improve. However, if combination treatments are administered without maintaining refugia, multiple drug resistance could develop quite rapidly.

Using TSTs to select for resistance to parasites

Targeted selective treatment can be used to identify small ruminants that are more resistant

and especially more resilient to internal parasites. Resistant animals are more immune to parasitic infection. Resilient animals maintain good health and performance while harboring a parasite load.

It goes without saying that animals that require frequent deworming should be culled—sent for slaughter, not sold to other producers. The frequency standard will depend on the level of parasite challenge and the success of other parasite control measures. The culling standard should be applied more stringently to breeding males, as they contribute the majority of genetics to the flock/herd, especially if they are bred to a lot of females and/or used in multiple breeding seasons.

The downside to using TST to select for parasite resistance is that resilient animals, i.e. those not requiring deworming, may still be shedding a lot of worm eggs onto the pasture and thereby exposing the more susceptible members of the flock/herd, especially young stock. Genetic correlations between FEC and FAMACHA© score are variable, but generally only low to moderate. The same is usually true of other clinical parameters.

Fecal egg counts are the best measure of parasite resistance and are recommended to producers who want to make more rapid genetic improvement. Some central performance tests evaluate rams/bucks for parasite resistance. In some countries (and breeds), estimated breeding values (EBVs) are available for fecal egg counts (parasite resistance) (National Sheep Improvement Program (NSIP), 2024). On-farm performance testing is another option for identifying more resistant animals. Producers can determine which animals in their flocks/herds are more resistant to internal parasites by comparing fecal egg counts of animals in the same contemporary (age and management) groups.

Conclusion

Modern anthelmintics made it easier to control gastrointestinal nematode infections in small ruminants. For many years, sheep/goats and especially lambs/kids were dewormed frequently and prophylactically, depending on challenge (climate + management), with little regard for treatment need of the individual animal. This strategy was effective for a long time, as anthelmintics were available, inexpensive, safe, and effective. But over the years, the situation changed, as the worms, especially *H. contortus*, began to develop resistance to the drugs. Today, most countries have some level of resistance to dewormers and the chemical classes from which they derive.

Refugia-based strategies are now recommended to reduce selection for resistant worms and prolong effectiveness of anthelmintic drugs. Targeted selective treatment is recommended. It involves only deworming animals that require treatment (or would benefit from treatment) based on certain criteria. Untreated animals serve as a reservoir for susceptible worms (refugia). Tools for implementing TST include the FAMACHA© eye anemia system, the Five Point Check, the Happy Factor (weight gain), and other performance and combined criteria. Failure to adopt such refugia-based strategies could eventually result in complete anthelmintic failure (on a farm), accompanied by increased morbidity and mortality, especially in situations where parasite risk is high.

References

Bath, G. and Van Wyk, J. (2009) The five point check© for targeted selective treatment of internal parasites in small ruminants. *Small Ruminant Research* 86, 6–13. DOI: 10.1016/j.smallrumres.2009.09.009.

Battini, M., Peric, T., Ajuda, A., Vieira, A., Grosso, L *et al.* (2015) Hair coat condition: A valid and reliable indicator for on-farm welfare assessment in adult dairy goats. *Small Ruminant Research* 123(2–3), 197–203. DOI: 10.1016/j.smallrumres.2014.11.014.

Burke, J. and Morgan, J. (2015) Changing dogma: Changes to parasite management in the 2000's to keep your dewormers working. American Consortium for small ruminant parasite control. Available at: www.wormx.info/changingdogma (accessed 9 July 2025).

Cantón, L., Lanusse, C. and Moreno, L. (2022) Chemical agents of special concern in livestock meat production. In: Purslow, P. (ed.) *New Aspects of Meat Quality*. Woodhead Publishing, Cambridge, UK, pp. 785–808.

Cobb, R. and Boeckh, A. (2009) Moxidectin: A review of chemistry, pharmacokinetics, and use in horses. *Parasites & Vectors* 2(Suppl 2), S5.

Dilrukshi Herath, H.M.P., Taki, A.C., Sleebs, B.E., Hofmann, A., Nguyen, N. *et al*. (2021) Advances in the discovery and development of anthelmintics by harnessing natural product scaffolds. In: Rollinson, D. and Stothard, R. (eds) *Advances in Parasitology*. Academic Press, Cambridge, USA, pp. 203–251.

FDA (2023) New antiparasitic drugs needed for sheep and goats. Available at: http://www.fda.gov/animal-veterinary/safety-health/new-antiparasitic-drugs-needed-sheep-and-goats (accessed 9 July 2025).

Fissiha, W. and Kinde, M.Z. (2021) Anthelmintic resistance and its mechanism: A review. *Infectious Drug Resistance* 14, 5403–5410. DOI: 10.2147/idr.s332378.

George, M.M., Paras, K.L., Howell, S.B. and Kaplan, R. (2017) Utilization of composite fecal samples for detection of anthelmintic resistance in gastrointestinal nematodes of cattle. *Veterinary Parasitology* 240, 24–29. DOI: 10.1016/j.vetpar.2017.04.024.

Howell, S. and Storey, B. (2012) The DrenchRite™ assay. American Consortium of small ruminant parasite control. Available at: www.wormx.info/drenchriteassay (accessed 9 July 2025).

Kaplan, R. and Miller, J. (2002) FAMACHA© information guide. Available at: https://smallruminants.ces.ncsu.edu/wp-content/uploads/2013/04/FAMACHA-Info-Guide.pdf?fwd=no (accessed 9 July 2025).

Kaplan, R.M. (2015) How and why resistance to worms develops. In: Kaplan, R.M. (ed.) *Proceedings of W4: What Works with Worms Congress Pretoria, South Africa*, American Association of Small Ruminant Parasite Control.

Kaplan, R. (2018) Combination treatments: The time is now. American Consortium for Small Ruminant Parasite Control. Available at: www.wormx.info/combinations (accessed 9 July 2025).

Kaplan, R.M. (2009) Anthelmintic treatment in the era of resistance. In: Anderson, D.E. and Rings, D.M. (eds) *Food Animal Practice*. Elsevier, St Louis, USA, pp. 470–478.

Kenyon, F., Rinaldi, L., McBean, D., Pepe, P., Bosco, A. *et al*. (2016) Pooling sheep faecal samples for the assessment of anthelmintic drug efficacy using McMaster and Mini-FLOTAC in gastrointestinal strongyle and nematodirus infection. *Veterinary Parasitology* 225, 53–60. DOI: 10.1016/j.vetpar.2016.03.022.

Kaplan, R.M., Denwood, M.J., Nielsen, M.K., Torgerson, P. *et al.* (2023) World association for the advancement of veterinary parasitology (W.A.A.V. P.) guideline for diagnosing anthelmintic resistance using the faecal egg count reduction test in ruminants, horses and swine. *Veterinary Parasitology* 318, 109936. DOI: 10.1016/j.vetpar.2023.109936.

Kaplan, R.M., Burke, J.M., Terrill, T.H., Miller, J., Getz, W. *et al.* (2004) Validation of the FAMACHA© eye color chart for detecting clinical anemia in sheep and goats on farms in the southern United States. *Veterinary Parasitology* 123, 105–120. DOI: 10.1016/j.vetpar.2004.06.005.

Leathwick, D. (2017) Worms in refugia: A tool to delay drench resistance. Beef + Lamb New Zealand. Available at: https://beeflambnz.com/sites/default/files/factsheets/pdfs/fact-sheet-151-worms-in-re fugia.pdf (accessed 9 July 2025).

McBean, D., Nath, M., Lambe, N., Morgan-Davies, C. and Kenyon, F. (2016) Viability of the Happy Factor™ targeted selective treatment approach on several sheep farms in Scotland. *Veterinary Parasitology* 218, 22–30. DOI: 10.1016/j.vetpar.2016.01.008.

Merola, V.M. and Eubig, P.A. (2012) Toxicology of avermectins and milbemycins (macrocyclic lactones) and the role of P-glycoprotein in dogs and cats. *Veterinary Clinics of North American Small Animal Practice* 42(2), 313. DOI: 10.1016/j.cvsm.2018.07.002.

National Sheep Improvement Program (NSIP) (2024). Available at: https://nsip.org (accessed 9 July 2025).

Nipane, S.F., Mishra, B. and Panchbuddhe, A.N. (2008) Anthelmintic resistance – clinician's present concern. *Veterinary World* 1(9), 281–284.

O'Brien, D. (2018) Managing dewormer resistance. American Consortium of Small Ruminant Parasite Control. Available at: https://wormx.info/_files/ugd/6ef604_2433e77f4321478d91939c160854a0ed .pdf (accessed 11 July 2025).

Olah, S., Wyk, J., Wall, R. and Morgan, E. (2015) FAMACHA©: A potential tool for targeted selective treatment of chronic fasciolosis in sheep. *Veterinary Parasitology* 212, 188–192. DOI: 10.1016/j. vetpar.2015.07.012.

Petersson, K. (2016) Do's and don'ts of FAMACHA© scoring. American Consortium for Small Ruminant Parasite Control. Available at: www.wormx.info/dosdonts (accessed 9 July 2025).

Prichard, R., Ménez, C. and Lespine, A. (2012) Moxidectin and the avermectins: Consanguinity but not identity. *International Journal for Parasitology: Drugs and Drug Resistance* 2, 134–153. DOI: 10.1016/j.ijpddr.2012.04.001.

Rizzon Cinta, M.C., Ollhoff, R.D., Weber, S.H. and Sotomaior, C. (2019) Is the FAMACHA© system always the best criterion for targeted selective treatment for the control of haemonchosis in growing lambs. *Veterinary Parasitology* 266, 67–72.

Schoenian, S. (2020) Targeted selective treatment. American Consortium for Small Ruminant Parasite Control. Available at: www.wormx.info/_files/ugd/6ef604_20b98181b0434502847a8d308957c422. pdf (accessed 11 July 2025).

Sharma, S. and Anand, N. (1997) Tetrahydropyrimidines. In: *Approaches to Design and Synthesis of Antiparasitic Drugs*. 167, Amsterdam, The Netherlands, pp. 171–180.

Soto-Barrientos, N., Chan-Perez, J., Espana-Espana, E., Novelo-Chi, L. *et al.* (2018) Comparing body condition score and FAMACHA© to identify hair-sheep ewes with high faecal egg counts of gastrointestinal nematodes in farms under hot tropical conditions. *Small Ruminant Research* 167, 92–99. DOI: 10.1016/j.smallrumres.2018.08.011.

Storey, B., Williamson, L., Howell, S., Terrlll, T., Berghaus, R. *et al.* (2017) Validation of the FAMACHA© system in south American camelids. *Veterinary Parasitology* 243, 85–91.

Torres-Acosta, J.F.J., Perez-Cruz, M., Canul-Ku, H., Soto-Barrientos, N., Camara-Sarmiento, R. *et al.* (2014) Building a combined targeted selective treatment scheme against gastrointestinal nematodes in tropical goats. *Small Ruminant Research* 121, 27–35. DOI: 10.1016/j.smallrumres.2014.01.009.

Westers, T., Jones-Bitton, A., Menzies, P., Vanleeuwen, J., Poljak, Z. *et al.* (2017) Comparison of selective and whole flock treatment of periparturient ewes for controlling *Haemonchus* spp. on sheep farms in Ontario, Canada. *Small Ruminant Research* 150, 102–110. DOI: 10.1016/j.smallrumres.2017.03.013.

WormBoss (2022) Assessing faecal consistency score for sheep and goats. Available at: https:// wormboss.com.au/tests-tools/assessing-faecal-consistency-score/ (accessed 9 July 2025).

Zajac, A. (2016) White eyes and bottle jaw: Are there zebras? American Consortium for Small Ruminant Parasite Control. Available at: www.wormx.info/zebra (accessed 9 July 2025).

4 Alternative Methods for the Control of Gastrointestinal Nematodes in Small Ruminants

Joan M. Burke[1]* and James E. Miller[2]

[1]*USDA, ARS, Dale Bumpers Small Farms Research Center, Booneville, Arkansas USA; [2]Department of Pathobiological Sciences, School of Veterinary Medicine, Louisiana State University, Baton Rouge, Louisiana, USA*

Abstract

Due to the wide prevalence of anthelmintic-resistant gastrointestinal nematodes (GIN) and the pathogenicity of *Haemonchus contortus*, alternative control methods have been studied by the American Consortium for Small Ruminant Parasite Control and conditions in which to optimize their use via effective presentation to farmers. Such methods include copper oxide wire particles with anthelmintic properties, nematode trapping fungus to forestall nematodes from becoming infective on pasture, and *Bacillus thuringiensis* (Bt) crystal proteins, a biological dewormer. Other alternative approaches are discussed. Methods such as the above should be applied in relation to farm conditions and used alongside targeted selective treatment and paired with anthelmintics as appropriate.

Introduction

Alternatives to anthelmintics for the control of gastrointestinal nematodes (GIN) are necessary because of the poor efficacy of dewormers. Anthelmintic resistance to all classes of dewormers is prevalent in the US and globally. Also, organic and grass-fed farming systems aim to minimize use of chemicals or pharmaceuticals to increase the sustainability of the soil microbiome and meet the desires of consumers for 'clean' food sources. Alternative methods to be discussed include copper oxide wire particles, nematode trapping fungus, diatomaceous earth, herbal and horticultural products, and *Bacillus thuringiensis* (Bt) crystal proteins. Some of these methods should be thought of as tools in the toolbox of solutions to manage GIN and resulting infections while others serve little purpose, as will be discussed. Tools should be combined according to farm conditions and used alongside targeted selective treatment, paired with anthelmintics as appropriate.

Copper Oxide Wire Particles

Copper oxide wire particles (COWP) were developed commercially to alleviate copper deficiency in livestock, including sheep (Dewey, 1977; Whitelaw *et al.*, 1980; Suttle, 1987) and goats (Winter *et al.*, 2004), which can be a problem, for instance when copper is deficient in soils and

*Corresponding author: joan.burke@usda.gov

forages or an excess of dietary molybdenum, sulfur, iron, or zinc (Borobia *et al.*, 2022) antagonizes copper availability to the animal. Copper oxide wire particles administered orally in gelatin capsules, as loose particles in feed, or in pelleted feed (Bang *et al.*, 1990a, b; Knox, 2002; Burke *et al.*, 2010a, bBurke and Miller, 2006b) are swallowed and traverse the rumen to the abomasum, where they are either retained or passed through feces. When free copper is released in the abomasum, it increases concentrations of copper in the abomasal digesta and is subsequently stored in the liver (Dewey, 1977; Bang *et al.*, 1990b). It was postulated that when administered to sheep, COWP led to a reduction in serum pepsinogen activity, perhaps with an anthelmintic effect (Judson *et al.*, 1982). Since then, several papers have been published on safe use of COWP as an anthelmintic in small ruminants.

Mode of action against gastrointestinal nematodes

Copper oxide wire particles appear to be effective primarily against adult-stage *H. contortus* (Knox, 2002; Waller *et al.*, 2004) and to some degree L4 stages (Waller *et al.*, 2004). Furthermore, there was a reduction in *Teladorsagia circumcincta* to a lesser degree than *H. contortus* (Bang *et al.*, 1990a; Waller *et al.*, 2004), but not *Trichostrongylus colubriformis* (Bang *et al.*, 1990a).

The abomasum is where both *H. contortus* and *T. circumcincta* develop to the adult stage. After the administration of COWP, copper ions become available in the gastrointestinal tract which is sensitive to pH. It was proposed that COWP could be acting on adult nematodes through the increased copper in the abomasum. Bremner (1961) found a positive correlation between copper content in abomasal fluid and abomasal nematodes sampled; thus, copper could be absorbed through the cuticle of the nematode or host blood consumption. Alternatively, the physical presence of the COWP in the abomasum could potentially penetrate the cuticle of *H. contortus* (Bang *et al.*, 1990b). In addition, Moscona *et al.* (2008) found evidence of a direct effect of COWP on *H. contortus* by viewing *H. contortus* extracted from abomasum-cannulated lambs administered COWP.

Transmission electron microscopy showed that cuticle lesions were present, with the greatest frequency of lesions observed within 12 hours post treatment and still present 84 hours later. Concentrations of copper were also higher in *H. contortus* from COWP-treated than untreated lambs (Moscona *et al.*, 2008). Even though particles can be found in the abomasum for several weeks after administration (Judson *et al.*, 1984a; Burke *et al.*, 2004), anthelmintic activity does not persist more than 21 days (Burke *et al.*, 2007b) or 41 days (Vatta *et al.*, 2012).

Despite increased hepatic copper concentrations in goats dosed with COWP or copper sulfate, a more soluble form of copper, developing *H. contortus* larvae (Burke and Miller, 2008; Vatta *et al.*, 2009) were not affected. Thus, it seems the physical or prolonged presence of the particles in the abomasum, along with the lower abomasal pH, is essential in the demise of *H. contortus*.

The source of COWP may be important, possibly due to diameter and length of the particles (Burke *et al.*, 2016). In this study, COWP as Copasure® (Animax Ltd) or Ultracruz™ (Santa Cruz Animal Health) led to a reduction in FEC, but not an Australian formula (Pharmplex). In another study, an industrial form of COWP failed to reduce FEC of predominantly *H. contortus* (Burke, unpublished).

Copper oxide wire particles are not always effective against GIN. Typically, abomasal pH of uninfected lambs is less than 3, but can increase above 3.4 in GIN-infected lambs (Bang *et al.*, 1990b). This increase in pH may lead to less soluble copper from COWP in the abomasum and possibly less of an effect of COWP as an anthelmintic. In addition, if digesta passes through the gastrointestinal tract too quickly, such as when an animal has diarrhea, COWP may pass through the abomasum without being retained, thus failing to reduce fecal e.g.g counts (FEC) of *H. contortus* (Burke, unpublished observations).

Efficacy against GIN

The efficacy of COWP against adult *H. contortus* was reported to be between 75% (Chartier *et al.*, 2000) and 97% (Bang *et al.*, 1990a; Burke *et al.*, 2004), and similar between lambs and kids (Soli *et al.*, 2010). In contrast, Knox (2002) observed an anthelmintic effect of COWP against developing larvae, but other studies showed limited or no effect (Waller *et al.*, 2004; Burke *et al.*, 2007b; Vatta *et al.*, 2009). In addition, COWP was found either to be only 56% effective (Bang *et al.*, 1990a) or ineffective (Chartier *et al.*, 2000) against *T. circumcincta*, but also, when administered by itself, lacks an anthelmintic effect on intestinal worms (Chartier *et al.*, 2000; Burke *et al.*, 2016). In other words, it is important to consider the proportion of *H. contortus* within a GIN population when using COWP as a dewormer. For instance, assess the presence of anemia within a herd by recording FAMACHA© scores or measuring blood packed cell volume as an indication of the appropriateness of use of COWP over other methods of deworming. Notably, Burke *et al.* (2010b) determined that efficacy was similar whether COWP was administered as a capsule or directly in the feed, though the latter mode of delivery risks providing too much or too little.

The efficacy of COWP against GIN burden and/or FEC reduction was greater when administered to small ruminants while either fed or grazing on sericea lespedeza, a forage rich in condensed tannins (Burke *et al.*, 2007b, 2012). COWP was also more effective when used in combination with an anthelmintic compared with either strategy used alone, not only when there was a mixed GIN population but in a flock with known resistance to albendazole (Burke *et al.*, 2016). For instance, administering both COWP (2 g) and albendazole (15 mg/kg body weight) led to a FEC reduction of 99.1% compared with 12–58% or 20% with respective use of either COWP or albendazole alone. Similarly, a combination of COWP and levamisole administered to lambs with a mixed GIN population was more effective than either treatment alone (Burke *et al.*, 2020). This was exemplified by improved efficacy even when the GIN population comprised nearly 100% *hour. contortus*, in that the combination of COWP with albendazole improved efficacy, in contrast to COWP and levamisole in combination, which were less consistent in improving efficacy (Whitley *et al.*, 2021). In a mixed GIN population with the presence of anthelmintic resistance, the combination of COWP and anthelmintic provides control of both *H. contortus* and other GIN which offers

hope for small ruminant farmers in the age of complete anthelmintic failures.

Dose and frequency of treatment

Doses of COWP as low as 0.5 g administered to lambs (Burke and Miller, 2006a) or kids (Burke *et al.*, 2007b), and 1 g to mature ewes (Burke *et al.*, 2007a) were effective in reducing an infection of *H. contortus*. In general, to minimize risk of copper toxicity especially under conditions of relatively high levels of copper in the soil, forage or feed, a lower dose should be used. As a rule of thumb, that would be 0.5–1 g of COWP to lambs or kids less than 1 year of age, and 1–2 g of COWP to adult sheep and goats. In the case of camelids, more research is necessary to determine dose or frequency, though Needleman *et al.* (2022) did observe a reduction in FEC in adult alpacas administered 2 g COWP.

As regards safety, Burke and Miller (2006a) reported that administration of COWP at a low dose (0.5 or 1 g) every 6 weeks for 126 days to lambs did not exceed concentrations of hepatic copper considered unsafe. However, administration of COWP does lead to an increase in hepatic copper and producers need to be careful in overdosing. Often, due to convenience, US producers are inclined to administer the readily available 4 g doses to sheep or goats as an anthelmintic in which case each successive dose will increase the risk of copper toxicity.

Stocking rate and contamination level of the pasture with GIN may require greater frequency of COWP (or dewormer) administration for control of GIN, or *H. contortus* will quickly become pathogenic in susceptible animals. Goats that were highly stocked required an additional deworming within 3 weeks of initial treatment (Burke *et al.*, 2007b). Frequency also depends on other preventive and/or control measures employed on the farm including use of parasite resistance genetics, as part of multiple tools, described below, as aids for minimizing reinfection.

Other forms of copper

Copper sulfate was used as a dewormer before synthetic anthelmintics were developed

(Wright and Bozicevich, 1931). However, no value was found in including copper sulfate either in the mineral or feed of growing goats (Burke and Miller, 2008) or lambs (Waller *et al.*, 2004) or as a drench in lambs for control of *H. contortus* (Miller *et al.*, 2011). A reduction in FEC occurred in goats treated with a sustained-release multi-trace element/vitamin ruminal bolus that lodged in the reticulum and contained 3.7 g copper as copper oxide along with other trace minerals (Burke and Miller, 2006b). The reduction in FEC was likely mostly *H. contortus* and not *Trichostrongylus* spp., lending to the hypothesis that not just the physical presence of COWP in the abomasum but the increase in copper contributes to reduced GIN in the animal. However, the multimineral bolus is not available in the US.

Avoiding copper toxicity

It is well known that administration of COWP will increase the copper status of sheep and goats as evidenced by a linear increase in concentrations of copper in the liver of lambs relative to dosing with COWP (Langlands *et al.*, 1983; Judson *et al.*, 1984b; Suttle, 1987; Burke *et al.*, 2004). Toxicity can be measured by the liver enzyme aspartate aminotransferase (AST) in plasma (Buckley and Tait, 1981). Use of low doses (0.5 or 1 g) of COWP resulted in maintenance of a normal plasma enzyme activity (Burke and Miller, 2006a, 2007a). Other consequences of giving COWP included an initial increase in plasma AST activity of offspring from treated pregnant ewes, along with a reduction in body weight of twin born lambs (Burke *et al.*, 2005a).

Breed differences may also influence flock susceptibility to copper toxicity. Liver concentrations of copper in the North Ronaldsay breed of sheep were increased in response to COWP treatment more than the Cheviot breed (Suttle, 1987), and Scottish Blackface were more susceptible to copper toxicity than Finnish Landrace sheep (Suttle, 1977). Copper status is also influenced by other factors, such as dietary sources of copper (water, forage, feeds, trace mineralized salt), antagonistic interactions of dietary minerals (molybdenum, sulfur, iron, zinc

in feed, mineral, or water), and other environmental sources, which should all be considered before using COWP.

While the risk of copper toxicity should always be evaluated before a decision to use COWP as an anthelmintic, low doses of COWP, as well as COWP used in combination with anthelmintics, are an effective means to control *H. contortus* and GIN in the age of anthelmintic resistance.

At present, COWP is allowed as an anthelmintic by at least some organic certifiers in the US, giving an alternative to organic producers and those wishing to minimize chemical use in small ruminants. Producers should always consult a veterinarian, livestock specialist, or professional in formulating a GIN control strategy best suited to their production system. COWP is commercially available (Fig. 4.1) and, at the time of writing, costs as little as 11¢/treatment for 1 g if purchasing in bulk, or more than $1 per ready-made 2 g bolus. The ACSRPC fact sheet (Coffey, 2018) includes tips on how to use COWP (see Box 4.1).

Nematode Trapping Fungus (*Duddingtonia flagrans*)

As discussed in Chapter 3, anthelmintic resistance has already increased to the extent that dewormers are no longer generally reliable in relation to their claims of efficacy, as stated on their labels. There are, however, other methods to reduce the number of worm eggs that contaminate pastures when passed in the feces, including COWP (above), condensed tannin containing forages (see Chapter 7), and genetic selection for worm resistance (see Chapter 6), but they too have some limitations. Since worms have demonstrated such high levels of ability to become resistant to anthelmintics when targeted, they could perhaps develop tolerance to other alternative methods. In other words, reliance on dewormers for limiting levels of worm burden within the animal and on the pasture may prove to be unsustainable if applied in such a way that high levels of prophylaxis ensue. Until recently, there were no proven products on the market to specifically target the worm burden on pasture.

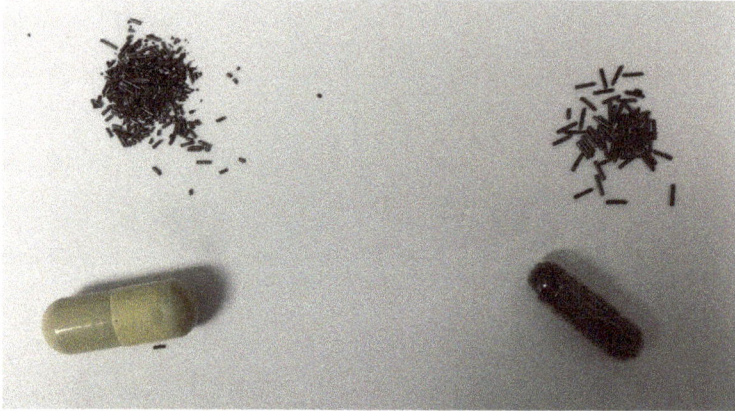

Fig. 4.1. Two commercially available sources of copper oxide wire particles.

Box 4.1. Use of COWP as dewormer.

- Administer COWP selectively based on need (i.e. using the FAMACHA©)
- Economically use cattle boluses (12.5–25 g) in gel capsules to provide the effective lowest dose: (0.5–1 g for lambs and kids less than 1 year of age; 1–2 g for adults).
- Combine COWP with an anthelmintic to increase efficacy against mixed populations of GIN.

The only practical method to control GIN larvae on pasture is through the action of a nematode-trapping fungus. Fungi include *Duddingtonia flagrans* and other genera of nematophagous fungi, though *D. flagrans* is unique in its formation of traps and adhesive networks (Balbino *et al.*, 2022), thus being capable of cleaning pastures to reduce transmission of GIN larvae (Healey *et al.*, 2018).

It is important to have some basic knowledge of the worm life cycle. Briefly, the cycle consists of two parts: in the animal and on the pasture. The adult worms reside in the gastrointestinal tract of the animal and after mating, female worms lay eggs that are passed out in the feces. Eggs then hatch in the feces and develop through two larval stages to the third larval stage (infective) that then migrates out of feces, once moistened, onto the surrounding forage whereupon they are ready to be consumed by grazing animals. Ingested larvae develop to adult worms and the life cycle is complete.

Mode of action

Nematode-trapping fungi have been shown to be an efficient biological control agent against the worm larvae in livestock feces. These fungi are found worldwide and occur at low levels naturally in soil and other environments rich in organic matter where they normally feed on a variety of nonparasitic soil nematodes (Faedo *et al.*, 2002; Knox *et al.*, 2002; Yeates *et al.*, 2002; Saumell *et al.*, 2016). *D. flagrans* has no adverse effect on these beneficial nematodes and was no longer detectable in the environment 2 months after initiation of nematophagous fungal treatment. Spores of various species of these fungi have been isolated, concentrated, tested for efficacy and fed to livestock, passing through the gastrointestinal tract intact or introduced into feces that contain developing GIN larvae.

Of those fungi investigated in livestock (including sheep, goats, cattle, and horses), *D. flagrans* spores (Fig. 4.2A) have the best ability to survive passage through the ruminant gastrointestinal tract. When passed in the feces,

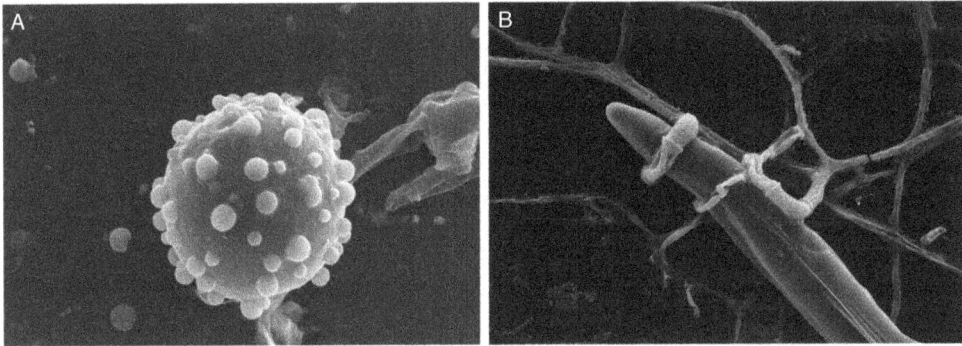

Fig. 4.2. (A) Spore of *Duddingtonia flagrans* in BioWorma. (B) *D. flagrans* fungal trapping system illustrating an ensnared gastrointestinal nematode larvae. Photos courtesy of International Animal Health, used with permission from Elsevier.

D. flagrans spores germinate and mycelia grow rapidly into sticky, sophisticated traps/loops with a high affinity for trapping and digesting larvae. The trapping structures are usually present within the first few hours after defecation and a sticky substance occurs within 48 hours to help with larval contact followed by hyphal cuticle penetration (Fig. 4.2B). Once the larvae are trapped by the structures of the mycelium, hyphae penetrate the larval cuticle, grow and fill the body of the larvae, whereupon they digest the contents. Most importantly, trapped larvae are unable to migrate out of the fecal mass and onto plant material that may be consumed by the grazing host animal. Thus, fewer larvae migrate onto pasture, resulting in healthier animals. This form of control has been successfully applied under field conditions and is an environmentally safe biological approach for forage-based feeding systems, i.e. nonconfinement.

While *D. flagrans* has mainly been targeted at trichostrongylid nematodes, it has been shown to be effective in controlling *Strongyloides papillosus in vitro* (Campos *et al.*, 2009; Braga *et al.*, 2020) and *Fasciola hepatica* (liver fluke; Braga *et al.*, 2008). There is no expectation of controlling other worms such as tapeworm, or coccidia.

Delivery to the animal

The primary delivery system of the spore material is thorough mixing with supplemental feedstuffs, which then provides a continuous source of the fungus in the feces. Daily feeding is essential so that each animal has the opportunity consistently to consume an adequate amount of the feed/spore mixture. The spores cannot be incorporated into pellets or cooked blocks as the heat of the pelleting process will kill them. However, a dried nutritional pellet containing chlamydospores, resembling a tortilla, was developed by researchers in Mexico (Fitz-Aranda *et al.*, 2015; Aguilar-Marcelino *et al.*, 2017), though not for commercial production. An individual single pellet or cookie formulation may be easier to administer in some farming systems, including those for dairy goats.

To achieve adequate control of larvae in the feces during the transmission season (May–October for most US areas), spores need to be fed for a period of 60–120 days. This usually starts at the beginning of the grazing season, especially for young, freshly weaned livestock. Similarly, to help curb the periparturient rise in FEC phenomenon, feeding spores to dams during late pregnancy and lactation will also help to reduce pasture contamination, especially for nursing growing young that will graze the same pasture with their dams. Feeding studies with sheep, goats, and cattle have shown high reduction (80–90%) of larvae in feces and on pasture, and that FEC can be expected to decrease over time due to the reduced reinfection. During periods of drought or low transmission (winter, nongrazing), it would not be necessary to feed spores as attrition of larvae in feces would occur naturally.

Pasture or range-based systems may not feed supplement to sheep and would need an alternate delivery system of fungal spores. Recently, we conducted a controlled study in which spores were thoroughly mixed into a loose mineral supplement eliminating the need to provide concentrate feeds (Burke, unpublished). Feeding the spores in the loose mineral mix worked as well or better than when mixed in a feed supplement. Lesser controlled field studies also indicate the efficacy of including spores in mineral for on-farm use (A.F. Vatta, personal communication; Paraud *et al.*, 2007). The mineral needs to be kept covered, dry and available for regular consumption by the animal to provide a constant source of spores for the duration of the treatment period.

The two products on the market for livestock producers in the US are BioWorma® and Livamol® with BioWorma (International Animal Health Products, Huntingwood, NSW, Australia). BioWorma is a feed additive labeled for grazing livestock which contains *D. flagrans* in the form of chlamydospores. Livamol with BioWorma is a more diluted formula and considered a protein supplement. BioWorma is available through veterinarians, premix companies, and feed mills. BioWorma and Livamol with BioWorma are available through consumer outlets. The product is not certified organic and contains grain products though less so in BioWorma, thus may not be used for organic or grass-finished farms.

The cost of feeding these BioWorma products is relatively high compared to dewormers, but the long-term benefit of reduced pasture contamination is a factor that needs consideration. Furthermore, with increased acceptance and use, the cost is expected to come down, making it more cost-effective. The above-mentioned products embrace the only control method that specifically targets the worm population on pasture, where an estimated majority of more than 90% of the total population reside during the parasite season. In Brazil, there is a similar product available (Bioverm®; Balbino *et al.*, 2022) and other strains of *D. flagrans* with similar efficacy have been developed in other countries but not commercialized.

Factors that influence efficacy

Earlier research showed that *D. flagrans* could be combined with COWP without any antagonistic activity (Burke *et al.*, 2005b). However, some anthelmintics could interfere with *D. flagrans*, at least in the short term. For instance, benzimidazoles, including fenbendazole and albendazole, have antifungal activity and have been shown to have an antagonistic effect on *D. flagrans* survival when fed to sheep (Sanyal *et al.*, 2004; Zegbi *et al.*, 2019) and ivermectin slowed *in vitro* growth of *D. flagrans* (Zegbi *et al.*, 2019). Efficacy of *D. flagrans* was maintained in sheep dewormed with levamisole (Vilela *et al.*, 2018). Thus, providing *D. flagrans* after initial deworming may inhibit fungal activity, although it should be restored once the anthelmintic is cleared. At present, it is not known if other products or feed supplements, such as coccidiostats or probiotics, could interact with the spores in the gastrointestinal tract and this merits further research.

Certain managed grazing can improve the efficacy of *D. flagrans*. For instance, the combination of *D. flagrans* and rotational grazing led to markedly reduced worm burdens and FEC (Chandrawathani *et al.*, 2004). Rotational grazing often promotes frequent rotation of animals among forage plots, so that they are returned to the original plot from as little as 2–4 weeks to as long as a year, depending on land availability (Burke *et al.*, 2009a). When combined with *D. flagrans*, such a system will lead to greater reductions in residual GIN larvae.

Since heat and excess moisture can affect the viability of the chlamydospores, it is important, especially in research studies, to make use of diagnostics of nematophagous fungi, such as spore count and viability. Viability or predatory activity of chlamydospores can be examined by plating on water agar (Ojeda-Robertos *et al.*, 2008a). To this end, fecal pellets from GIN-free animals, to which chlamydospores had been administered or fed, are placed on an agar petri dish and GIN larvae added the next day. Thereupon, the presence or absence of three-dimensional adhesive nets or trapped larvae can be visualized by microscopy, followed by Baermannization of the culture up to 10 days later to determine the proportion of recovered or untrapped larvae. Ojeda-Robertos *et al.* (2008b) demonstrated that *D. flagrans* chlamydospores could be counted using a modified McMaster technique with a sugar flotation solution and would be helpful to verify that spores reach feces in adequate numbers.

Summary

- *D. flagrans* is the only viable method of GIN control that targets infective larvae on pasture.
- Spores of *D. flagrans* must be fed daily.
- *D. flagrans* should be provided to susceptible animals (periparturient females; weaned offspring) during times when GIN infection is high (summers with rainfall).

Bacillus thuringiensis Crystal Proteins

Crystal toxin (Cry) proteins, released upon sporulation by Bt, a soil bacterium, have been used against insect pests by organic application. The lack of any negative effects of these Cry proteins in vertebrate species makes this an appealing choice for biological control. The proteins target intestinal receptors of invertebrates, and in nematodes are invertebrate-specific glycolipids present on the intestinal mucosa of nematodes. Kotz et al. (2005) reported on two Bt strains that contained Cry proteins, Cry5A and Cry5B, or Cry13, with nematocidal activity against both adult and larval development of *H. contortus*, *T. colubriformis*, and *Teladorsagia circumcincta*, at a level of toxicity similar to or greater than that of thiabendazole and levamisole. Cry5B was also found to act as an anthelmintic against *Ascaris suum*, an intestinal nematode of swine (Urban et al., 2013), and *Heligmosomoides bakeri*, an intestinal nematode of mice (Hu et al., 2010).

Orally administered Cry5B comprises spore crystal lysates, i.e. a mix of Bt spores and Cry protein crystals (Li et al., 2021). To increase the shelf-life of Cry5B and protect the crystals from harsh rumen conditions (Sanders et al., 2020), the crystals were expressed in asporogenous Bt during the vegetative phase to form cytosolic crystals. Inactivated bacteria with cytosolic crystal (IBaCC) were treated with essential oils to inactivate Bt, maintaining efficacy in pigs and horses (Urban et al., 2021). This formulation, which could be more readily mass-produced, retained activity against nematodes in hamsters and mice. Further increasing scalability, the IBaCC Cry5B were purified to yield purified cytosolic crystals (PCC) which maintained *in vivo* activity against nematodes of humans (hookworms), rodents (*Ascaris*), and horses (*Parascaris* spp.; Chicca et al., 2022). Of particular interest, IBaCC Cry5B reduced FEC of *H. contortus*-infected sheep by 90% and adult worms by 72% and female worms by 96% (Sanders et al., 2020). This is an exciting area of research that may offer a viable alternative or combination with anthelmintics, though being able to mass-produce Cry5B and obtain FDA approval will not be a quick process.

Diatomaceous Earth

Diatomaceous earth (DE) has long captured the interest of farmers to control parasites, including GIN. Diatomaceous earth is a natural siliceous sedimentary rock that can be crushed to a particle size of 3 mm to 1 micrometer that is formed from the fossilized remains of diatoms or hard-shelled microalgae which have microscopically rough edges. DE is sold commercially for a number of uses including as a mild abrasive, absorbent for liquids, and a filler in plastics. Finely crushed DE is commercially available as an insecticide, acting to adsorb lipids from the exoskeleton of insects, increasing evaporation and leading to dehydration (Fields et al., 2002). Large spiny diatoms work best for control of slugs and snails, lacerating the epithelium, and may have an effect on nematodes that have a shedding cuticle (such as the L3 stage of strongyles).

Unfortunately, studies on cattle (Fernandez et al., 1998; Lartigue and Rossanigo, 2004) and sheep (Ahmed et al., 2013; Jones et al., 2020) reported no reduction in FEC after feeding 2% of diet as DE for 7 days. However, there was a benefit to including 2% DE in the diet of organically managed poultry, with a reduction in

Capillaria egg counts and northern fowl mites (*Ornithonyssus sylviarum*) (Bennett *et al.*, 2011). Many farmers will state that they believe in the ability of DE to control worms in sheep and goats. It may be that these farmers already possess excellent management, nutrition, and/or genetics for parasite resistance, thus maintaining low levels of worms in their flocks/herds.

Herbal Products

Another class of product often claimed as effective by producers is herbal dewormers which contain various mixtures of dried plants or plant products such as *Allium sativum* (garlic), *Artemisia absinthium* (wormwood), *Artemisia vulgaris* (mugwort), *Cucurbita pepo* (field pumpkin), *Foeniculum vulgare* (fennel), *Hyssopus officinalis* (hyssop), *Juglans nigra* (black walnut), and *Thymus vulgaris* (thyme). Many of these plants have demonstrated various levels of activity against nematodes and other parasites of humans and animals (Soffar and Mokhtar, 1991; Guarrera, 1999; Waller *et al.*, 2001; El Shenawy *et al.*, 2008). However, research studies have failed to show any efficacy in reducing FEC or GIN infection in small ruminants using doses recommended by manufacturers (Luginbuhl *et al.*, 2006; Burke *et al.*, 2009b, c). Caution should be used because higher doses of some herbs such as *Artemisia absinthium* could be toxic or cause abortion in pregnant animals due to the presence of santonin (Waller *et al.*, 2001).

Anthelmintic properties have also been reported for latex and seeds from *Carica papaya* when used in humans and mice (Satrija *et al.*, 1995; Okeniyi *et al.*, 2007) and tested *in vitro* against *H. contortus* (Hounzangbe-Adote *et al.*, 2005). Unfortunately, garlic juice or bulbs or papaya seeds administered to goats were ineffective in reduction of GIN (Burke *et al.*, 2009b). The seeds of squash (*Cucurbita moshata*) and pumpkins (*Cucurbita maxima*) are thought to contain an anthelmintic compound cucurbitacin and were fed to lambs (Strickland *et al.*, 2009) with varying results in GIN control. Matthews *et al.* (2016) found no reduction in FEC or worms in lambs or kids although they did not measure cucurbitacin content. Ginger (*Zingiber officinale*) has also been used as an anthelmintic purge for cattle, horses (Duval, 1997), and lambs (Iqbal *et al.*, 2006), but was ineffective in lambs and goat kids (Matthews *et al.*, 2016). Other Ayurvedic interventions have not been documented to show reductions in GIN infection in small ruminants but are still being explored by scientists worldwide.

Conclusion

It is important to understand and emphasize that the products described are just one component of an integrated control program and should not be relied on alone for GIN worm control. COWP should be used for control of GIN in sheep or goats only as needed. Using the FAMACHA© system, scores of 1 or 2 do not need deworming, scores of 3 may depending on age, stocking rate, and other factors, and scores of 4 and 5 indicate dire need for deworming (Kaplan *et al.*, 2004). COWP targets *H. contortus* but not other GIN that could cause weight loss or diarrhea. A nematode-trapping fungus should be used during times when animals are more susceptible to GIN, such as around time of weaning in young animals or the periparturient period for dams. Products advertised that seem too good to be true likely are and should be used with caution, particularly when animals become extremely parasitized.

Of resounding importance is that minimal use of chemical interventions for GIN control is good for the environment, gut biodiversity of animals, and consumers wishing for clean protein sources. These alternatives offer these advantages as well as options for farms with high anthelmintic resistance.

More information can be found at www.wormx.info and www.iahp.com.au.

References

Aguilar-Marcelino, L., Mendoza-de-Gives, P., Torres-Hernandez, G., Lopez-Arellano, M., Becerril-Perez, C. *et al.* (2017) Consumption of nutritional pellets with *Duddingtonia flagrans* fungal chlamydospores reduces infective nematode larvae of *Haemonchus contortus* in faeces of Saint Croix lambs. *Journal of Helminthology* 91, 665–671.

Ahmed, M.A., Laing, M.D. and Nsahlai, I.V. (2013) Studies on the ability of two isolates of *Bacillus thuringiensis*, an isolate of *Clonostachys rosea f. rosea* and a diatomaceous earth product to control gastrointestinal nematodes of sheep. *Biocontrol Science and Technology* 23, 1067–1082.

Balbino, H.M., de Souza Gouviea, A., Monteiro, T.S.A., Morgan, T. and Grassi de Freitas, L. (2022) Overview of the nematophagous fungus *Duddingtonia flagrans*. *Biocontrol Science and Technology* 32, 911–929.

Bang, K.S., Familton, A.S. and Sykes, A.R. (1990a) Effect of copper oxide wire particle treatment on establishment of major gastrointestinal nematodes in lambs. *Research in Veterinary Science* 49, 132–137.

Bang, K.S., Familton, A.S. and Sykes, A.R. (1990b) Effect of ostertagiasis on copper status in sheep: A study involving use of copper oxide wire particles. *Research in Veterinary Science* 49, 306–314.

Bennett, D.C., Yee, A., Rhee, Y.-J. and Cheng, K. (2011) Effect of diatomaceous earth on parasite load, egg production, and egg quality of free-range organic laying hens. *Environmental Well-Being and Behavior* 90, 1416–1426.

Borobia, M., Villanueva-Saz, S., Ruiz de Arcaute, M., Fernandez, A., Verde, M. *et al.* (2022) Copper poisoning, a deadly hazard for sheep. *Animals* 12, 2388.

Braga, F.R., Araujo, J.V., Campos, A.K. and Araujo, J. (2008) *In vitro* evaluation of the action of the nematophagous fungi *Duddingtonia flagrans*, *Monacrosporium sinense* and *Pochonia chlamydosporia* on *Fasciola hepatica* eggs. *World Journal of Microbiology and Biotechnology* 24, 1559–1564.

Braga, F.R., Ferraz, C.M., Silva, E.N. and Araujo, J.V. (2020) Efficiency of the bioverm® (*Duddingtonia flagrans*) fungal formulation to control *in vivo* and *in vitro Haemonchus contortus* and *Strrongyloides papillosus* in sheep. *Biotechnmology* 10, 62.

Bremner, K.C. (1961) The copper status of some helminth parasites, with particular reference to host-helminth relationships in the gastro-intestinal tract of cattle. *Australian Journal of Agricultural Research* 12, 1188–1199.

Buckley, W.T. and Tait, R.M. (1981) Chronic copper toxicity in lambs: A survey of blood constituent responses. *Canadian Journal of Animal Science* 61, 613–624.

Burke, J.M. and Miller, J.E. (2006a) Evaluation of multiple low dose copper oxide wire particles compared with levamisole for control of *Haemonchus contortus* in lambs. *Veterinary Parasitology* 139, 145–149.

Burke, J.M. and Miller, J.E. (2006b) Control of *Haemonchus contortus* in goats with a sustained-release multi-trace element/vitamin ruminal bolus. *Veterinary Parasitology* 141, 132–137.

Burke, J.M. and Miller, J.E. (2008) Dietary copper sulfate for control of gastrointestinal nematodes in goats. *Veterinary Parasitology* 154, 289–293.

Burke, J.M., Miller, J.E., Olcott, D.D., Olcott, B. and Terrill, T. (2004) Effect of copper oxide wire particles dosage and feed supplement level on *Haemonchus contortus* infection in lambs. *Veterinary Parasitology* 123, 235–243.

Burke, J.M., Miller, J.E. and Brauer, D.K. (2005a) The effectiveness of copper oxide wire particles as an anthelmintic in pregnant ewes and safety to offspring. *Veterinary Parasitology* 131, 291–297.

Burke, J.M., Miller, J.E., Larsen, M. and Terrill, T. (2005b) Interaction between copper oxide wire particles and *Duddingtonia flagrans* in lambs. *Veterinary Parasitology* 134, 141–146.

Burke, J.M., Morrical, D. and Miller, J.E. (2007a) Control of gastrointestinal nematodes with copper oxide wire particles in a flock of lactating Polypay ewes and offspring in Iowa. *Veterinary Parasitology* 146, 372–375.

Burke, J.M., Terrill, T.H., Kallu, R.R., Miller, J. and Mosjidis, J. (2007b) Use of copper oxide wire particles to control gastrointestinal nematodes in goats. *Journal of Animal Science* 85, 2753–2761.

Burke, J.M., Miller, J.E. and Terrill, T.H. (2009a) Impact of rotational grazing on management of gastrointestinal nematodes in weaned lambs. *Veterinary Parasitology* 163, 67–72.

Burke, J.M., Wells, A., Casey, P. and Kaplan, R. (2009b) Herbal dewormer fails to control gastrointestinal nematodes in goats. *Veterinary Parasitology* 160, 168–170.

Burke, J.M., Wells, A., Casey, P. and Miller, J. (2009c) Garlic and papaya lack control over gastrointestinal nematodes in goats and lambs. *Veterinary Parasitology* 159, 171–174.

Burke, J.M., Orlik, S., Miller, J.E. and Terrill, T. (2010a) Using copper oxide wire particles or sericea lespedeza to prevent a peri-parturient gastrointestinal nematode infection in sheep and goats. *Livestock Science* 132, 13–18.

Burke, J.M., Soli, F., Miller, J.E. and Terrill, T.H. (2010b) Administration of copper oxide wire particles in a capsule or feed for gastrointestinal nematode control in goats. *Veterinary Parasitology* 168, 346–350.

Burke, J.M., Miller, J.E., Mosjidis, J.A., Terrill, T., Wildeus, S. *et al.* (2012) Use of a mixed sericea lespedeza pasture system for control of gastrointestinal nematodes lambs and kids. *Veterinary Parasitology* 186, 328–336.

Burke, J.M., Miller, J.E., Terrill, T.H., Smyth, E. and Acharya, M. (2016) Examination of commercially available copper oxide wire particles in combination with albendazole for control of gastrointestinal nematodes in lambs. *Veterinary Parasitology* 215, 1–4.

Burke, J.M., Miller, J.E., Acharya, M. and Wood, E. (2020) Copper oxide wire particles to complement control of gastrointestinal nematodes with levamisole and/or albendazole in lambs. *Journal of Animal Science* 98(Suppl. 2), 73.

Campos, A.K., Araujo, J.V., Guimaraes, M.P. and Dias, A. (2009) Resistance of different fungal structures of *Duddingtonia flagrans* to the digestive process and predatory ability on larvae of *Haemonchus contortus* and *Strongyloides papillosus* in goat feces. *Parasitology Research* 105, 913–919.

Chandrawathani, P., Jamnah, O., Adnan, M., Waller, P., Larsen, M. *et al.* (2004) Field studies on the biological control of nematode parasites of sheep in the tropics, using the microfungus *Duddingtonia flagrans*. *Veterinary Parasitology* 120, 177–187.

Chartier, C., Etter, E., Hoste, H., Pors, I., Koch, C. *et al.* (2000) Efficacy of copper oxide needles for the control of nematode parasites in dairy goats. *Veterinary Research Communications* 24, 389–399.

Chicca, J., Cazeault, N.R., Rus, F., Abraham, A., Garceau, C. *et al.* (2022) Efficient and scalable process to produce novel and highly bioactive purified cytosolic crystals from *Bacillus thuringiensis*. *Microbiology Spectrum* 10, 1–10.

Coffey, L. (2018) Copper oxide wire particles. Available at: www.wormx.info/_files/ugd/6ef604_fb60b9b8f cdc415eacd23a3dc5bd6de5.pdf (accessed 10 July 2025).

Dewey, D.W. (1977) An effective method for the administration of trace amounts of copper to ruminants. *Search* 8, 326–327. DOI: 10.1016/j.vetpar.2003.07.016.

Duval, J. (1997) The control of internal parasites in cattle and sheep. Available at: http://eap.mcgill.ca/publications/EAP70.htm (accessed 10 July 2025).

El Shenawy, N.S., Soliman, M.F.M. and Reyad, S.I. (2008) The effect of antioxidant properties of aqueous garlic extract and Nigella sativa as anti-schistosomiasis agents in mice. *Journal of the Institute of Tropical Medicine of São Paulo* 50, 29–36.

Faedo, M., Larsen, M., Dimander, S.O., Yeates, G., Hoglund, J. *et al.* (2002) Growth of the fungus *Duddingtonia flagrans* in soil surrounding feces deposited by cattle or sheep fed the fungus to control nematode parasites. *Biological Control* 23, 64–70.

Fernandez, M.I., Woodward, B.W. and Stromberg, B.E. (1998) Effect of diatomaceous earth as an anthelmintic treatment on internal parasites and feedlot performance of beef steers. *Animal Science* 66, 635–641.

Fields, P., Allen, S., Korunic, Z. and McLaughlin, A. (2002) Standardized testing for diatomaceous earth. In: *Proceedings of the 8th International Working Conference on Stored-Product Protein*, York, UK.

Fitz-Aranda, J.A., Mendoza-de-Gives, P., Torres-Acosta, J.F.J., Liebano-Hernandez, E., Lopez-Arellano, M. *et al.* (2015) *Duddingtonia flagrans* chlamydospores in nutritional pellets: Effect of storage time and conditions on the trapping ability against *Haemonchus contortus* larvae. *Journal of Helminthology* 89, 13–18.

Guarrera, P.M. (1999) Traditional antehelmintic, antiparasitic and repellent uses of plants in Central Italy. *Journal of Ethnopharmacology* 68, 183–192.

Healey, K., Lawlor, C., Knox, M.R., Chambers, M. and Lamb, J. (2018) Field evaluation of *Duddingtonia flagrans* IAH 1297 for the reduction of worm burden in grazing animals: Tracer studies in sheep. *Veterinary Parasitology* 253, 48–54.

Hounzangbe-Adote, M.S., Paolini, V., Fouraste, I., Moutairou, K. and Hoste, H. (2005) *In vitro* effects of four tropical plants on three life-cycle stages of the parasitic nematode, *Haemonchus contortus*. *Research in Veterinary Science* 78, 155–160.

Hu, Y., Georghiou, S.B., Kelleher, A.J. and Aroian, R. (2010) *Bacillus thuringiensis* Cry5B protein is highly efficacious as a single-dose therapy against an intestinal roundworm infection in mice. *PLOS Neglected Tropical Disease* 4, e614.

Iqbal, Z., Lateef, M., Akhtar, M.S., Ghayur, M. and Gilani, A. (2006) *In vivo* anthelmintic activity of ginger against gastrointestinal nematodes of sheep. *Journal of Ethnopharmacology* 106, 285–287. DOI: 10.1016/j.jep.2005.12.031.

Jones, O., Burke, J.M., Miller, J.E. and Rosenkrans, C. (2020) Use of diatomaceous earth and copper oxide wire particles to control gastrointestinal nematodes in lambs. *Journal of Animal Science* 98(Suppl. 2), 72.

Judson, G.J., Brown, T.H., Gray, D., Dewey, D. and Babidge, P. (1984a) Oxidized copper wire as a copper supplement for sheep: A study of some variables which may alter copper availability. *Australian Veterinary Journal* 61, 294–295.

Judson, G.J., Brown, T.H., Gray, D., Dewey, D., Edwards, J. *et al.* (1982) Oxidized copper wire particles for copper therapy in sheep. *Australian Journal of Agricultural Research* 33, 1073–1083.

Judson, G.J., Trengove, C.L., Langman, M.W. and Vandergraaff, R. (1984b) Copper supplementation of sheep. *Australian Veterinary Journal* 61, 40–43.

Kaplan, R.M., Burke, J.M., Terrill, T.H., Miller, J., Getz, W. *et al.* (2004) Validation of the FAMACHA© eye color chart for detecting clinical anemia on sheep and goat farms in the southern United States. *Veterinary Parasitology* 123, 105–120.

Knox, M.R. (2002) Effectiveness of copper oxide wire particles for *Haemonchus contortus* control in sheep. *Australian Veterinary Journal* 80, 224–227.

Knox, M.R., Josh, P.F. and Anderson, L.J. (2002) Deployment of *Duddingtonia flagrans* in an improved pasture system: Dispersal, persistence, and effects on free-living soil nematodes and microarthropods. *Biological Control* 24, 176–182.

Kotz, A.C., O'Grady, J., Gough, J.M., Pearson, R., Bagnall, N. *et al.* (2005) Toxicity of *Bacillus thuringiensis* to parasitic and free-living life-stages of nematode parasites of livestock. *International Journal for Parasitology* 35, 1013–1022.

Langlands, J.P., Bowles, J.E., Donald, G.E., Smith, A., Paull, D. *et al.* (1983) Copper oxide particles for grazing sheep. *Australian Journal of Agricultural Research* 34, 751–765.

Lartigue, E. del C. and Rossanigo, C.E. (2004) Insecticide and anthelmintic assessment of diatomaceous earth in cattle. *Veternaria Argentina* 21, 660–674.

Li, H., Abraham, A., Gazzola, D., Hu, Y., Beamer, G. *et al.* (2021) Recombinant paraprobiotics as a new paradigm for treating gastrointestinal nematode parasites of humans. *Antimicrobial Agents and Chemotherapy* 21, e01469–20.

Luginbuhl, J.-M., Pietrosemoli Castagni, S. and Howell, J.M. (2006) Use of an herbal dewormer for the control of gastric intestinal tract nematodes in meat goats. *Archives of Latin America Production Animals* 14, 88–89.

Matthews, K.K., O'Brien, D.J., Whitley, N.C., Burke, J., Miller, J. *et al.* (2016) Investigation of possible pumpkin seeds and ginger effects on gastrointestinal nematode infection indicators in meat goat kids and lambs. *Small Ruminant Research* 136, 1–6.

Miller, J.E., Burke, J.M., Garza, J., Callahan, S. and Terrill, T.H. (2011) Comparison of copper oxide wire particles, copper sulfate and anthelmintic treatment for controlling gastrointestinal nematode infection in lambs. *Journal of Animal Science* 89(E-Suppl. 2), 16.

Moscona, A.K., Borkhsenious, O., Sod, G.A., Leibenguth, B.A. and Miller, J.E. (2008) Mechanism of action of copper oxide wire particles (COWP) as an anthelmintic agent. *Proceedings of the 53rd Annual Meeting of the American Association of Veterinary Parasitologists* 39.

Needleman, A.L., Wright, M.C., Schaefer, J.J., Videla, R. and Lear, A. (2022) Copper oxide wire particles effective against gastrointestinal nematodes in adult alpacas during a randomized clinical trial. *American Journal of Veterinary Research* 83, 1–5.

Ojeda-Robertos, N.F., Torres-Acosta, J.F.J., Aguilar-Caballero, A.J., Ayala-Burgos, A., Cob-Galera, L. *et al.* (2008a) Assessing the efficacy of *Duddingtonia flagrans* chlamydospores per gram of faeces to control *Haemonchus contortus* larvae. *Veterinary Parasitology* 158, 329–335.

Ojeda-Robertos, N.F., Torres-Acosta, J.F.J., Ayala-Burgos, A., Cob-Galera, L. and Mendoza-de-Gives, P. (2008b) A technique for the quantification of *Duddingtonia flagrans* chlamydospores in sheep faeces. *Veterinary Parasitology* 152, 339–343.

Okeniyi, J.A., Ogunlesi, T.A., Oyelami, O.A. and Adeyemi, L. (2007) Effectiveness of dried *Carica papaya* seeds against human intestinal parasitosis: A pilot study. *Journal of Medicinal Food* 10, 194–196.

Paraud, C., Pors, I. and Chartier, C. (2007) Efficiency of feeding *Duddintonia flagrans* chlamydospores to control nematode parasites of first-season grazing goats in France. *Veterinary Research Communications* 31, 305–315.

Sanders, J., Xie, Y., Gazzola, D., Li, H., Abraham, A. *et al.* (2020) A new paraprobiotic-based treatment for control of *Haemonchus contortus* in sheep. *International Journal for Parasitology: Drugs and Drug Resistance* 14, 230–236.

Sanyal, P.K., Chauhan, J.B. and Mukhopadhyaya, P.N. (2004) Implications of fungicidal effects of benzimidazole compounds on *Duddingtonia flagrans* in integrated nematode parasite management in livestock. *Veterinary Research Communications* 28, 375–385.

Satrija, F., Nansen, P., Murtini, S. and He, S. (1995) Anthelmintic activity of papaya latex against patent *Heligmosomoides polygyrus* infections in mice. *Journal of Ethnopharmacology* 48, 161–164.

Saumell, C.A., Fernández, A.S., Echevarria, F., Goncalves, I., Iglesias, L. *et al.* (2016) Lack of negative effects of the biological control agent *Duddingtonia flagrans* on soil nematodes and other nematophagous fungi. *Journal of Helminthology* 90, 706–711.

Soffar, S.A. and Mokhtar, G.M. (1991) Evaluation of the antiparasitic effect of aqueous garlic (*Allium sativum*) extract in hymenolepiasis and giardiasis. *Journal of the Egyptian Society of Parasitology* 21, 497–502.

Soli, F., Terrill, T.H., Shaik, S.A., Getz, W., Miller, J. *et al.* (2010) Efficacy of copper oxide wire particles against gastrointestinal nematodes in sheep and goats. *Veterinary Parasitology* 168, 93–96.

Strickland, V.J., Krebs, G.L. and Potts, W. (2009) Pumpkin kernel and garlic as alternative treatments for the control of *Haemonchus contortus* in sheep. *Animal Production Science* 49, 139–144.

Suttle, N.F. (1977) Reducing the potential copper toxicity of concentrates to sheep by the use of molybdenum and sulphur supplements. *Animal Feed Science Technology* 2, 235–246.

Suttle, N.F. (1987) Safety and effectiveness of cupric oxide particles for increasing liver copper stores in sheep. *Research in Veterinary Science* 42, 219–223.

Urban, J.F., Jr, Hu, Y., Miller, M.M., Scheib, U., Yiu, Y.Y. *et al.* (2013) *Bacillus thuringiensis*-derived Cry5B has potent anthelmintic activity against *Ascaris suum*. *PLOS Neglected Tropical Diseases* 7, e2263. DOI: 10.1371/journal.pntd.0002263.

Urban, J.F.Jr., Nielsen, M.K., Gazzola, D., Xie, Y., Beshah, E. *et al.* (2021) An inactivated bacterium (paraprobiotic) expressing *Bacillus thuringiensis* Cry5B as a therapeutic for *Ascaris* and *Parascaris* spp. infections in large animals. *One Health* 12, 100241.

Vatta, A.F., Waller, P.J., Githiori, J.B. and Medley, G. (2009) The potential to control *Haemonchus contortus* in indigenous South African goats with copper oxide wire particles. *Veterinary Parasitology* 162, 306–313.

Vatta, A.F., Waller, P.J., Githiori, J.B. and Medley, G. (2012) Persistence of the efficacy of copper oxide wire particles against *Haemonchus contortus* in grazing South African goats. *Veterinary Parasitology* 190, 159–166.

Vilela, V.L.R., Feitosa, T.F., Braga, F.R., Vieira, V., de Lucena, S. *et al.* (2018) Control of sheep gastrointestinal nematodes using the combination of *Duddingtonia flagrans* and levamisole hydrochloride 5%. *Brazilian Journal of Veterinary Parasitology* 27, 26–31.

Waller, P.J., Bernes, G., Thamsborg, S.M., Sukura, A., Richter, S. *et al.* (2001) Plants as de-worming agents of livestock in the Nordic countries: Historical perspective, popular beliefs and prospects for the future. *Acta Veterinaria Scandinavica* 42, 31–44.

Waller, P.J., Bernes, G., Rudby-Martin, L., Ljungstrom, B. and Rydzik, A. (2004) Evaluation of copper supplementation to control *Haemonchus contortus* infections of sheep in Sweden. *Acta Veterinaria Scandinavica* 45, 149–160.

Whitelaw, A., Armstrong, R.H., Evans, C.C., Fawcett, A., Russel, A. *et al.* (1980) Effects of oral administration of copper oxide needles to hypocupraemic sheep. *Veterinary Record* 107, 87–88.

Whitley, N.C., Dykes, G., Vazquez, J., Burke, J. and Terrill, T. (2021) Effect of copper oxide wire particles with and without anthelmintic treatment or anthelmintic treatment alone on gastrointestinal nematode (GIN) fecal egg counts in goats. *Journal of Animal Science* 99, 43.

Winter, P., Hochsteiner, W. and Chizzola, R. (2004) Use of copper oxide wire particles (Copinox) for the prevention of congenital copper deficiency in a herd of German Improved Fawn breed of goat. *Deutsche Tierärztliche Wochenschrift* 111, 395–397.

Wright, W.H. and Bozicevich, J. (1931) Control of gastrointestinal parasites of sheep by weekly treatments with various anthelmintics. *Journal of Agricultural Research* 43, 1053–1069.

Yeates, G.W., Dimander, S.-O., Waller, P.J. and Hoglund, J. (2002) Environmental impact on soil nematodes following the use of the ivermectin sustained release bolus or the nematophagous fungus
Duddingtonia flagrans to control nematode parasites of cattle in Sweden. *Acta Agriculturae
Scandinavica Section A. Animal Science* 52, 233–242.
Zegbi, S., Saumell, C.A., Sagüés, M.F., Ceballos, L., Dominguez, P. *et al.* (2019) Effect of different concen-
trations of anthelmintics on mycelial growth of the biological control agent *Duddingtonia flagrans*. In:
27th Conference of the World Association for the Advancement of Veterinary Parasitology, Madison,
WI, USA, pp. 1–2.

5 Genetics of Gastrointestinal Nematode Parasite Resistance in Small Ruminants

Scott A. Bowdridge[1]*, James L.M. Morgan[2] and Andrew R. Weaver[3]
[1]School of Food and Agriculture, West Virginia University, Morgantown, West Virginia, USA; [2]Round Mountain Consulting, Fayetteville, Arkansas, USA; [3]Department of Animal Science, North Carolina State University, Raleigh, North Carolina, USA

Abstract

This chapter will explore genetic strategies of parasite control using fecal egg count (FEC) as the means to identify superior individuals. Significant variation exists among breeds and between individuals to permit selection strategies to improve parasite resistance. No single marker or group of markers has been identified to consistently select parasite-resistant sheep, yet these studies identify immunity as the key mechanism of parasite resistance. An improved understanding of immune response to parasitism is needed to ultimately identify a single trait or marker. Quantitative forms of genetic selection have been shown to be an effective strategy in reducing the impact of parasitism. In the US, FEC-estimated breeding values (EBV) have incorporated molecular techniques to enhance the accuracy of selection for parasite resistance. These FEC-EBVs have become the standard for parasite resistance selection in the US and are a durable and effective means to reduce the impact of gastrointestinal nematode (GIN) parasitism.

Introduction

Breeding for parasite resistance depends on the identification of highly resistant individuals. A convenient measurement of parasite resistance to *Haemonchus contortus*, and other strongylid parasites, is the fecal egg output. An indirect measurement of infection can be done by quantifying the number of eggs in a known quantity of cleanly collected feces. The McMaster's fecal egg count (FEC) is a convenient exam that measures the number of worm eggs per gram of feces (Whitlock, 1948). While not a sensitive exam (1 egg counted = 50 eggs/g), this assay requires less time than repeated individual sampling, which is where the power of this exam lies. Fecal egg output is an indirect measurement of actual infection, but it indicates relative levels of infection (Gray, 1997). Measurements that are more specific to *H. contortus* are the hematocrit or packed cell volume (PCV), which provides a measurement of anemia, and the FAMACHA© score, a visual measure of anemia based on a five-point scale. Selection criteria to improve parasite

*Corresponding author: scott.bowdridge@mail.wvu.edu

DOI: 10.1079/9781800623767.0005

resistance have commonly been based on FEC. Although PCV and FAMACHA© score may be utilized in some scenarios, these traits identify resilience rather than resistance.

Heritability of Parasite Resistance

Selection for parasite resistance has been conducted for many years worldwide, through selection for low FEC in response to both natural and artificial infections (Kemper et al., 2009). Within-breed selection based on FEC has improved parasite resistance. If improvement in parasite resistance can be made through selection for lower FEC, then parasite resistance is a genetically mediated trait. Genetic selection strategies for parasite resistance discussed in this section will only be based on selection for low FEC lambs whereas selection based on other traits associated with parasitism, FAMACHA© scores, and PCV focus on resilience. These measures of anemia only work to identify specific species of parasites and do not represent more global trichostrongylid parasite resistance. These measures can be a valuable tool in determining the need for anthelmintic treatment and maybe as an adjunctive selection metric.

Prediction of the potential response to selection requires knowledge of genetic parameters such as heritability estimates and genetic correlations. Heritability is defined as the proportion of phenotypic variation within a population that is attributable to genetic variation among individuals (Falconer and Mackay, 1996). The genetic correlation is the proportion of variance that two traits share due to common genetic factors. Research has focused on FEC and its relationship to growth and maternal traits to determine whether selection for parasite resistance will have positive or negative impact on growth rate, number of lambs born, and number of lambs weaned.

Heritability of FEC, or parasite resistance, has been calculated for different breeds of sheep. In Polish Longwool sheep, the heritability of parasite resistance varied between 0.20 and 0.33 depending on the time of year (Bouix et al., 1998), with a favorable negative genetic correlation (−0.61) between FEC and average daily gain. Selection for growth in an infected

environment would be expected to indirectly also improve parasite resistance of lambs (Bouix et al., 1998). In France, researchers evaluated differences in parasite resistance of Rhön and Merinoland sheep (Gauly et al., 2002). Rhön sheep had a higher heritability (0.35) of FEC than Merinoland (0.17) (Gauly and Erhardt, 2002). These studies and others note that animals that have lower FEC early in the grazing season also have lower FEC later in the season (Bouix et al., 1998; Gauly and Erhardt, 2002; Gauly et al., 2002).

In the UK, Scottish Blackface sheep were used to estimate heritability of parasite resistance. Heritability estimates varied with the age of the lamb, slowly increasing from an average of 0.01 at 1 month to 0.22 at 6 months (Bishop et al., 1996). Heritability determined from mean FEC from month 3 to month 6 was 0.33, indicating a moderate level of heritability. The genetic correlation between FEC and live weight in lambs older than 3 months of age was close to −1.0 (Bishop et al., 1996), which is consistent with results in the Polish Longwool sheep (Bouix et al., 1998).

In Australia, the estimated heritability of FEC in Merino sheep divergently selected for parasite resistance was 0.29 across sexes, years, and infection levels (Woolaston and Piper, 1996). Heritability of FEC in Merino sheep selected for parasite resistance since 1988 was 0.24 and a virtual null genetic correlation of FEC and growth was reported (Kemper et al., 2009). These data indicate that selection for parasite resistance should not impact expression of other economically important traits.

In the US, heritability estimates for FEC are very consistent with those from other countries and those found in the recent metaanalysis. In a group of crossbred sheep, not selected for parasite resistance, heritability for FEC was 0.31 at the peak of infection (Vanimisetti et al., 2004a). Genetic correlation data from this study indicated that lambs with high genetic merit for body weight had a higher level of parasite resistance. Data from 12,869 Katahdin lambs born between 2003 and 2015 indicate heritability of weaning FEC (WFEC) and postweaning FEC (PFEC) to be 0.18–0.26 and 0.23–0.46, respectively, depending on the model used. In this study, genetic correlations between WFEC and PFEC were positive and strong (0.82), indicating that selection for low FEC at 8 weeks of age will be associated with resistance at 16 weeks of age. Genetic correlations (-0.29 to −0.38) between WFEC and body weight support Vanimisetti *et al.* (2004a), with decreased WFEC associated with increased body weight. However, relationships between PFEC and body weight were weak (Ngere *et al.*, 2018). Notter *et al.* (2018) reported heritability estimates of 0.35 and 0.24 for periparturient rise at lambing and 30 days postpartum, respectively, in NSIP Katahdin data from ewes born 2007–2013. Increased litter size had a small positive (unfavorable) relationship (0.12–0.18) with increased periparturient FEC and a moderate positive relationship (0.27–0.40) with lamb WFEC and PFEC. There was a relatively strong positive relationship (0.56–0.77) between ewe periparturient rise and lamb FEC, indicating that selection of replacement females based on low FEC should result in mature ewes with improved parasite resistance and decreased fecal egg shedding.

Heritability estimates for FEC in lambs ranging from 0.20 to 0.35 can be considered to have moderate heritability. A recent metaanalysis utilizing 591 estimates of heritability, incorporating much of the data reviewed to this point, has determined a comprehensive heritability estimate of 0.25 for FEC, with a genetic correlation to production traits to be +0.10 (Hayward, 2022). Meaningful genetic improvement will therefore require multiple generations of selection for low FEC. However, there are sources of concentrated genetics for parasite resistance, located in breeds that have developed in equatorial climates. The incorporation of those breeds into a program selecting for parasite resistance would have promise. For example, the heritability of FEC in Suffolk × Gulf Coast Native crossbred lambs was 0.22, but heritability in their purebred Suffolk ancestors was only 0.12 (Miller *et al.*, 2006).

Selection for other traits associated with parasitism, such as FAMACHA© scores and PCV, is possible. FAMACHA© scoring has a limited range and heritability estimates of 0.26 (Arisman *et al.*, 2023), 0.06 (low worm challenge) to 0.24 (high worm challenge) in Merino sheep (Riley and Van Wyk, 2009), and 0.33 in Dorper sheep (Ngere *et al.*, 2018). Selection has also been attempted based on PCV, but has also been less effective than selection based on FEC with heritability estimated

of 0.39 in lambs and 0.15 in ewes (Vanimisetti *et al.*, 2004b). FAMACHA© and PCV reflect anemia status, are only relevant for *H. contortus* infections, and do not indicate fecal egg shedding or total strongylid worm burden. Thus, their use in a selection scheme would identify resilience, not resistance, and may distract from the primary goal of decreasing infection rates as indicated by FEC.

Another test of gastrointestinal nematode (GIN) resistance or immunity is the carbohydrate larval antigen or CarLA® Saliva test (AgResearch, NZ) developed in New Zealand (Shaw *et al.*, 2013). The test measures the amount of salivary IgA against a lipoglycan on the cuticular surface of the infective stage GIN larvae. There is a negative correlation between salivary anti-CarLA IgA concentrations and FEC in New Zealand sheep. The trait is considered moderately heritable at 0.2–0.4. Recently, researchers at the University of Guelph have been exploring the use of CarLA for selection of GIN resistance in Canadian sheep and found similar results (DeWolf *et al.*, 2025). There may be promise in using CarLA in the US, the advantage being that a high GIN infection level is not required to detect resistance in a flock, and even animals that have been dewormed can be tested. Evidence shows the saliva test can also be used in goats (Shaw *et al.*, 2023).

Genetic Markers for Parasite Resistance

Breeding for parasite resistance can bring about changes within a flock in a relatively short period of time, especially if breeds like the St Croix are introduced into the flock. However, crossbreeding is not applicable in purebred flocks, and purebred producers must rely on the identification of parasite-resistant individuals within their breed. Identification of parasite-resistant sheep is a difficult task that requires multiple FEC to reliably confirm reduced infection levels through seasons of high and low parasite infectivity. Over the past two decades, there has been a trend in livestock selection to focus on the identification of genetic markers and implementation of genetic marker-assisted selection (GMAS). This principle of GMAS relies on identification of variable alleles in regions of DNA that are specifically associated with the desired phenotype. The use of GMAS to identify parasite-resistant individuals would be very helpful and may eliminate the need for labor-intensive FEC determinations.

Resistance to parasites is a highly variable quantitative trait which researchers lack the ability to divide into discrete genetic units and therefore it has been described statistically as heritability (Beh and Maddox, 1996). The additive effect of many genes is responsible for the phenotype of quantitative traits (Falconer and Mackay, 1996) but the question is: what gene controls parasite resistance? The resulting parasite-resistant phenotype could be due to small actions from many genes or major genes whose effects may be obfuscated by additive genetic variation and environmental effects (Beh and Maddox, 1996).

QTLs of parasite resistance

Fecal egg counts and hematological measurements have proven to be reasonably accurate at identifying parasite-resistant and/or -resilient individuals and there is clear variation among breeds for parasite resistance. The first attempts at genetic marker identification used quantitative trait loci (QTL) analysis to locate markers for parasite resistance (Charon, 2004). A QTL is a genomic region that affects the phenotypic variation of a trait (Powder, 2020). Most of such studies have yielded similar results, suggesting that QTLs for resistance to strongyle-type parasites are located on chromosome 3 near the interferon-(IFN) γ gene (Gasbarre et al., 2001; Coltman et al., 2001; Beh et al., 2002; Davies et al., 2006), and on chromosome 20 near the major histocompatibility complex (MHC) (Schwaiger et al., 1995; Paterson, 1998; Charon, 2004; Davies et al., 2006). The cumulative effect of these QTLs has been associated with 98% reduction in FEC among resistant genotypes in some studies (Schwaiger et al., 1995) but to have no significant effect on FEC reduction in others (Marshall et al., 2009). These QTL studies have consistently indicated that the regions of the genome associated with parasite resistance are typically also involved in immune response.

Microarray technology used to discover parasite-resistant genes

Microarray technology has allowed researchers to evaluate which genes are differentially expressed during infection. These microarray assays have typically been conducted on bovine cDNA microchips as no ovine cDNA microchips were available. The first published report using this technology stated that over 100 genes were differentially expressed in susceptible and resistant sheep. Two pathways that were represented by differentially expressed genes were involved in development of the acquired immune response and related to the structure of intestinal smooth muscle (Diez-Tascon et al., 2005). Many upregulated genes were associated with MHC class II components, which are a critical aspect in antigen presentation. Studies using QTL and microarray analyses have found that immunity-related genes are involved in parasite resistance.

A later microarray study attempted to reduce variation in gene up- or downregulation by evaluating parasite-naïve sheep that were also genetically resistant to parasites. In this particular scenario, it was expected that different genes would be upregulated since these individuals had not been exposed to parasites and had not developed immune memory response (Keane et al., 2006). This study was the first to use an ovine cDNA microarray. The authors indicate that intestines of resistant sheep do not appear to become stressed due to parasitic infection, whereas the intestines of susceptible sheep expressed significantly more stress genes (Keane et al., 2006). The gene ontology (GO) terms associated with resistance were cellular processes, whereas the GO term associated with susceptibility was response to stress. However, both of these studies are limited because responses were not assessed until 84 days (Keane et al., 2006) and 120 days (Diez-Tascon et al., 2005) after initial infection.

Two reports compared infection at 3 versus 27 days (MacKinnon et al., 2009) or from 1 to 45 days after infection (Rowe et al., 2009). MacKinnon et al. (2009) reported increased expression of genes related to neutrophil cell markers, migration of immune cells, blood flow to site of infection and expression of IL-4Rα and IL-12Rβ1 at 3 days after infection (MacKinnon *et al.*, 2009). By 27 days, the profile of expressed genes in the resistant sheep had shifted from inflammatory or innate genes to genes responsible for protective responses, including increased expression of IL-4 and decreased expression of IFNγR. There was also an increase in the expression of smooth muscle genes in the resistant sheep and the authors speculated that those individuals may have been attempting to physically expel the parasite. Rowe and colleagues reported that intelectin 2 was upregulated over all time points, and has a variety of functions ranging from effects on mucus viscosity (Arranz-Plaza *et al.*, 2002) to a protective antibacterial role (Tsugi *et al.*, 2001) and phagocyte activation (Abe *et al.*, 1999). Other differentially expressed genes shifted in expression from being associated with innate immune responses at 3–10 days after infection to a later expression profile consistent with the protective effects of an acquired immune response. Immunoglobulin genes dominated the expression profile on 22 and 45 days after infection, supporting development of an acquired response (Rowe *et al.*, 2009). Although these two reports used sheep that have natural parasite resistance (MacKinnon *et al.*, 2009) and sheep that are susceptible to parasites (Rowe *et al.*, 2009), both authors reported consistent results in that the substantial numbers of genes related to the immune response were activated during both the prepatent and patent periods of parasite infection.

Genome-wide analysis methods

Copy number variant (CNV) evaluates the number of copies of a particular gene; it varies from one individual to another and has been utilized in discovery of genes associated with parasite resistance. Recent studies utilizing this technology have found that CNVs associated with desirable FEC and PCV were like those found in other QTL studies and many of these genes are linked to immune response (Estrada-Reyes *et al.*, 2022). Single nucleotide polymorphisms (SNP) have been identified in genome-wide analysis studies (GWAS) using a 50K SNP chip. During artificial and natural infection with *H. contortus*, this study found a total of 26 significant SNP, of which 21 were located

within 20 kb of genes involved in immune cell development, mucin production, and cellular signaling for wound healing and coagulation (Thorne *et al.*, 2023). Using a 388K SNP on progeny-tested Katahdin sires enrolled in the National Sheep Improvement Program (NSIP), Notter *et al.* (2022) reported chromosome-wide significance on chromosome 5 for FEC EBV. The IL12B gene at 68.5 Mb on chromosome 5 codes for a subunit of interleukins 12 and 23, and other immunoregulatory genes are located in areas of significance possibly leading to additive or associative effects (Notter *et al.*, 2022). Becker *et al.* (2022) identified significant SNPs associated with lower FEC using high-density genotype data from Katahdin lambs enrolled in the NSIP. The SNP were within introns of the gene adhesion G protein-coupled receptor B3. Among various studies on genetic resistance to GIN using genomic techniques among several breeds, there is little consensus on major genes involved (Cunha *et al.*, 2024).

Molecular approaches to identify specific genetic markers for parasite resistance have provided clear and consistent evidence about the type of genes involved in parasite resistance. However, identification of a small number of major genes or reliable markers associated with reduced FEC has yet to be determined. Thus, a better understanding of genetic differences among various sheep types will benefit from enhanced understanding of differences in immune function to assist in identification of logical pathways and potential candidate genes. To date, molecular genetic techniques have not been commercially deployed.

Immune Mechanism of Parasite Resistance

Immunity to helminth parasites is complex and varies widely based on parasite species, route of transmission, parasite life stage, host, and tissue niche within the host. A great deal of research has focused on initiation of immune response in the murine host and how those responses predicate adaptive responses. In small ruminant hosts, the timing and observation, in a production setting, may leave producers and researchers blind to the initial exposure to helminth parasites. To discover the immunobiology of parasite resistance, scientists will often raise small ruminants in an environment devoid of helminth parasites to study these responses. Results of these experiments inform biological processes but fail to provide a means by which to improve parasite resistance. Analysis of challenge immune responses is more relevant to immune processes that occur on-farm and as such provide a potential means to understand genetic contribution to differences in immune response to helminth parasite infection.

T helper cell type 2 (Th2) immune activation, in response to *H. contortus* larval stages, reduces adult establishment and fecundity. Innate immune cell influx (eosinophils, mast cells, neutrophils, globule leukocytes), cytokine production (IL-4, IL-5, IL-13), and increased parasite-specific antibody (IgA, IgE) production are all implicated in parasite expulsion (Balic *et al.*, 2000; Lacroux *et al.*, 2006). The gastrointestinal environment during a Th2 response is characterized by increased luminal flow coupled with intestinal muscle contractility, and these responses are driven by IL-4 and IL-13 cytokine production (Harris, 2011).

In the context of *H. contortus* infection in sheep, research has demonstrated a correlation between elevated IL-4 and IL-13 expression during early infection and prevention of parasite establishment. Initial IL-4 expression was detected in St Croix abomasal tissue by day 3 and in Suffolk sheep at day 10 post infection. These data indicate a delay in IL-4 expression in susceptible sheep (Jacobs *et al.*, 2016). IL-13 expression at 3 days post infection (DPI) was significantly increased in both STC abomasum and lymph node tissue but was markedly reduced in susceptible sheep (MacKinnon *et al.*, 2015). Delayed SUF IL-4 expression and reduced IL-13 expression to *Haemonchus* larval stages in susceptible hosts permit the establishment of adults. Bowdridge *et al.* (2015) identified cellular infiltrate of abomasal tissue during the first 7 days of *H. contortus* infection and found a significant increase of neutrophils in STC abomasum when compared to SUF sheep at 3 DPI.

An *in vitro* model of *H. contortus* larval antigen stimulation of ovine neutrophils revealed an ability to produce IL-4 as early as 30 min after antigen stimulation, with no breed differences observed. Neutrophils preferentially produced significant amounts of IL-4 after stimulation with larval but not adult *H. contortus* antigen. When culturing larval antigen-primed neutrophils with naïve peripheral blood mononuclear cells (PBMC), primed neutrophils were able to induce the production of IL-4 in naïve cell populations (Middleton *et al.*, 2020). From these data, it is reasonable to conclude that early neutrophil infiltration, IL-4 production, and increased early IL-4 and IL-13 expression in abomasal tissue of STC lambs drive activation of early Th2 responses. *H. contortus*-infected STC PBMC (composed of monocytes and lymphocytes) cultured with larvae led to a reduction in larval motility (Holt *et al.*, 2015). Quantifying larval death after culture with PBMC by ATP quantification further found a greater reduction in larval ATP when cultured with STC PBMC compared to culture with SUF PBMC (Shepherd *et al.*, 2017).

Taken together, these studies demonstrate the significance of early IL-4/IL-13 signaling in promoting parasite expulsion. Interleukin-4 acting on Th2 cells causes the subsequent production of IL-4, creating a positive feedback loop and promoting the differentiation of B cells to plasma cells, necessary for both IgE and IgG production (Armitage *et al.*, 1992). Differences between resistant and susceptible sheep have been documented with emphasis on a delay in response to larval stages observed in susceptible sheep.

Breeds with Natural Resistance to Gastrointestinal Nematodes

Breeds of sheep originating from humid, tropical climates arc hypothesized to have evolved parasite resistance in order to survive under constant exposure to *H. contortus*. In the US, the Florida Native has demonstrated higher weight gains and lower establishment of adult parasites when compared to Rambouillet sheep (Bradley *et al.*, 1973). The Gulf Coast Native, another breed indigenous to the US, also had lower FEC and higher PCV when naturally infected with *H. contortus* compared to other wool sheep (Miller *et al.*, 1998). Many studies have been conducted using these breeds but breeds originating from the Caribbean also provide a useful model for studying natural parasite resistance.

The Barbados Blackbelly (Yazwinski *et al.*, 1979), St Croix (Courtney *et al.*, 1985), and Katahdin (Burke and Miller, 2002; Vanimisetti *et al.*, 2004a) breeds have been noted for their resistance to GIN. When compared to the Dorset (Yazwinski *et al.*, 1979) or Rambouillet-Dorset crossbred (Zajac *et al.*, 1990), Barbados Blackbelly sheep had consistently lower FEC and higher PCV. St Croix sheep have shown similar results to those reported for Barbados Blackbelly and therefore these Caribbean hair-type sheep are superior in parasite resistance to domesticated sheep originating from Europe or the UK (Zajac *et al.*, 1990; Vanimisetti *et al.*, 2004a). Concerns over use of Caribbean hair sheep in crossbreeding programs arise due to their small mature size, slow growth rate, and lower carcass weights (Wildeus, 1997).

In the late 1950s, a commercial sheep breeder in northern Maine created a breed using Caribbean hair sheep and British wool sheep (Parker *et al.*, 1991). After years of breeding for a similar phenotype, the resulting breed was named Katahdin. The intention behind the creation of the Katahdin breed was to produce a meat animal that did not require shearing. However, the Katahdin has gained favor in the south-eastern US as a low-input maternal ewe breed (Burke and Miller, 2002). The mature size of the Katahdin ewe is significantly larger than that of Caribbean breeds and Katahdin lambs typically have better carcass merit (Wildeus, 1997; Vanimisetti *et al.*, 2004b). In practical lamb production scenarios, Katahdin ewes would be mated to terminal sires to produce offspring that can both survive on infected pastures and maintain carcass merit. The Katahdin breed is a very functional ewe breed as they have complementarity with black-faced terminal sires and are nearly as parasite resistant as Caribbean breeds (Burke and Miller, 2002; Vanimisetti *et al.*, 2004b). The breed has grown to become the most frequently registered breed in the US (Morgan, 2019). In the last 20 years, hair sheep as a percentage of the US sheep flock have risen from less than 1 to 26%. In the south-east alone, the number of farms raising sheep has increased by 167% (Newton, 2019). Clearly, the influence of hair sheep and the Katahdin breed has been pronounced.

Development and Application of Estimated Breeding Value for Parasite Resistance in the US Sheep Industry

Estimated breeding values (EBV) predict differences in genetic merit between two individuals. Assuming environmental effects are the same, i.e. within the same contemporary group, these values would predict the difference in phenotypic performance. On average, an individual passes half of their genetics to their offspring. Thus, expected progeny differences (EPD) are half of an EBV and predict performance differences between two individuals' progeny. The prediction of EBV and EPD incorporates pedigree records, individual performance records, progeny performance records, and genetic relationships between traits. This multitude of data contributing to the breeding value for each trait makes EBV and EPD the most accurate selection tools available.

History of FEC breeding value development in the US

Dr Charles Parker's early advocacy of selecting sheep genetically resistant to GIN led to development of a FEC EPD in the USA. Parker was influenced by graduate thesis work at Ohio State University (Courtney *et al.*, 1985) which documented that certain sheep breeds had innate resistance to GIN parasites that could be measured by 8 weeks of age. Courtney *et al.* (1985) also documented significant breed differences in parasitism, indicating a genetic component for GIN resistance. In the absence of an EBV for producers, Parker (1998, 2000) advocated that producers do on-farm testing of ram lambs to identify potential sires with GIN resistance. The protocol included selecting newly weaned ram lambs to place on a worm-infected pasture for the summer. There was an initial recommendation to deworm infected lambs, place them on a highly infected pasture and monitor their subsequent FEC for several weeks. By the end of the summer, ram lambs with low FEC would have a significant probability of being more resistant to GIN.

Parker's advocacy led to two efforts in the Katahdin breed to select for resistance to GIN. In 2003 and 2004, two separate projects were started that, when combined, resulted in the release of the first EPD for FEC in the USA (Notter *et al.*, 2007). One set of projects was two North Central Region Sustainable Agriculture Research and Education (NCR-SARE USDA) Farmer-Rancher Grants to Kathy Bielek in 2005 and 2007 (Bielek, 2005, 2007). A second project involved three Katahdin flocks in the NSIP that submitted data as a pilot study with the objective of development of a FEC EPD.

Bielek recruited 10 flocks, primarily Katahdins, from Missouri, Ohio, and Pennsylvania and with the guidance of Parker and William Shulaw, DVM, designed protocols for flocks to do FEC on groups of lambs with at least two sires and at least 10 offspring per sire represented in each contemporary group. Results were published as a final report to NC-SARE in 2005 and 2007. Notter provided genetic and statistical analyses for the 2007 report. Besides providing FEC that were used in the first published Katahdin FEC EPD (Notter *et al.*, 2007), Bielek's project provided several guidelines that are still used in the FEC EBV provided by the NSIP in the USA. First, that age of lamb on first detection of genetic resistance to GIN is less important than level of infection. Basically, if most or all lambs in the contemporary group have low FEC (small phenotypic range), the accuracy of using FEC to differentiate genetic resistance to GIN is lower. Second, the mean FEC of the contemporary group needs to have a minimum of 500 eggs/g. Depending on month of lambing and pasture conditions, a 500 eggs/g mean in the contemporary group can be detected at 8 weeks of age but more often at 13–15 weeks of age (Bielek, 2007; Notter *et al.*, 2007). Third, there were preliminary indications of nongenetic factors impacting FEC, including differences in individual lamb growth rates and litter size at birth and weaning (Bielek, 2007).

In the second project, Notter was approached by the Katahdin breed representative of the NSIP to develop an EPD for parasite resistance. At a 2003 regional meeting at the Appalachian Farming Systems Research Center (USDA-ARS) in Beaver, West Virginia, Notter approached an *AD hoc* group (Charles Parker,

James Morgan, Anne Zajac, Henry Zerby, Paul Rodgers) to discuss a pilot FEC EPD project. The discussion group assigned Parker, Notter, and Morgan to develop the protocol for a pilot project. Parker advocated for doing FEC at 8 weeks (Courtney *et al.*, 1985) and Notter said international publications had not reported heritability of FEC until lambs were a minimum of 12–16 weeks of age. A compromise resulted and producers collected fecal samples when the contemporary group averaged 8 weeks of age, then all lambs were dewormed and fecal samples collected again at both 12 and 13 weeks of age. Three flocks were recruited and after 2 years, results showed that a FEC EPD could be implemented (Notter *et al.*, 2007). Notter *et al.* (2007) found that the mean progeny FEC at 8 weeks of age for three sires had the same relative rankings across two consecutive years (Fig. 5.1). Similar results were observed for the same rank of sires based on progeny FEC later in the grazing season. Further analyses found that the two sires used in two separate flocks had the same relative rank in progeny FEC (Fig. 5.2).

Combining the lamb FEC data from the Bielek NCR-SARE projects and the proof-of-concept NSIP project provided enough lambs and sires to publish the first FEC EPD for the US sheep industry. The first FEC EPD sire summary had 26 Katahdin sires. Mean FEC between flocks was adjusted to 2000 eggs/g, and sire EPD at 8 weeks of age ranged from −1000 eggs/g to +2000 eggs/g (Fig. 5.3).

FEC EBV in the USA

In 2010, the NSIP contracted with Meat & Livestock Australia for genetic evaluations through the LambPlan. This contract provided twice-monthly genetic evaluations which allowed each flock to receive FEC EBV on lambs within a month of sampling. This greatly increased the rate of genetic improvement in parasite resistance by allowing more accurate selection of replacement ram and ewe lambs based on FEC EBV. Also, the analysis of lamb FEC resulted in calculation of FEC EBV for the sires and dams. With the transition to LambPlan, two changes were made. First, EPD were replaced with EBV. Second, sheep evaluated for parasite

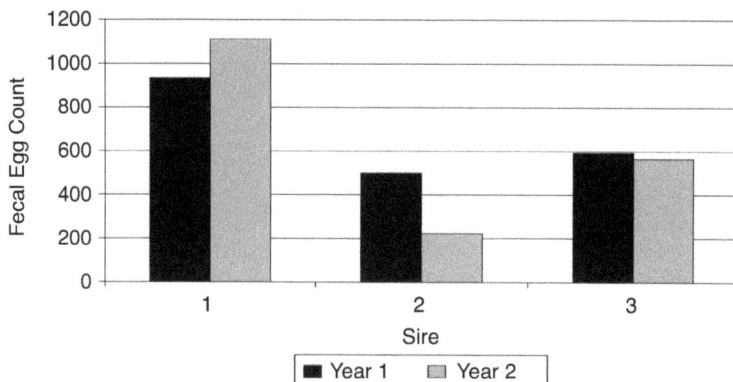

Fig. 5.1. Average progeny fecal egg counts at 8 weeks of age for three sires evaluated in the same Katahdin flock in 2 years (Notter *et al.*, 2007). Courtesy of David Notter and used with permission.

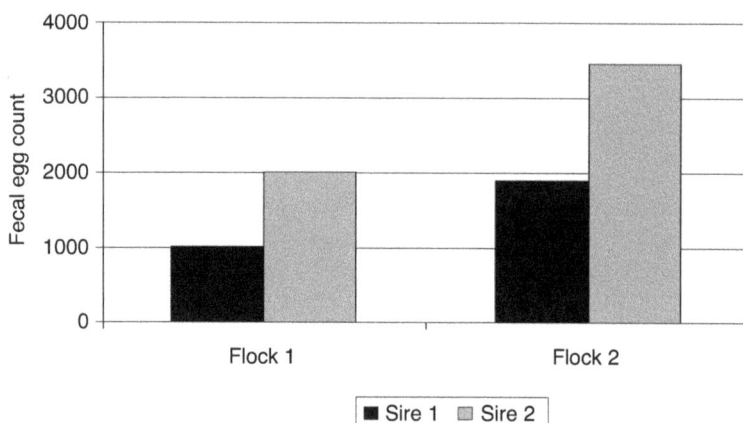

Fig. 5.2. Average progeny fecal egg counts at 2 weeks of age for Katahdin sires evaluated in two flocks in 2 years (Notter *et al.*, 2007). Courtesy of David Notter and used with permission.

resistance received both a WFEC and a PFEC, increasing the accuracy of the EBV by using two measures. The twice-monthly updates in FEC EBV and the development of two measures (WFEC and PFEC) have greatly increased the rate of flock improvement of genetic resistance to GIN (Fig. 5.4).

Dr Joan Burke implemented studies with 14 Katahdin NSIP flocks from 2010 to 2014 to determine the genetic components of the periparturient rise in fecal egg counts in Katahdin ewes (USDA, NIFA, Organic Agriculture Research and Extension Initiative grant #2010–01884). The periparturient period along with young lambs are when sheep are most susceptible to GIN and when the most GIN eggs are shed.

When the periparturient data were analyzed, the researchers also updated the genetic parameters for WFEC and PFEC in Katahdin lambs at weaning and postweaning, (Ngere *et al.*, 2018; Notter *et al.*, 2018) and genetic parameters for FAMACHA© in lambs (Notter *et al.*, 2017a). These publications definitively showed that in at least some breeds, in this case Katahdins, genetic resistance to GIN can be detected as early as 8 weeks of age. Heritability of the periparturient rise in Katahdin ewes is higher than that of Katahdin lambs (Notter *et al.*, 2017b, 2018). The potential for the implementation of a FEC EBV for the periparturient rise exists. With the genetic correlations between lamb FEC EBV and a periparturient FEC EBV, producers would have

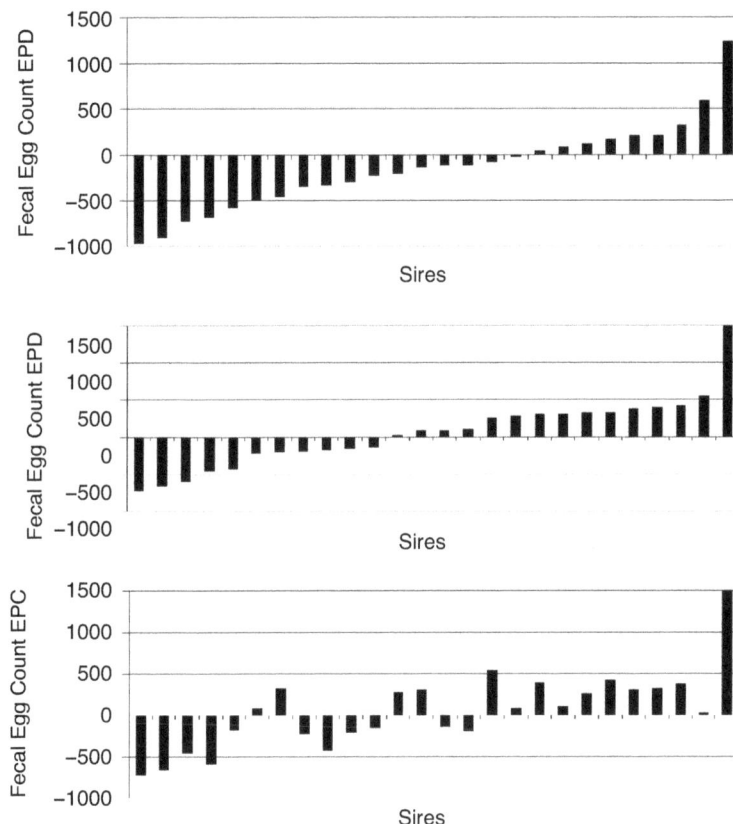

Fig. 5.3. FEC EPDs for Katahdin sires at 8 weeks (top panel) and 22 weeks (middle panel). In each case, EPDs are ranked from lowest to highest. The bottom panel shows 22-week FEC EPDs of the sires ranked from highest to lowest on 8-week FEC EPD, thus showing correspondence between FEC EPDs at the two ages (Notter *et al.*, 2007). Courtesy of David Notter and used with permission.

access to increased accuracy of selection. Also, a periparturient FEC EBV would be a further tool to decrease pasture contamination.

The next stage in using EBV to improve selection for parasite resistance was the release of genomically enhanced estimated breeding values (GEBV). More than 4300 Katahdins were genotyped using the GeneSeek Genomic Profiler Ovine 50k array (Neogen Corp., Lincoln, NE, USA) with most genotyped animals being born 2016–2019. These 50k SNPs were incorporated into the LambPlan genetic evaluation to improve prediction accuracy of FEC EBV, resulting in the name change to GEBV. This occurred for Katahdins in October 2021 (McMillan *et al.*, 2022). This improvement in FEC EBV accuracy provides the opportunity to increase the rate of

genetic change for improvement of FEC and consequently parasite resistance. The DNA samples collected were also used to identify regions that were associated with resistance to GIN in Katahdins (Becker *et al.*, 2022).

While most of the research on FEC EBV in the USA has been conducted in Katahdins, there have been efforts by researchers and producers to identify GIN resistance in other breeds. Currently, the NSIP searchable database includes FEC EBVs for Polypays. FEC data have been submitted to the NSIP for other breeds including Texels, Suffolks, Dorsets, Dorpers, and a few goat herds. Due to lack of significant genetic connections between flocks/herds, participants are receiving within-flock FEC EBV which are not published on the searchable NSIP database

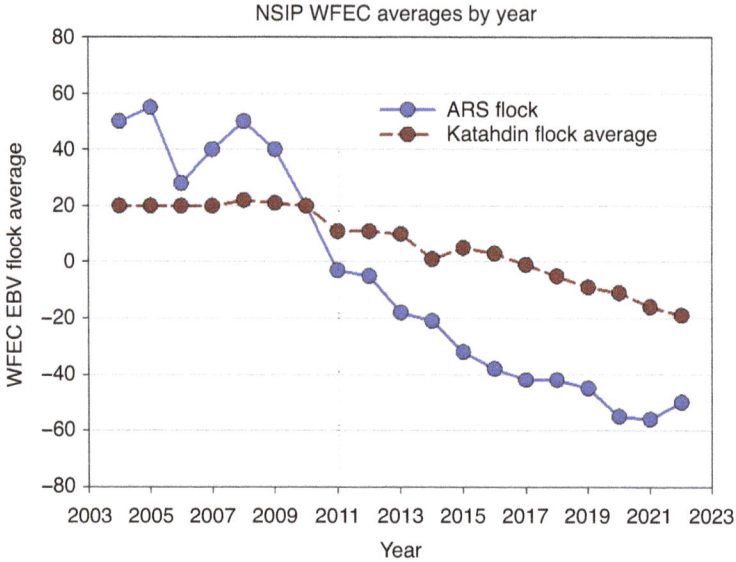

Fig. 5.4. Weaning FEC (WFEC) EBVs for the NSIP Katahdin breed average and for a USDA Agricultural Research Station (ARS) flock actively selecting for parasite-resistant sires and dams. Adapted by Joan M. Burke from SheepGenetics MLA.

(http://nsipsearch.nsip.org/#!/search). With more data and sharing of sires, the expansion of EBVs for more sheep and goat breeds is expected.

Conclusion

Due to the global prevalence of anthelmintic resistance, alternatives are highly valuable for sustained small ruminant production. Genetic and possibly genomic selection for parasite resistance and resilience represents the most promising technology that in some instances can divert the need for pharmaceuticals. Because immune function related to GIN infection occurs across many genes, currently there are no genetic markers available to farmers to aid in animal selection. Organized breeding programs such as the NSIP allow selection for parasite resistance through FEC EBV, and have the potential to include measures of resilience such as FAMACHA© and changes in body weight over time. At the same time, producers can also consider selection for other heritable and economically important traits.

Acknowledgment

We thank the NSIP Katahdin breeders starting in 2004 who collected thousands of fecalfecal samples, FAMACHA© scores, and later DNA samples and made sure their lambs had significant GIN exposure. Without them, the development of the FEC EBV in the USA would not have occurred.

References

Abe, Y., Tokuda, M., Ishimoto, R., Asumi, K. and Yokosawa, H. (1999) A unique primary structure, cDNA cloning and function of a galactose-specific lectin from ascidian plasma. *European Journal of Biochemistry* 261, 33–39.

Arisman, B.C., Burke, J.M., Morgan, J.L.M. and Lewis, R. (2023) Genotype by environment interaction and heteroscedasticity influence the expression of parasite resistance in Katahdin sheep. *Journal of Animal Science* 101, skad228.

Armitage, R.J., Fanslow, W.C.S.L., Strockbine, L., Sato, T., Clifford, K. *et al.* (1992) Molecular and biological characterization of a murine ligand for CD40. *Nature* 357(6373), 80–82.

Arranz-Plaza, E., Tracy, A.S., Siriwardena, A., Pierce, J. and Boons, G.J. (2002) High-avidity, low-affinity multivalent interactions and the block to polyspermy in *Xenopus laevis*. *Journal of the American Chemistry Society* 124, 13035–13046.

Balic, A., Bowles, V.M. and Meeusen, E.N.T. (2000) Cellular profiles in the abomasal mucosa and lymph node during primary infection with *Haemonchus contortus* in sheep. *Veterinary Immunology and Immunopathology* 75, 109–120.

Becker, G.M., Burke, J.M., Lewis, R.M., Miller, J., Morgan, J. *et al.* (2022) Variants within wenes EDIL3 and ADGRB3 are associated with divergent fecal egg counts in Katahdin sheep at weaning. *Frontiers in Genetics* 13, 817319.

Beh, K.J. and Maddox, J.F. (1996) Prospects for development of genetic markers for resistance to gastrointestinal parasite infection in sheep. *International Journal for Parasitology* 26, 879–897.

Beh, K.J., Hulme, D.J., Callaghan, M.J., Leish, Z., Lenane, I. *et al.* (2002) A genome scan for quantitative trait loci affecting resistance to *Trichostrongylus columbriformis* in sheep. *Animal Genetics* 33, 97–106.

Bielek, K. (2005) Sustainable internal parasite control for sheep in a forage based system. Available at: https://projects.sare.org/project-reports/fnc04-523/ (accessed 11 July 2025).

Bielek, K. (2007) Selecting sheep for parasite resistance. Available at: https://projects.sare.org/project-reports/fnc05-583/ (accessed 11 July 2025).

Bishop, S.C., Birden, K., McKellar, Q.A., Park, M. and Stear, M. (1996) Genetic parameters for faecal egg count following mixed, natural, predominantly *Ostertagia circumcincta* infection and relationships with live weight in young lambs. *Animal Science* 63, 423–428.

Bouix, J., Krupinski, J., Rzepecka, J., Nowosad, B., Skrzyzala, I. *et al.* (1998) Genetic resistance to gastrointestinal nematode parasites in Polish long-wool sheep. *International Journal for Parasitology* 28, 1797–1804.

Bowdridge, S.A., Zajac, A.M. and Notter, D.R. (2015) St. Croix sheep produce a rapid and greater cellular immune response contributing to reduced establishment of *Haemonchus contortus*. *Veterinary Parasitology* 208, 204–210.

Bradley, R.E., Radhakrishnan, C.V., Patil-Kulkarni, V.G. and Loggins, P. (1973) Responses in Florida native and Rambouillet lambs exposed to one and two oral doses of *Haemonchus contortus*. *American Journal of Veterinary Research* 34, 729–735.

Burke, J.M. and Miller, J.E. (2002) Relative resistance of Dorper crossbred ewes to gastrointestinal nematode infection compared with St. Croix and Katahdin ewes in the southeastern United States. *Veterinary Parasitology* 109, 265–275.

Charon, K.M. (2004) Genes controlling resistance to gastrointestinal nematodes in ruminants. In: *Gene Polymorphisms Affecting Health and Production Traits in Farm Animals*. Jastrzebiec, Poland, pp. 135–139.

Coltman, D.W., Wilson, K., Pilkington, J.G., Stear, M. and Pemberton, J. (2001) A microsatellite polymorphism in the gamma interferon gene is associated with resistance to gastrointestinal nematodes in a naturally-parasitized population of Soay sheep. *Parasitology* 122, 571–582.

Courtney, C.H., Parker, C.F., McClure, K.E. and Herd, R. (1985) Resistance of nonlambing exotic and domestic ewes to naturally acquired gastrointestinal nematodes. *International Journal for Parasitology* 15, 239–243.

Cunha, S.M.F., Willoughby, O., Schenkel, F. and Cánovas, Á. (2024) Genetic parameter estimation and selection for resistance to gastrointestinal nematode parasites in sheep—A review. *Animals* 14(4), 613.

Davies, G., Stear, M.J., Benothman, M., Abuagob, O., Kerr, A. *et al.* (2006) Quantitative trait loci associated with parasitic infection in Scottish blackface sheep. *Heredity* 96, 252–258.

DeWolf, B.D., Bauman, C.A., Menzies, P.I., Borkowski, E.A., Shaw, R.J. *et al.* (2025) Evaluating the use of salivary anti-carLA IgA testing to reduce gastrointestinal parasitism in Canadian pastured sheep. *Veterinary Parasitology* 335, 110417.

Diez-Tascon, C., Keane, O.M., Wilson, T., Zadissa, A., Hyndman, D. *et al.* (2005) Microarray analysis of selection lines from outbred populations to identify genes involved with nematode parasite resistance in sheep. *Physiological Genomics* 21, 59–69.

Estrada-Reyes, Z.M., Ogunade, I.M., Pech-Cervantes, A.A. and Terrill, T. (2022) Copy number variant-based genome-wide association study reveals immune-related genes associated with parasite resistance in a heritage sheep breed from the United States. *Parasite Immunology* 44, e12943.

Falconer, D.S. and Mackay, T.F.C. (1996) *Introduction to Quantitative Genetics*, 4th edn. Pearson Education Limited, Harlow, UK.

Gasbarre, L.C., Leighton, E.A. and Sonstegard, T. (2001) Role of bovine immune system and genome in resistance to gastrointestinal nematodes. *Veterinary Parasitology* 98, 51–64.

Gauly, M. and Erhardt, G. (2002) Changes in faecal trichostrongyle egg count and haematocrit in naturally infected Rhon sheep over two grazing periods and associations with biochemical polymorphisms. *Small Ruminant Research* 44, 103–108.

Gauly, M., Kraus, M., Vervelde, L., Van Leeuwen, M. and Erhardt, G. (2002) Estimating genetic differences in natural resistance in Rhon and Merinoland sheep following experimental *Haemonchus contortus* infection. *Veterinary Parasitology* 106, 55–67.

Gray, G.D. (1997) The use of genetically resistant sheep to control nematode parasitism. *Veterinary Parasitology* 72, 345–366.

Harris, J. (2011) Autophagy and cytokines. *Cytokines* 56, 140–144.

Hayward, A.D. (2022) Genetic parameters for resistance to gastrointestinal nematodes in sheep: A meta-analysis. *International Journal for Parasitology* 52(13–14), 843–853.

Holt, R.M., Shepherd, E.A., Ammer, A.G. and Bowdridge, S. (2015) Effects of peripheral blood mononuclear cells on *Haemonchus contortus* larval motility *in vitro*. *Parasite Immunology* 37, 553–556.

Jacobs, J.R., Sommers, K.N., Zajac, A.M., Notter, D. and Bowdridge, S. (2016) Early IL-4 gene expression in abomasum is associated with resistance to *Haemonchus contortus* in hair and wool sheep breeds. *Parasite Immunology* 38, 333–339.

Keane, O.M., Zadissa, A., Wilson, T., Hyndman, D., Greer, G. *et al.* (2006) Gene expression profiling of naive sheep genetically resistant and susceptible to gastrointestinal nematodes. *BMC Genomics* 7, 42.

Kemper, K.E., Elwin, R.L., Bishop, S.C., Goddard, M. and Woolaston, R. (2009) *Haemonchus contortus* and *Trichostrongylus colubriformis* did not adapt to long-term exposure to sheep that were genetically resistant or susceptible to nematode infections. *International Journal for Parasitology* 39, 607–614.

Lacroux, C., Nguyen, T.H., Andreoletti, O., Prevot, F., Grisez, C. *et al.* (2006) *Haemonchus contortus* (Nematoda: Trichostrongylidae) infection in lambs elicits an unequivocal Th2 immune response. *Veterinary Research* 37, 607–622.

MacKinnon, K.M., Burton, J.L., Zajac, A.M. and Notter, D. (2009) Microarray analysis reveals difference in gene expression profiles of hair and wool sheep infected with *Haemonchus contortus*. *Veterinary Immunology Immunopathology* 130, 210–220.

MacKinnon, K.M., Bowdridge, S.A., Kanevsky-Mullarky, I., Zajac, A. and Notter, D. (2015) Gene expression profiles of hair and wool sheep reveal importance of Th2 immune mechanisms for increased resistance to. *Journal of Animal Science* 93, 2074–2082.

Marshall, K., Maddox, J.F., Lee, S.H., Zhang, Y., Kahn, L. *et al.* (2009) Genetic mapping of quantitative trait loci for resistance to *Haemonchus contortus* in sheep. *Animal Genetics* 40, 262–272.

McMillan, A.J., Brown, D.J., Burke, J.M. and Morgan, J. (2022) Cross-validation of single-step genetic evaluation in U.S. Katahdin sheep. In: *Proceedings of 12th World Congress on Genetics Applied to Livestock Production (WCGALP)*, p. 2964. DOI: 10.3920/978-90-8686-940-4_71.

Middleton, D., Garza, J.J., Greiner, S.P. and Bowdridge, S. (2020) Neutrophils rapidly produce Th2 cytokines in response to larval but not adult helminth antigen. *Parasite Immunology* 42, e12679.

Miller, J.E., Bahirathan, M., Lemarie, S.L., Hembry, F., Kearney, M. *et al.* (1998) Epidemiology of gastrointestinal nematode parasitism in Suffolk and Gulf Coast Native sheep with special emphasis on relative susceptibility to *Haemonchus contortus* infection. *Veterinary Parasitology* 74, 55–74.

Miller, J.E., Bishop, S.C., Cockett, N.E. and McGraw, R. (2006) Segregation of natural and experimental gastrointestinal nematode infection in F2 progeny of susceptible Suffolk and resistant Gulf Coast Native sheep and its usefulness in assessment of genetic variation. *Veterinary Parasitology* 140, 83–89.

Morgan, J.L.M. (2019) 2018 KHSI statistics: Comparing with other breeds. *Katahdin Hairald* 31, 3.

Newton, R. (2019) World shepherd: A model for grass-fed Katahdin meat production in the south. *Katahdin Hairald* 31, 3–4.

Ngere, L., Burke, J.M., Morgan, J.L.M., Miller, J. and Notter, D. (2018) Genetic parameters for fecal egg counts and their relationship with body weights in Katahdin lambs. *Journal of Animal Science* 96, 1590–1599.

Notter, D.R., Morgan, J.L.M. and Vanimisetti, H.B. (2007) Tools for genetic improvement of parasite resistance: Development of a fecal egg count EPD. Katahdin NSIP Notebook #8.

Notter, D.R., Burke, J.M., Miller, J.E. and Morgan, J. (2017a) Association between FAMACHA© scores and fecal egg counts in Katahdin lambs. *Journal of Animal Science* 95.

Notter, D.R., Burke, J.M., Miller, J.E. and Morgan, J. (2017b) Factors affecting fecal egg counts in peri-parturient Katahdin ewes and their lambs. *Journal of Animal Science* 95, 103–112.

Notter, D.R., Ngere, L., Burke, J.M., Miller, J. and Morgan, J. (2018) Genetic parameters for ewe reproductive performance and peri-parturient fecal egg counts and their genetic relationships with lamb body weights and fecal egg counts in Katahdin sheep. *Journal of Animal Science* 96, 1579–1589.

Notter, D.R., Heidaritabar, M., Burke, J.M., Shirali, M. and Murdoch, B.M. (2022) Single nucleotide polymorphism effects on lamb fecal egg count estimated breeding values in progeny-tested Katahdin sires. *Frontiers in Genetics* 13, 866176.

Parker, C.F. (1998) Presentation to the membership at the Katahdin Hair Sheep International, Annual Meeting. Petit Jean Mountain, Arkansas, USA.

Parker, C.F. (2000) Presentation to the membership at the Katahdin Hair Sheep International. Annual meeting, Waynesboro, Virginia, USA.

Parker, C.F., McClure, K.E. and Herd, R.P. (1991) Hair sheep potential for specific environmental conditions and production systems in North America. In: *Proceedings Hair Sheep Research Symposium*, University of Virgin Islands, St Croix, p. 155.

Paterson, S. (1998) Evidence for balancing selection at the major histocompatibility complex in a free-living ruminant. *Journal of Heredity* 89, 289–294.

Powder, K.E. (2020) Quantitative trait loci (QTL) mapping. *Methods in Molecular Biology* 2082, 211–229.

Riley, D.G. and Van Wyk, J.A. (2009) Genetic parameters for FAMACHA© score and related traits for host resistance/resilience and production at differing severities of worm challenge in a Merino flock in South Africa. *Veterinary Parasitology* 164(1), 44–52.

Rowe, A., Gondro, C., Emery, D. and Sangster, N. (2009) Sequential microarray to identify timing of molecular responses to *Haemonchus contortus* infection in sheep. *Veterinary Parasitology* 161, 76–87.

Schwaiger, F.W., Gostomski, D., Stear, M.J., Duncan, J., McKellar, Q. *et al.* (1995) An ovine major histocompatibility complex DRB1 allele is associated with low faecal egg counts following natural, predominantly *Ostertagia circumcincta* infection. *International Journal for Parasitology* 25, 815–822.

Shaw, R.J., Morris, C.A. and Wheeler, M. (2013) Genetic and phenotypic relationships between carbohydrate larval antigen (CarLA) IgA, parasite resistance and productivity in serial samples taken from lambs after weaning. *International Journal for Parasitology* 43, 661–667.

Shaw, R.J., Wheeler, M. and Leathwick, D.M. (2023) Carbohydrate larval antigen (CarLA IgA) responses to mixed species nematode infection in pasture grazed Angora goats. *Veterinary Parasitology* 315, 109883.

Shepherd, E.A., Garza, J.J., Greiner, S.P. and Bowdridge, S. (2017) The effect of ovine peripheral blood mononuclear cells on *Haemonchus contortus* larval morbidity *in vitro*. *Parasite Immunology* 39.

Thorne, J.W., Redden, R., Bowdridge, S.A., Becker, G., Stegemiller, M. *et al.* (2023) Genome-wide analysis of sheep artificially or naturally infected with gastrointestinal nematodes. *Genes* 14, 1342.

Tsugi, S., Uehori, J., Matsumoto, M., Suzuki, Y., Matsuhisa, A. *et al.* (2001) Human intelectin is a novel soluble lectin that recognizes galactofuranose in carbohydrate chains of bacterial cell wall. *Journal of Biological Chemistry* 276, 23456–23463.

Vanimisetti, H.B., Greiner, S.P., Zajac, A.M. and Notter, D. (2004a) Performance of hair sheep composite breeds: Resistance of lambs to *Haemonchus contortus*. *Journal of Animal Science* 82, 595–604.

Vanimisetti, H.B., Andrew, S.L., Zajac, A.M. and Notter, D. (2004b) Inheritance of fecal egg count and packed cell volume and their relationship with production traits in sheep infected with *Haemonchus contortus*. *Journal of Animal Science* 82, 1602–1611.

Whitlock, H.V. (1948) Some modifications of the McMaster helminth egg-counting technique apparatus. *Journal for Council of Scientific Industry Research* 21, 177–180.

Wildeus, S. (1997) Hair sheep genetic resources and their contribution to diversified small ruminant production in the United States. *Journal of Animal Science* 75, 630–640.

Woolaston, R.R. and Piper, L.R. (1996) Selection of Merino sheep for resistance to *Haemonchus contortus*: Genetic variation. *Animal Science* 62, 451–460.

Yazwinski, T.A., Goode, L., Moncol, D.J., Morgan, G. and Linnerud, A. (1979) Parasite resistance in straightbred and crossbred Barbados Blackbelly sheep. *Journal of Animal Science* 49, 919–926.

Zajac, A.M., Krakowka, S., Herd, R.P. and McClure, K. (1990) Experimental *Haemonchus contortus* infection in three breeds of sheep. *Veterinary Parasitology* 36, 221–235.

6 Benefits of Grazing Management and Pasture Species Rotation Systems for Integrated Gastrointestinal Nematode Parasite Management in Small Ruminant Production

Richard A. Ehrhardt[1]* and Heather Glennon[2]

[1]*Department of Animal Science, College of Agriculture and Natural Resources, Michigan State University, East Lansing, Michigan, USA, and Department of Large Animal Clinical Sciences, College of Veterinary Medicine, Michigan State University, East Lansing, Michigan, USA; [2]Agricultural Sciences Department, University of Mount Olive, Mount Olive, NC USA*

Abstract

A key component of a sustainable parasite control program for small ruminants is grazing management methods that reduce pasture infectivity and provide a high plane of nutrition to build host immunity against gastrointestinal nematode (GIN) infection. Complementary forage systems, multispecies grazing, and rotational grazing practices can reduce an animal's exposure to infective GIN larvae as part of an evasive grazing strategy. This need becomes especially important in grazing programs with high stocking rates and/or in highly susceptible animals where GIN management is very challenging. Complementary forage systems can also fill gaps in forage quality and availability compared to those consisting exclusively of perennial forages, thus also improving whole-farm forage utilization. The use of forage species that contain secondary compounds with antiparasitic properties provides yet another arm of GIN control through pasture management. Together, these practices form a major part of an integrated approach to GIN control in small ruminants.

Introduction

Grazing management practices provide a critical tool of control against gastrointestinal nematode (GIN) parasite infection in small ruminants. Grazing management practices that decrease an animal's exposure to (and ingestion of) infective larvae such as rotational grazing, multispecies grazing, and the use of pasture species rotations are key to decreasing parasite burdens (Barger, 1999; Colvin et al., 2008) . These practices have additional benefits in improving animal nutrition and whole-farm forage utilization and offer opportunities for provision of forage species with protective benefits against GIN infection (Garcia et al.,

*Corresponding author: ehrhard5@msu.edu

© CAB International 2026. *Management Practices for Controlling Nematode Parasites of Small Ruminants* (eds James E. Miller and Joan M. Burke)
DOI: 10.1079/9781800623767.0006

2008; Houdijk *et al.*, 2012). Collectively, these benefits can improve the profitability, health, and wellbeing of small ruminant production systems (Ehrhardt, 2016).

Grazing Management Practices and GIN Control

In any grazing management system, optimizing forage intake is key to the health and performance of animals. Intake can be optimized via different grazing practices that have unique parasite management concerns.

Continuous grazing (or set-stocking) is the practice of allowing animals to remain in the same pasture every day. In this system, forages are not grazed uniformly throughout the pasture and manure is not evenly distributed. Sheep have a grazing preference for shorter, younger forage and have been known to repeatedly spot-graze certain areas of the pasture. This can result in a highly contaminated pasture where animals have an increased risk of reinfection, especially in areas where they congregate such as watering sites, supplemental feeding areas, and shade or resting spots. The high concentration of animals and their feces in these areas can lead to the build-up of infective L3 larvae. In addition, forages that are continually grazed will often become weak and have slower regrowth, forcing animals to graze closer to the ground. These plants will eventually die, allowing for less desirable and less nutritious weeds to dominate (Barger, 1997).

Rotational grazing involves regularly moving animals to different pastures or paddocks within a pasture and then returning them to the previously grazed plots at varied time periods based on forage availability. In this system, producers control the length of the grazing period, the length of the rest period, and the grazing height of the plants. As a result, rotational grazing can lead to a decrease in pasture contamination, a decrease in the animals' exposure to infective L3 larvae and, most importantly, a decrease in the need for deworming (Barger *et al.*, 1994; Burke *et al.*, 2009).

To prevent reinfection, the length of the grazing period should be shorter than the time it takes an egg to develop into an infective L3 larvae. While this developmental period is dependent upon temperature and moisture levels, it can occur in as few as 3–4 days in warm, wet weather (O'Connor *et al.*, 2006; Burke *et al.*, 2009). Under cooler and/or drier conditions, this developmental period could take 1–2 weeks (Besier *et al.*, 2016). While the minimum temperature for parasite eggs to hatch is 10°C, the ideal range for *Haemonchus contortus* to hatch and develop is 30–35° F. Short-duration grazing events (1–2 days), such as practiced in strip grazing, would provide a high level of protection against rapid reinfection (Smith *et al.*, 2009).

Producers utilizing rotational systems also control the rest period (length of time between grazing events). A longer rest period could decrease the parasite load on the pasture as the larvae desiccate due to unfavorable environmental conditions or use their stored energy and eventually die. Unfortunately, that could take 6–18 months in temperate climates (Torres-Acosta and Hoste, 2008). Nematode larvae in tropical climates have been shown to deplete their body reserves and die within 1–2 months on pasture, allowing animals to safely return to paddocks sooner (O'Connor *et al.*, 2006; Mahieu *et al.*, 2008). Hence, lambs under hot humid conditions can be included in a rotational system with a grazing period of 3–7 days and a rest period of 28–35 days and this may result in lower worm infections and fewer anthelmintic treatments than lambs in a continuous system (Barger *et al.*, 1994; Chandrawathani *et al.*, 2004; Burke *et al.*, 2009). The same results were seen in rotationally grazed goats with a 5 day grazing period and a 65 day rest period (Min *et al.*, 2004).

Meanwhile, cool-season forage grasses and legume pastures are usually ready to graze again and of the highest quality within 21–35 days. Unfortunately, in temperate climates, parasite larvae may reach peak infectivity during the same period post grazing (Barger, 1999). Returning animals to a pasture after only 3–4 weeks of rest could potentially increase their parasite burden under those temperate conditions. The producer must weigh their options as a longer rest period will also result in decreased forage quality due to the plants maturing (Barger, 1999).

Cograzing of Different Livestock Species

Pasture contamination may also be reduced if cograzing of different livestock species is implemented. In general, cattle and horses do not share the same gastrointestinal parasites as sheep and goats (Rocha *et al.*, 2008). Grazing cattle or horses in the same area as small ruminants could decrease the pasture's overall infection level because ingested L3 larvae are unable to reproduce in the foreign host, effectively stopping the cycle.

Cograzing livestock species at the same time can be challenging due to their differences in mineral nutrition and fencing requirements. An alternate or leader-follower grazing system is commonly used, with small ruminants grazing first. This allows the sheep and goats to graze higher up on the plant and access the most nutritious vegetation. Then, cattle or horses will follow and graze the remaining forage closer to the ground while "cleaning" up parasite larvae emerging from sheep and goat feces, residing at that lower level of the grass. Grazing multiple livestock species in succession can also increase the time in between small ruminant grazing events. If this rest period is long enough, a proportion of the larvae may die due to desiccation or use of stored energy. An added benefit to multispecies grazing is improved forage production and utilization due to differences in the animals' grazing behaviors and preferences (Jordan *et al.*, 1988; Luginbuhl *et al.*, 2000). Cattle are considered grazers and prefer grass. Goats are considered browsers and prefer taller woody plants and broadleaf forbs/weeds. Sheep eat a mix of grass, legumes, and forbs (Torres-Fajardo *et al.*, 2024).

Much of this research has been conducted when grazing sheep and cattle together. Improved weight gain and/or decreased parasitism has been seen in lambs alternately grazed with cattle when short grazing periods and long rest periods were implemented (Colvin *et al.*, 2008; Mahieu and Aumont, 2009). Even under a continuously grazed system, lambs grazed with cattle had increased weight gain compared to lambs grazed with sheep only (Jordan *et al.*, 1988). Because there is a risk for calves to become infected with *Haemonchus contortus*

from small ruminants, it is recommended to only use adult cattle in multispecies grazing systems (Amarante *et al.*, 1997). Adult cattle are generally unaffected by GIN. Calves grazed with sheep either had no difference in weight gain (Abaye *et al.*, 1994) or had increased worms and lower weight gains (Jordan *et al.*, 1988) when compared to calves grazing with cattle alone (Cellier *et al.*, 2022).

Use of Browse in Small Ruminant Grazing Systems

There are several benefits associated with allowing animals to browse woodlot vegetation (brush, vines, trees) regarding parasite control. First and foremost, it will decrease their exposure to infective larvae as it encourages them to eat higher up in the canopy. Goats prefer browse and instinctively choose to eat taller plants (Cellier *et al.*, 2022). Second, certain browse species and trees are known to contain condensed tannins which can decrease the effects of *H. contortus* in small ruminants (Hoste *et al.*, 2015). Ground pine bark supplementation has been shown to decrease FEC and increase weight gain in goats (Min *et al.*, 2012). Finally, when animals are removed from permanent pastures even for a few weeks during the warmer months, the pasture's rest period increases which could lead to a decrease in infective L3s and an increase in forage production. Silvopastoralism, or agroforestry, integrates livestock, forage production, and forestry to provide high-quality feed to ruminants while keeping animals from continuously grazing near the ground (Griffiths and Carr, 2022). Producers should be careful not to overstock woodlot areas as vegetation biomass and regrowth time could be decreased compared to that of pastures.

Machine Harvest of Excess Pasture to Reduce Parasite Contamination

Another way to increase the time between grazing events and decrease the larval contamination of a pasture is to harvest excess forage as hay or silage (Anderson, 1983; Vlassoff *et al.*, 2001; Cabaret *et al.*, 2002a). Producers who implement rotational grazing may end up with extra forage due to increased utilization. If excess forage is harvested on these areas instead of by grazing animals, the rest period will be increased, potentially killing some of the larvae. Additionally, machine harvest will remove many of the infective L3 larvae from the pasture. It will also open the canopy, allowing sunlight and heat to reach the soil surface and desiccate the L1 and L2 larvae. Machine harvest will also tend to increase forage quality for subsequent grazing events by reducing the maturity of the stand. Simply mowing excess forage after grazing animals rotate off pastures will create the same effect.

Pasture Species Rotation Systems for Small Ruminants

Pasture species rotation systems can increase the biodiversity of a farm forage system by incorporating many different functional groups of forage species (forbs, legumes, and grasses) into the rotation. This has benefits for both livestock and soil health while improving seasonal availability and quality of forage (Reed and Morrissey, 2022). An added benefit is that the establishment of new plantings offers an opportunity to reduce pasture contamination and the infectivity risk of GIN as part of an evasive grazing strategy (Barger, 1997; Thamsborg *et al.*, 1999; Cabaret *et al.*, 2002b). Pasture species rotations can consist of several types of combinations. For this chapter, the focus will be on complementary forage rotation systems and cover crop grazing.

Complementary forage systems

Complementary forage systems can be a combination of annual, short-term perennial, and long-term perennial plantings. These have been evaluated most extensively in pasture-based dairy production (Garcia *et al.*, 2008; Pembleton *et al.*, 2008; Chapman *et al.*, 2015). The inclusion of annual and short-term perennial pastures can augment a long-term perennial pasture base providing either grazing or harvested forage to fill in seasonal deficits in forage

mass and quality. These systems have been demonstrated to improve total forage production and quality compared to production systems relying entirely on perennial pasture. This is achieved by improving the seasonal availability and persistence of forage production (Garcia *et al.*, 2008; Pembleton *et al.*, 2008). By using a complement of forages with distinctly different growth habits, the availability of forage over the year can be improved compared to perennial pastures which have clear seasonal deficits in forage production. For example, brassica species accumulate dry matter during cool, wet periods and annual grasses with the C4 photosynthetic pathway will accumulate dry matter during warm, dry periods at greater rates than that of a perennial pasture composed principally of grass species of the C3 pathway over the same period (Ehrhardt, 2016).

By developing a pasture rotation system consisting of annuals, short-term perennial pastures, and long-term perennial pastures, whole-farm forage utilization can be improved while simultaneously improving parasite management. An example of such a system is shown in Fig. 6.1. In this example, the arable land of a farm was divided into ten parcels (paddocks) with half of the land in long-term perennial pasture. Any farm can modify this system depending on forage needs, soil type, and climatic factors. Some farms may have a sizable proportion of the farm in nonarable perennial pasture and in that instance, the arable land could rotate between annual and short-term perennial forage species.

It is possible to utilize a double cropping system during certain years of this rotation as well. For example, corn (*Zea mays*) can be grown in some climates for silage followed by cereal rye (*Secale cereale* L.), or perennial pasture terminated in early summer followed by a brassica seeding (see Fig. 6.1). This creates an opportunity to increase seasonal biomass while creating additional evasive grazing opportunities. For example, in a small ruminant spring pasture lambing or kidding system (pasture birth system), it is possible to terminate the perennial pasture used as a spring birth system ground after lambs and kids are several weeks post birth. Pastures used for this purpose typically have a high degree of GIN infectivity due to the periparturient rise in fecal egg output (Barger, 1993; Beasley *et al.*, 2010) (Fig. 6.2). In many

Paddock	Year of rotation									
	1	2	3	4	5	6	7	8	9	10
A	Perennial	Perennial	Perennial	Perennial	Perennial	Perennial/Brassica	ST Perennial	ST Perennial	Corn silage/Rye	Corn silage/Rye
B	Corn silage/Rye	Perennial	Perennial	Perennial	Perennial	Perennial	Perennial/Brassica	ST Perennial	ST Perennial	Corn silage/Rye
C	Corn silage/Rye	Corn silage/Rye	Perennial	Perennial	Perennial	Perennial	Perennial	Perennial/Brassica	ST Perennial	ST Perennial
D	ST Perennial	Corn silage/Rye	Corn silage/Rye	Perennial	Perennial	Perennial	Perennial	Perennial	Perennial/Brassica	ST Perennial
E	ST Perennial	ST Perennial	Corn silage/Rye	Corn silage/Rye	Perennial	Perennial	Perennial	Perennial	Perennial	Perennial/Brassica
F	Perennial/Brassica	ST Perennial	ST Perennial	Corn silage/Rye	Corn silage/Rye	Perennial	Perennial	Perennial	Perennial	Perennial
G	Perennial	Perennial/Brassica	ST Perennial	ST Perennial	Corn silage/Rye	Corn silage/Rye	Perennial	Perennial	Perennial	Perennial
H	Perennial	Perennial	Perennial/Brassica	ST Perennial	ST Perennial	Corn silage/Rye	Corn silage/Rye	Perennial	Perennial	Perennial
I	Perennial	Perennial	Perennial	Perennial/Brassica	ST Perennial	ST Perennial	Corn silage/Rye	Corn silage/Rye	Perennial	Perennial
J	Perennial	Perennial	Perennial	Perennial	Perennial/Brassica	ST Perennial	ST Perennial	Corn silage/Rye	Corn silage/Rye	Perennial

Fig. 6.1. Complementary pasture rotation plan for a 10-year period for a farm with ten paddocks. Paddocks are rotated between a 5-year planting of perennial pasture, an annual brassica pasture planted following termination of perennial pasture, a 2-year planting of a short-term perennial pasture (ST perennial), consecutive annual plantings of corn (*Zea mays*) for silage with a cereal rye (*Secale cereale*) cover crop, and then back to the 5-year planting of perennial pastures to complete the 10-year rotation.

temperate climates, nonirrigated long-term perennial pastures with a dominant cool-season grass base typically produce more than half of their seasonal biomass by early summer (Oates *et al.*, 2011). Therefore, terminating these birth system pastures shortly after the birth period allows utilization of the majority of seasonal biomass, and an opportunity to reduce pasture infectivity as well as to establish a new pasture with an annual species that can outproduce the biomass of a long-term perennial pasture during summer and fall (see Figs 6.1 and 6.2). This annual pasture planted mid-summer would constitute a double crop with the terminated perennial pasture earlier in the season. The annual pasture would provide an evasive grazing opportunity as a pasture rested from grazing with low parasitic infectivity (Ehrhardt, 2016).

Short-term perennial rotations may last 2–3 years and have the advantage of superior forage quality which is important for certain classes of sheep and goats in highly productive states (Kemp *et al.*, 2010; Golding *et al.*, 2011) (Fig. 6.3). Animals in these states include lactating prolific sheep and goats and their offspring as well as sheep and goats in the postweaning phase of growth. Both forage quality and availability

in long-term perennial systems may be limited in meeting the nutritional requirements of these animals in pasture-based systems consisting of only long-term perennial pastures.

In New Zealand, a very successful and popular short-term perennial pasture consists of forbs and clover, principally chicory (*Cichorium intybus*), plantain (*Plantago* spp.), and red clover (Kemp *et al.*, 2010; Cranston *et al.*, 2015). These pastures have been demonstrated to have superior animal performance compared to long-term perennial stands of white clover and ryegrass, with the added benefit of more consistent availability and greater preference during much of the grazing season (Pain *et al.*, 2014). These pastures excel in digestibility and have been adapted in other regions, including the north temperate zone (Ehrhardt, 2016), and can be used in a complementary forage system to add diversity to existing perennial and annual pastures. They tend to be short term in nature due to a lack of persistency, particularly in northern temperate regions (Ehrhardt, 2016).

Complementary forage systems work well in small ruminant production and hold the promise of being highly adaptable to many climates and livestock production systems (Thomas *et al.*,

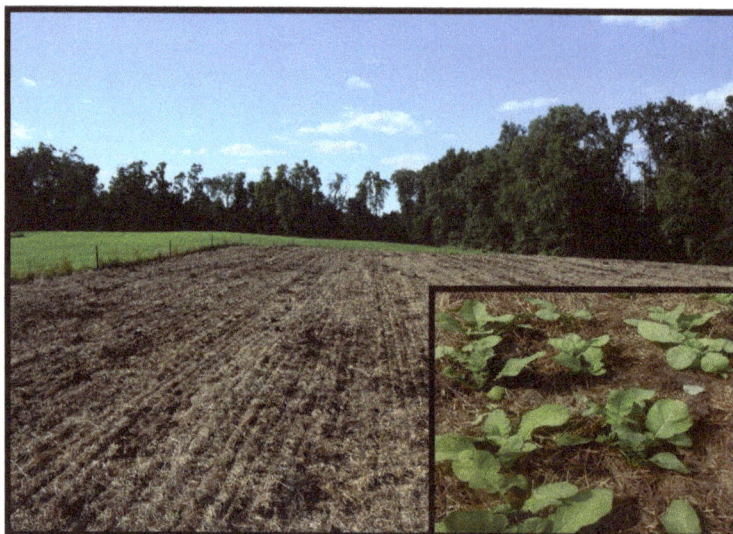

Fig. 6.2. New pasture establishment offers opportunity to break the parasitic life cycle within a perennial pasture. This photo shows a perennial pasture used as a pasture lambing area that has been terminated with herbicide in early summer after most of the seasonal forage mass has accumulated. A new seeding of summer/fall annuals has been planted into the existing sod using no-till methods (inset photo shows forage brassica seedlings 14 days after planting). This establishment cycle allowed 60 days of rest from grazing and desiccation of an existing, highly infected pasture. These practices are predicted to reduce parasite infectivity in the newly established annual pasture.

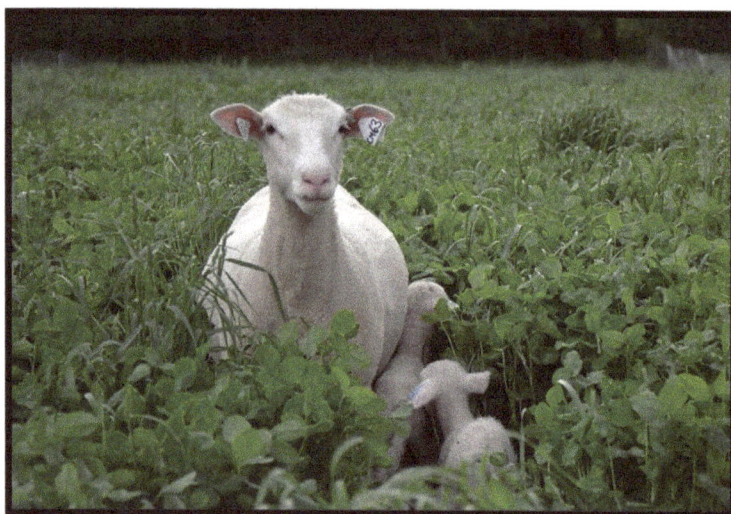

Fig. 6.3. Short-term perennial pastures, such as this red clover (*Trifolium pratense*) and Italian ryegrass (*Lolium multiflorum*) stand, offer nutrient-dense forage that improves resilience against GIN infection. This is particularly important in grazing systems with classes of animals highly susceptible to GIN infection, such as this 13-month-old ewe rearing twins.

2009; Alves *et al.*, 2020). The principle of using a diverse complement of forages with distinctly different seasonal growth patterns to outcompete, in yearly forage mass, that of a single perennial system would hold for most climatic regions of the world. The disadvantage of complementary forage systems is that they require a greater degree of management and labor as well as greater risk for crop failure given the more frequent need for new crop establishment compared to an exclusively perennial-based system. These factors may cause the cost of forage per unit DM to be greater in these systems compared to perennial-based systems. Despite these negatives, these systems are advantageous for optimizing on-farm forage utilization and are particularly useful in farms that have high stocking rates that are naturally more prone to production losses to GIN infection (Thamsborg *et al.*, 1999). Furthermore, animal performance as expressed as gain per unit of land can be high in these systems compared to perennial systems (Table 6.1), offsetting their higher establishment costs and thereby creating a cost of gain comparable to perennial-based systems.

A complementary forage system provides a means of generating areas of low infectivity pastures as well as pastures with superior forage quality (Golding *et al.*, 2011) that can enhance immunity against GIN infection (Houdijk *et al.*, 2012). Complementary forage systems are particularly helpful in creating evasive grazing opportunities in regions with more intensified small ruminant grazing systems that have high stocking rates (Ehrhardt, 2016).

Inclusion of annual forages as cover crops into a small ruminant farming system

Annual forages can also be integrated into livestock and crop farming systems when grazed as cover crops (Carvalho *et al.*, 2010; Planisich *et al.*, 2021). The use of annual forages as cover crops has clear benefits for a crop production system as they can protect the soil from erosion, maintain beneficial soil microbial activity, scavenge nutrients to retain them within the soil for future need, alleviate soil compaction, suppress weeds, and break plant disease cycles (Derpsch *et al.*, 1986; Baggs *et al.*, 2000; Kruidhof *et al.*,

2008; Schipanski *et al.*, 2014). They can also benefit livestock production when grazed or harvested for feed and provide high-quality and inexpensive feed (Planisich *et al.*, 2021). Like complementary forage systems, cover crop grazing can provide quality forage when perennial pasture growth has slowed or ceased completely, thus filling gaps in forage availability and extending the grazing season. They also offer an opportunity to rest perennial pastures in fall to allow them to improve persistence and productivity. Cover crops are particularly valued for grazing during late fall, winter, and early spring when perennial pastures have limited growth or are dormant.

Cover crop species for grazing should be chosen based on ability to grow well during cool weather (fall or spring) and retain their quality when grazed as stockpiled forage during winter. Species in the Brassicaceae family, commonly referred to as brassicas, tend to grow well during cool weather and can be stockpiled into winter as their roots and herbage can withstand cool weather, partly explained by their phenolic content (Fletcher and Kott, 1999; Liu *et al.*, 2022). The extent to which brassicas can withstand cold varies according to the variety so varieties should be chosen with this in mind when the goal is to extend grazing into winter (Warwick, 2011). Certain small grain cereals can also grow well during cool weather, with some surviving into spring and offering grazing forage availability early in the season before perennial pastures return from winter dormancy. Examples of such cereals include winter wheat (*Triticum aestivum*) and barley (*Hordeum vulgare* L.). Cover crop mixtures that contain species with fibrous root systems like cereal grains along with species in the Brassicaceae family, such as forage radish (*Raphanus* L.) and forage rape (*Brassica napus* L.), provide a complement of ecosystem services including immobilizing nitrogen in the soil from previous crops (Li *et al.*, 2020) and efficient penetration of highly compacted soil (Blanco-Canqui and Ruis, 2020). This combination also has potential advantages in minimizing soil erosion while providing favorable animal nutrition given its complement of energy sources for the rumen with a balance of soluble carbohydrate from brassicas and digestible fiber from cereal grain species.

Cover crop grazing can also serve to expand grazing opportunities beyond the borders of

Table 6.1. Compilation of field studies evaluating annual yield of annual, short-term perennial, and perennial pastures and growth performance of lambs grazing these pastures in Ingham County, MI, USA.

Study year(s)	Forage specie(s)	Date planted[a]	Seasonal biomass, kg/ha[b]	Grazing period, days	Gain per lamb, g/dc[c]	Gain per hectare, kg
2014	Annual: forage radish (*Raphanus sativus*)	June 30	12,083	66	154	568
2014	Annual: forage brassica (*Brassica rapa*)	June 30	8877	66	129	497
2013	Annual: BMR-6[d] Sudan grass (*Sorghum bicolor × Sorghum arundinaceum*)	June 10	12,944	86	137	788
2013	Annual: BMR-6 Sorghum (*Sorghum bicolor*)	June 10	16,936	86	92	750
2014	Annual: forage brassica (*Brassica napus × Brassica rapa*)	June 18	10,977	112	310	817
2014	Annual: BMR-6 Sudan brachytic dwarf (*Sorghum bicolor × Sorghum arundinaceum*)	June 18	8799	112	206	509
2013–2014	Short-term perennial pasture: red clover (*Trifolium pratense*) and Italian ryegrass (*Lolium multiflorum*)[e]	April 20	9961–12,556	150–190	265–295	1289–1614
2013–2014	Perennial pasture: tall fescue (*Festuca arundinacea*), orchard grass (*Dactylis glomerata*) and alfalfa (*Medicago sativa*)[e]	N/A[f]	13,215–13,680	185–195	84–92	684–723

[a]All annual pasture seedings were performed using no-till methods into perennial pasture sod terminated by glyphosate. Short-term perennial pasture was seeded using no-till methods into brassica pasture residue.
[b]Pasture mass was measured every 4–5 days just prior to grazing. Following grazing, available biomass was hand clipped to ground level from three randomly selected 0.33-m² quadrats.
[c]All lambs were Dorset crossbred lambs (equal proportion of wethers and ewe lambs) allotted a pasture mass at 10% of body mass in dry matter for 4–5-day grazing periods. Lambs began grazing at 0.3–0.4 maternal mature size.
[d]BMR-6 is brown mid rib gene 6 mutant with low lignin content (Rao *et al.*, 2012)
[e]Short-term perennial and perennial pastures were studied over 2 years with dates over a 2-year range indicated.
[f]N/A: not applicable. Perennial pasture was studied years four and five following establishment.

a farm when partnerships are formed with crop farmers. These integrated crop–livestock systems can reduce the cost of cover crops to the crop farmer while providing quality, inexpensive forage for livestock (Drewnoski *et al.*, 2018; Planisich *et al.*, 2021). Cover crop grazing also allows the possibility of flock/herd expansion without the constraint of land ownership, as it is possible to graze large tracts in a form of rental agreement with crop farmers owning the land and small ruminant producers grazing the land (Bowman *et al.*, 2024). In some instances, the small ruminant producer pays for the cover crop seed, thus lowering the cost of the cover crop to the crop producer (Ehrhardt, 2016). The small ruminant producer benefits from grazing quality, inexpensive forage that fills gaps in forage availability and quality found in perennial pasture systems with an added benefit of grazing forage essentially free of parasitic larvae.

There is a vast amount of cover crop grown in many parts of the world offering a large potential for livestock feed. Both sheep and goats are particularly well suited for grazing such crops when stockpiled for grazing during periods of pasture dormancy during late fall and winter (Pardo and Del Prado, 2020). The risk of soil compaction from grazing cover crops is minimized with smaller livestock species, such as small ruminants (Carvalho *et al.*, 2010), as damage by trampling of the crop is shallow and transient and does not appear to reduce subsequent crop yields or provide other negative impacts on physical aspects of the soil (Warren *et al.*, 1986; Hunt *et al.*, 2016). The practice of growing cover crops and grazing them appropriately also has benefits in the regenerative management of soils and in reducing the carbon footprint of integrated livestock and crop farming systems (Teague, 2018; Pardo and Del Prado, 2020; Recktenwald and Ehrhardt, 2024).

Pasture Establishment Practices and GIN Infectivity

Cover crop grazing and the use of annual and short-term perennial pastures in complementary forage pasture rotation systems offer opportunities to establish grazing forage with little to no GIN larval contamination. This opportunity provides great benefit as part of an integrated parasite management control program. Cover crops have essentially zero parasite infectivity as they have not been grazed previously, so they allow a "clean" grazing option at a time when perennial pasture systems typically are highly contaminated following a season of grazing. Therefore, cover crops are ideal for grazing livestock classes that have lower resilience/resistance to infection such as lambs and kids (Almeida *et al.*, 2018).

The use of annual and short-term perennial pastures as part of a complementary forage pasture rotation offers frequent opportunities for new pasture establishment. Pasture establishment typically provides a prolonged break from grazing, and this combined with tillage and/or herbicide application can reduce pasture infectivity to negligible levels (Ehrhardt, 2016; Almeida *et al.*, 2018; Ridler *et al.*, 2024). As introduced previously, these systems can be managed as part of a whole-farm pasture renovation scheme where perennial pastures at the end of the rotation (see Figs 6.1 and 6.2) can be used as a pasture birth ground and the high larval contamination of these pastures can be reduced to negligible levels following pasture termination via herbicide or tillage and subsequent reseeding of annual forage. Both tillage and desiccation of a contaminated pasture with herbicide will reduce contamination. In addition, the period from the last grazing of the contaminated perennial pasture to the first grazing of the annual pasture will vary depending on climate, annual forage species, establishment methods, and grazing goals but is typically greater than 60 days. This lengthy rest from grazing would in theory allow sufficient time for larvae that survive tillage and/or plant desiccation during pasture establishment to hatch, mature, and die. Therefore, new pasture establishment is an important part of a preventive or evasive grazing management strategy to prevent GIN infection (Michel, 1985; Barger, 1997; Thamsborg *et al.*, 1999; Cabaret *et al.*, 2002b).

Nutrition and Resistance to and Resilience against GIN Infection

Animal nutrition plays a critical protective role against GIN infection in small ruminants. The impact of nutrition in protection against GIN infection may be realized through both direct action from ingestion of antiparasitic plant secondary compounds (PSM) and indirect actions mediated through nutritional modulation of host immune responses (Hoste *et al.*, 2012; Houdijk *et al.*, 2012). Resistance to infection as well as host resilience can be improved by boosting immunity with improved nutrition to better withstand the negative effects of infection (Hoste *et al.*, 2005). GIN infections result in severe alterations in nutrient balance brought on at multiple levels through a depression in voluntary feed intake through pathways of inflammatory processes, through increased endogenous loss of protein and minerals via the gastrointestinal system, and by a drain on nutritional resources needed to support this heightened level of immunity (Knox *et al.*, 2006; Can-Celis *et al.*, 2022). Collectively, these alterations are quantitatively significant, and it has been estimated that infection may result in an increased requirement of metabolizable protein of 12 g/day in growing lambs (Liu *et al.*, 2003). The infection cost in metabolizable protein will be particularly apparent when protein availability may already be limiting production,

such as during lactation and both before and after weaning growth.

In temperate and tropical climates, forage energy availability is often more limiting than protein for ruminant animal performance, particularly in perennial pasture systems, as energy availability limits protein production within the rumen (Leng, 1991). Therefore, increasing the energy content of forage in these pasture systems can improve the amount of both energy and protein absorbed (Gárate-Gallardo *et al.*, 2015). Annual forages can be excellent sources of highly digestible, high-energy feed with sufficient protein (Table 6.2) and are therefore capable of providing the higher plane of nutrition needed to meet the

Table 6.2. Nutrient composition of common brassica species including kale (Brassica oleracea L. var. acephala), turnip (*Brassica septiceps*), radish (*Raphanus* L.), swede (*Brassica napus* ssp. *napobrassica*) and forage rape (*Brassica napus* L.) Forage quality estimates included dry matter (DM), crude protein (CP), metabolizable energy (ME), acid detergent fiber (ADF), and neutral detergent fiber (NDF).

Species	Component[a]	Study	DM, %	CP, %	ME, MJ/kg	ADF, %	NDF, %
Turnip	Herbage	Westwood and Mulcock, 2012	13.7	22.6	13.0	13.5	15.6
Turnip	Herbage	Koch *et al.*, 2002	–	14.6	–	19.8	23.8
Turnip	Herbage	NRC, 2007	18.0	16.0	10.5	13.0	–
Mean			15.8	17.7	11.8	15.4	19.7
Turnip	Tuber	NRC, 2007	9.0	12.0	13.0	34.0	44.0
Turnip	Tuber	Koch *et al.*, 2002	–	10.2	–	17.2	20.9
Turnip	Tuber	Westwood and Mulcock, 2012	10.1	14.2	11.7	18.9	22.5
Mean			9.6	12.1	12.4	23.4	29.1
Radish	Herbage	NRC, 2007	6.0	15.7	11.1	14.1	15.5
Radish	Herbage	Koch *et al.*, 2002	–	11.9	–	18.7	25.6
Radish	Herbage	Ehrhardt and Utsumi[b]	11.0	18.6	10.9	16.8	21.8
Mean			8.5	15.4	11.0	16.5	21.0
Rape	Herbage	Westwood and Mulcock, 2012	14.3	10.8	12.9	20.3	23.2
Rape	Herbage	Sun *et al.*, 2012	–	–	13.2	–	–
Rape	Herbage	Barry, 2013	12.6	19.3	–	16.3	23.4
Rape	Herbage	Ehrhardt and Utsumi[b]	12.7	18.4	10.5	20.2	26.9
Mean			13.2	16.2	12.2	18.9	24.5

[a]Component: herbage = above-ground portion of plant including stem and leaf; tuber = below-ground portion of plant including tuber; whole plant = herbage + tuber.
[b]Ehrhardt and Utsumi: unpublished variety trial replicated at three sites: Hickory Corners, Eaton Rapids, and East Lansing, MI.

high nutritional cost of immunological response to infection (Greer *et al.*, 2005) and demand for tissue repair and blood homeostasis (Coop and Holmes, 1996; Hoste *et al.*, 2016). By supporting a higher level of host immunity, a higher plane of nutrition may also improve resistance to infection by impacting aspects of egg hatching and larval development, although direct evidence is lacking (Houdijk *et al.*, 2012).

Feed or Nutritional Value of Annual Forages

In terms of feed value, many annual forages are highly digestible, high-energy crops. Therefore, the superior forage quality of many annual forages can also play an important protective role against GIN infection in small ruminants in addition to supporting phases of production requiring a higher plane of nutrition.

Brassicas are often considered a high-moisture, high-energy crop (Guillard and Allinson, 1988; Westwood and Mulcock, 2012) and are a common component of cover crop mixtures as well as part of a complementary forage rotation system due to their forage quality and growth characteristics. Brassicas excel in energy content with metabolizable energy (ME) concentration estimates ranging from 11.0 to 12.2 MJ of ME/kg dry matter with minor difference between species and between tubers vs herbage components (see Table 6.2). Comparatively, perennial ryegrass, considered a standard of cool-season pasture grass, has an ME concentration averaging 9.4 MJ/kg dry matter (Sun *et al.*, 2012). Brassica tubers tend to be much lower in dry matter concentration than herbage and their crude protein concentration follows similarly with lower concentration in tubers than in herbage (see Table 6.2). When compared to the perennial ryegrass standard, brassica herbage is similar in crude protein concentration, ranging from 15.4% to 17.7% making both high-protein forages. Standard measures of fiber concentration, both acid detergent fiber (ADF) and neutral detergent fiber (NDF), indicate that brassica species are much lower in fiber (<19% ADF and <30% NDF; see Table 6.2) and digestibility than the reference forage species, perennial ryegrass (28% ADF,

65% NDF). These attributes of high energy, high protein, low fiber, and high digestibility can confer important advantages in boosting immunity of animals challenged with GIN when compared to perennial pastures (Hoste *et al.*, 2005; Knox *et al.*, 2006). Improving the quality of grazing forage is especially important during times of parasitic challenge, and forage rotations using annuals are an effective means of providing high-quality forage in times of need.

Impact of nutritional value of annuals on animal performance

The high nutritional value of brassica species and other annual forages is such that they can support a high level of animal performance in grazing systems while also offering greater resilience against GIN parasites. Growing lambs/kids and lactating ewes/does have high energy and protein needs, with the high-energy need being particularly hard to meet in both tropical and temperate grazing systems. The energy content of forages within many grazing systems limits animal performance.

Annual forages are a high-energy forage crop that can support high levels of animal performance as shown in Table 6.2. In this compilation of grazing trials using Dorset crossbred lambs of similar maturity (0.3–0.4 of maternal mature size at the start of the trial), lamb performance can be considered a proxy for forage quality. As such, it is apparent that forage quality is high in most of these annual and short-term perennial forages and that high animal growth performance (300 g/day) can be achieved in these grazing systems. This level of performance is sufficient to provide enough dietary energy to promote fat deposition and to finish lambs (Macaluso, 2021). In addition to high individual animal gain, the high quality of forage in these pastures provides opportunities for superior gain on a land basis when compared to perennial pasture over the same period (see Table 6.2). These annual and short-term perennial pastures also exhibit different growth patterns than perennial pastures and can provide quality forage for animals with high requirements during periods when perennial forage is scarce.

Annual forages can fit many parts of small ruminant production systems in addition to pre- and postweaning growth. The high energy concentration is sufficient to meet the requirements of prolific breeds during late pregnancy when energy content and digestibility of the diet are particularly important in supporting fetal development and ensuring successful lactation. Another stage of production that benefits from a high-energy diet is during the prebreeding or flushing period. Grazing high-energy annuals can provide an excellent flushing diet and promote weigh gain, placing ewes and does in positive energy balance as they enter the breeding season and thus promoting a high ovulation rate and large lamb or kid crop (Downing and Scaramuzzi, 1991; Lassoued et al., 2004; Yıldırır et al., 2022).

Plant Secondary Metabolites with Antiparasitic Properties in Pasture Species

In addition to supporting heightened immunity to GIN infection, via greater supply of a more optimal balance of energy and protein to the rumen, annual and short-term perennial forages may also contain plant secondary metabolites (PSM) that have antiparasitic chemistry. The detrimental impacts of PSM on GIN have been demonstrated extensively *in vitro* (Torres-Fajardo et al., 2020). There are many grazing studies with plants containing PSM that have also supported this role; however, it is harder to separate out the direct role of PSM vs more indirect actions of these forages on parasite infection (boosting immunity) in grazing studies (Hoste et al., 2005; Houdijk et al., 2012).

The presence of PSM has been well documented in several perennial species that often lack persistence in pasture but can be used very effectively as short-term perennials in pasture mixes as part of a complementary forage system. Examples of such forages include chicory (*Chichorium intybus*) and sainfoin (*Onobrychis viciifolia*). Both forages struggle with persistency issues in cooler climates but work well in a pasture rotation as part of a short-term perennial pasture (2–3 year) mixture in rotation with either shorter (annual) or longer (long-term

perennial) pasture species (Carbonero et al., 2011; Houdijk et al., 2012).

Chicory is known to contain several compounds with antiparasitic chemistry but its sesquiterpene lactone content has been the best characterized as the basis for its antiparasitic properties (Molan et al., 2003; Peña-Espinoza et al., 2018). This action appears to be specific for abomasal nematodes (as demonstrated in *H. contortus* and *Teladorsagia circumcincta*) resulting in a suppression of fecal e.g.g count (FEC) and sometimes associated with a reduction in fourth-stage and adult larvae as evidenced in sheep studies (Peña-Espinoza et al., 2018). Sainfoin is a perennial forage legume rich in condensed tannin content and well adapted to many temperate zones (Carbonero et al., 2011). The condensed tannin content of sainfoin is widely considered to be the primary antiparasitic chemistry found in this species (Wang et al., 2015). Other pasture species high in condensed tannin content with demonstrated antiparasitic properties include birdsfoot trefoil (*Lotus cornicalus*) and sericea lespedeza (*Lespedeza cuneata*) (Marley et al., 2003; Mechineni et al., 2014). Extracts from these plants have been demonstrated to impede both egg hatching and larval development *in vivo* and *in vitro* (Brunet et al., 2007; Barone et al., 2019; Lonngren et al., 2020). Grazing studies with both sheep and goats indicate that these pasture species high in condensed tannin content tend to reduce FEC and improve blood packed cell volume (PCV), particularly in *H. contortus*-dominant infections without large impacts on the size of the adult larvae populations (Marley et al., 2003; Paolini et al., 2005; Burke et al., 2012). When sheep and goats are removed from pasture with rich content of these species or when supplements containing these species are withdrawn, FEC rises quickly and PCV declines, suggesting a suppression of fecundity but not necessarily viability of GIN species (Hoste et al., 2005; Lange et al., 2006). Condensed tannins also act to reduce degradation of protein in the rumen, thereby increasing the passage of undegraded dietary protein to the abomasum (Min et al., 2003). This may improve quantity and quality of metabolizable protein and support enhanced immunity as discussed earlier as a major indirect action of forage quality on the resilience against parasite infection by the host.

In addition to sesquiterpene lactones and tannins, other PSMs with documented antiparasitic properties include alkaloids (Satou *et al.*, 2002) and glycosides (Akhtar and Ahmad, 1992). There is increasing evidence that there are likely many additional PSMs to be characterized that have antiparasitic chemistry even in species with PSMs of known activity. For example, an *in vitro* assessment of 51 birdsfoot trefoil strains revealed that condensed tannin content was not a strong predictor of antiparasitic activity as extracts of these strains differed greatly in activity against egg hatching, larval motitlity, and exsheathment (Barone *et al.*, 2019). This suggests that other yet unknown PSMs are likely to explain part of many pasture species' antiparasitic activity.

Limitations in the use of bioactive forages include the challenge in providing sufficient PSM to control parasites while minimizing potential negative impacts on animal health and perfomance. Tannins, for example, can be benefical in reducing protein degradation in the rumen but may have negative impacts through a reduction in voluntary feed intake (Waghorn, 2008). There is a large literature on the detrimental impact of certain plant PSMs on animal health and productivity. Certain PSMs can reduce voluntary dry matter intake even at low levels (Barry, 2013) whereas others can result in photosensitivity symptoms (Quinn *et al.*, 2014) and anemia (Cox-Ganser *et al.*, 1994). Therefore pasture populations need to be established or managed to contain the appropriate level of PSM to impact parasites without detrimental impacts on animal health/performance. Grazing management and planting strategies can be used to manage PSM content by providing PSM-containing plants as mixtures in strips rather than perfectly intermingled, thereby allowing greater capacity for selection and choice in addition to limiting consumption when levels are high (Villalba *et al.*, 2019).

Interestingly, it appears that small ruminants may display preferences for forages that contain bioactive compounds in times of need, as evidenced by grazing lambs preferring sainfoin following parasite infection (Gaudin *et al.*, 2019.) Futhermore, goats browsing tannin-rich vegetations seem able to consume the tannin-rich vegetation as a preventive medication strategy, aiming to limit exsheathment of ingested L3 larvae (Torres-Fajardo *et al.*, 2019b).

Sward Structure Diversity in Pasture Rotation Systems

Sward structure may also impact the parasitic infectivity of a pasture. Pasture forages vary tremendously in sward structure, displaying large variation in both height and density from the top of the sward to the soil surface. The extent to which this impacts the parasitic infectivity of a pasture is challenging to evaluate, but there is evidence to suggest that certain sward structures may be less infective than others when stocking rate and biomass are controlled (Niezen *et al.*, 1998; Marley *et al.*, 2006; Gazda *et al.*, 2009). Stocking rate and pasture larval contamination level are closely associated, with stocking rate being a primary driver of pasture contamination (Barger, 1999). While differences can exist in larval concentration of a sward from soil surface to the distal end of plant (Moss and Vlassoff, 1993), they are not always consistent between forage species and are more apparent in temperate than subtropical and tropical climates (Moss and Vlassoff, 1993; Gasparina *et al.*, 2021). These gradients are clearly impacted by temperature, often tending to disappear over time following grazing events (Tontini *et al.*, 2015) and in pasture plots following inoculation (Amaradasa *et al.*, 2010; Gasparina *et al.*, 2021). When animals initially enter a forage stand, they tend to select the top horizon of the sward which may initially have a slightly lower concentration of larvae. Then as the animals continue to trample forage and consume the lower horizons of the sward, it is likely that the gradient of infectivity changes as the sward structure becomes compromised via trampling, thus changing over time. It is plausible that larval ingestion in contaminated swards is only minimized when highly selective grazing or browsing practices resulting in low forage utilization are employed.

Annual and short-term perennial forages often differ appreciably in sward structure compared to long-term perennial pasture and may also differ in stocking rate depending on the yield of these pastures and the type of grazing management applied. Limited evidence suggests that certain pasture species including chicory (Moss and Vlassoff, 1993) and birdsfoot trefoil (Niezen *et al.*, 1998; Marley *et al.*, 2006) tend to have lower larval contamination per unit of dry matter in grazing trials and there is speculation that this may relate in part to unique aspects of sward structure in these pasture species (Torres-Fajardo *et al.*, 2019a).

Conclusion

Grazing management practices are a critical part of an integrated approach to parasite control in small ruminants. Shorter duration grazing events minimize rapid reinfection, resulting in greater forage utilization and can improve animal nutrition. Multispecies grazing and machine harvest of excess forage can also reduce pasture contamination while maintaining pasture quality. The use of pasture species rotations utilizing annual and short-term perennial pastures offers more options for evasive grazing to minimize exposure of highly susceptible sheep and goats to GIN larvae. The need for evasive grazing management options becomes particularly important in grazing programs with high stocking rates and/or highly susceptible animals where GIN infection management in sheep and goats is especially challenging.

The forage quality of rotationally grazed pastures can exceed that of perennial pastures, providing a higher plane of nutrition which builds immunity to resist infection while also improving resilience against infection. Pasture rotations involving plant species with different growth profiles can fill gaps in forage quality and availability compared to forage systems consisting exclusively of perennial forages, thus also improving whole-farm forage utilization. The use of forage species within pasture rotations with beneficial plant secondary compounds that have antiparasitic properties may also provide an additional means of parasite control.

Collectively, these benefits indicate that grazing management and pasture rotations are key components of an effective and sustainable parasite control program.

References

Abaye, A.O., Allen, V.G. and Fontenot, J.P. (1994) Influence of grazing cattle and sheep together and separately on animal performance and forage quality. *Journal of Animal Science* 72, 1013–1022.

Akhtar, M. and Ahmad, I. (1992) Comparative efficacy of *Mallotus philippinensis* fruit (Kamala) or Nilzan® drug against gastrointestinal cestodes in Beetal goats. *Small Ruminant Research* 8, 121–128.

Almeida, F.A., Piza, M.L., Bassetto, C.C., Starling, R., Albuquerque, A. *et al.* (2018) Infection with gastrointestinal nematodes in lambs in different integrated crop-livestock systems (ICL). *Small Ruminant Research* 166, 66–72.

Alves, L.A., de Oliveira Denardin, L.G., Martins, A.P. and Bayer, C. (2020) The effect of crop rotation and sheep grazing management on plant production and soil C and N stocks in a long-term integrated crop-livestock system in Southern Brazil. *Soil and Tillage Research* 203, 104678.

Amaradasa, B.S., Lane, R.A. and Manage, A. (2010) Vertical migration of *Haemonchus contortus* infective larvae on *Cynodon dactylon* and *Paspalum notatum* pastures in response to climatic conditions. *Veterinary Parasitology* 170, 78–87.

Amarante, A.F., Bagnola, Jr.J., Amarante, M.R. and Barbosa, M. (1997) Host specificity of sheep and cattle nematodes in Sao Paulo state, Brazil. *Veterinary Parasitology* 73, 89–104.

Anderson, N. (1983) The availability of trichostrongylid larvae to grazing sheep after seasonal contamination of pastures. *Australian Journal of Agricultural Research* 34, 583–592.

Baggs, E.M., Watson, C.A. and Rees, R.M. (2000) The fate of nitrogen from incorporated cover crop and green manure residues. *Soil Use and Management* 16, 82–87.

Barger, I.A. (1993) Influence of sex and reproductive status on susceptibility of ruminants to nematode parasitism. *International Journal for Parsitology* 23, 463–469.

Barger, I.A. (1999) The role of epidemiological knowledge and grazing management for helminth control in small ruminants. *International Journal for Parsitology* 29, 41–47.

Barger, I.A., Siale, K., Banks, D.J. and Le Jambre, L. (1994) Rotational grazing for control of gastrointestinal nematodes of goats in a wet tropical environment. *Veterinary Parasitology* 53, 109–116.

Barger, I.A. (1997) Control by management. *Veterinary Parasitology* 72, 493–500. DOI: 10.1016/s0304-4017(97)00113-1.

Barone, C.D., Zajac, A.M., Ferguson, S.M., Brown, R., Reed, J. *et al.* (2019) *In vitro* screening of 51 birdsfoot trefoil (*Lotus corniculatus* L.; Fabaceae) strains for anti-parasitic effects against *Haemonchus contortus*. *Parasitology* 146, 828–836.

Barry, T. (2013) The feeding value of forage brassica plants for grazing ruminant livestock. *Animal Feed Science and Technology* 181, 15–25.

Beasley, A.M., Kahn, L.P. and Windon, R.G. (2010) The periparturient relaxation of immunity in Merino ewes infected with *Trichostrongylus colubriformis*: Endocrine and body compositional responses. *Veterinary Parasitology* 168, 51–59.

Besier, R.B., Kahn, L.P., Sargison, N.D. and van Wyk, J. (2016) The pathophysiology, ecology and epidemiology of *Haemonchus contortus* infection in small ruminants. *Advances in Parasitology* 93, 95–143. DOI: 10.1016/bs.apar.2016.02.022.

Blanco-Canqui, H. and Ruis, S.J. (2020) Cover crop impacts on soil physical properties: A review. *Soil Science Society of America Journal* 84, 1527–1576.

Bowman, M., Afi, M., Beenken, A., Boline, A., Drewnoski, M. *et al.* (2024) Cover crops on livestock operations: Potential for expansion in the United States. USDA Economic Research Service AP-120. Available at: https://ideas.repec.org/p/ags/uersap/342471.html (accessed 11 July 2025).

Brunet, S., Aufrere, J., El Babili, F., Fouraste, I. and Hoste, H. (2007) The kinetics of exsheathment of infective nematode larvae is disturbed in the presence of a tannin-rich plant extract (sainfoin) both *in vitro* and *in vivo*. *Parasitology* 134, 1253–1262.

Burke, J.M., Miller, J.E. and Terrill, T.H. (2009) Impact of rotational grazing on management of gastrointestinal nematodes in weaned lambs. *Veterinary Parasitology* 163, 67–72.

Burke, J.M., Miller, J.E., Mosjidis, J.A. and Terrill, T. (2012) Grazing sericea lespedeza for control of gastrointestinal nematodes in lambs. *Veterinary Parasitology* 186, 507–512.

Cabaret, J., Bouilhol, M. and Mage, C. (2002a) Managing helminths of ruminants in organic farming. *Veterinary Research* 33, 625–640.

Cabaret, J., Mage, C. and Bouilhol, M. (2002b) Helminth intensity and diversity in organic meat sheep farms in centre of France. *Veterinary Parasitology* 105, 33–47.

Can-Celis, A., Torres-Acosta, J., Mancilla-Montelongo, M., Gonzalez-Pech, P., Ramos-Bruno, E. *et al.* (2022) Effect of three feeding levels on the pathogenesis and establishment of *Haemonchus contortus* in parasite-naïve Pelibuey hair sheep lambs during their first infection. *Veterinary Parasitology* 311, 109811.

Carbonero, C.H., Mueller-Harvey, I., Brown, T.A. and Smith, L. (2011) Sainfoin (*Onobrychis viciifolia*): A beneficial forage legume. *Plant Genetic Resources* 9, 70–85.

Carvalho, P.C.D.F., Anghinoni, I., Moraes, A.D. and Souza, E. (2010) Managing grazing animals to achieve nutrient cycling and soil improvement in no-till integrated systems. *Nutrient Cycling in Agroecosystems* 88, 259–273.

Cellier, M., Nielsen, B.L., Duvaux-Ponter, C., Freeman, H., Hannaford, R. *et al.* (2022) Browse or browsing: Investigating goat preferences for feeding posture, feeding height and feed type. *Frontiers in Veterinary Science* 9, 1032631.

Chandrawathani, P., Jamnah, O., Adnan, M., Waller, P., Larsen, M. *et al.* (2004) Field studies on the biological control of nematode parasites of sheep in the tropics, using the microfungus *Duddingtonia flagrans*. *Veterinary Parasitology* 120, 177–187.

Chapman, D.F., Kenny, S.N., Beca, D. and Johnson, I. (2015) Pasture and forage crop systems for non-irrigated dairy farms in Southern Australia. 2. Inter-annual variation in forage supply, and business risk. *Animal Production Science* 55, 893–901.

Colvin, A.F., Walkden-Brown, S.W., Knox, M.R. and Scott, J. (2008) Intensive rotational grazing assists control of gastrointestinal nematodosis of sheep in a cool temperate environment with summer-dominant rainfall. *Veterinary Parasitology* 153, 108–120.

Coop, R.L. and Holmes, P.H. (1996) Nutrition and parasite interactions. *International Journal for Parsitology* 26, 951–962.

Cox-Ganser, J.M., Jung, G.A., Pushkin, R.T. and Reid, R. (1994) Evaluation of *Brassicas* in grazing systems for sheep: II Blood composition and nutrient status. *Journal of Animal Science* 72, 1832–1841.

Cranston, L., Kenyon, P., Morris, S. and Kemp, P. (2015) A review of the use of chicory, plantain, red clover and white clover in a sward mix for increased sheep and beef production. *Journal of New Zealand Grasslands* 77, 89–94.

Derpsch, R., Sidiras, N. and Roth, C.H. (1986) Results of studies made from 1977 to 1984 to control erosion by cover crops and no-tillage techniques in Parana, Brazil. *Soil and Tillage Research* 8, 253–263.

Downing, J.A. and Scaramuzzi, R.J. (1991) Nutrient effects on ovulation rate, ovarian function and the secretion of gonadotrophic and metabolic hormones in sheep. *Journal of Reproduction and Fertility Supplement* 43, 209–227.

Drewnoski, M., Parsons, J., Blanco, H., Redfearn, D., Hales, K. *et al.* (2018) Forages and pastures symposium: Cover crops in livestock production: Whole-system approach. Can cover crops pull double duty: Conservation and profitable forage production in the midwestern United States. *Journal of Animal Science* 96, 3503–3512.

Ehrhardt, R. (2016) Contribution of forage production systems to small ruminant profitability. *Journal of Animal Science* 94, 842.

Fletcher, R.S. and Kott, L.S. (1999) Phenolics and cold tolerance of *Brassica napus*. *Proceedings of the 10th International Rapeseed Congress* 26–29.

Gárate-Gallardo, L., de Jesús Torres-Acosta, J.F., Aguilar-Caballero, A.J., Sandoval-Castro, C., Camara-Sarmiento, R. *et al.* (2015) Comparing different maize supplementation strategies to improve resilience and resistance against gastrointestinal nematode infections in browsing goats. *Parasite* 22, 19.

Garcia, S.C., Fulkerson, W.J. and Brookes, S.U. (2008) Dry matter production, nutritive value and efficiency of nutrient utilization of a complementary forage rotation compared to a grass pasture system. *Grass and Forage Science* 63, 284–300.

Gasparina, J.M., Baby, R.G., Fonseca, L., Bricarello, P. and Rocha, R. (2021) Infective larvae of *Haemonchus contortus* found from the base to the top of the grass sward. *Revista Brasileira de Parasitologia Veterinária* 30, e028120.

Gaudin, E., Costes-Thire, M., Villalba, J.J., Hoste, H., Gerfault, V. *et al.* (2019) Relative abilities of young sheep and goats to self-medicate with tannin-rich sainfoin when infected with gastrointestinal nematodes. *Animal* 13, 1498–1507.

Gazda, T.L., Piazzetta, R.G., Dittrich, J.R. and Monteiro, A. (2009) Distribution of nematode larvae of sheep in tropical pasture plants. *Small Ruminant Research* 82, 94–98.

Golding, K., Wilson, E., Kemp, P. and Pain, R. (2011) Mixed herb and legume pasture improves the growth of lambs post-weaning. *Animal Production Science* 51, 717–723.

Greer, A., Stankiewicz, M., Jay, N., McAnulty, R. and Sykes, A. (2005) The effect of concurrent corticosteroid induced immuno-suppression and infection with the intestinal parasite *Trichostrongylus colubriformis* on food intake and utilization in both immunologically naïve and competent sheep. *Animal Science* 80, 89–99.

Griffiths, H. and Carr, A.M.N. (2022) Potential for silvopastoral systems to control nematode burden in livestock farming in winter rainfall areas of South Australia, Australia. *International Journal of Veterinary Science and Research* 8, 118–126.

Guillard, K. and Allinson, D.W. (1988) Yield and nutrient content of summer- and fall-grown forage brassica crops. *Canadian Journal of Plant Science* 68, 721–731.

Hoste, H., Torres-Acosta, J.F., Paolini, V., Aguilar-Caballero, A., Etter, E. *et al.* (2005) Interactions between nutrition and gastrointestinal infections in parasitic nematodes in goats. *Small Ruminant Research* 60, 141–151.

Hoste, H., Martinez-Ortiz-de-Montellano, C., Manolaraki, F., Brunet, S., Ojeda-Robertos, N. *et al.* (2012) Direct and indirect effects of bioactive tannin-rich tropical and temperate legumes against nematode infections. *Veterinary Parasitology* 186, 18–27.

Hoste, H., Torres-Acosta, J., Sandoval-Castro, C.A., Mueller-Harvey, I., Sotiraki, S. *et al.* (2015) Tannin containing legumes as a model for nutraceuticals against digestive parasites in livestock. *Veterinary Parasitology* 212, 5–17.

Hoste, H., Torres-Acosta, J., Quijada, J., Chan-Perez, I., Dakheel, M. *et al.* (2016) Interactions between nutrition and infections with *Haemonchus contortus* and related gastrointestinal nematodes in small ruminants. *Advances in Parasitology* 93, 239–351.

Houdijk, J.G., Kyriazakis, I., Kidane, A. and Athanasiadou, S. (2012) Manipulating small ruminant parasite epidemiology through the combination of nutritional strategies. *Veterinary Parasitology* 186, 38–50.

Hunt, J.R., Swan, A.D., Fettell, N.A. and Breust, P. (2016) Sheep grazing on crop residues do not reduce crop yields in no-till, controlled traffic farming systems in an equi-seasonal rainfall environment. *Field Crops Research* 196, 22–32.

Jordan, H.E., Phillips, W.A., Morrison, R.D., Doyle, J. and McKenzie, K. (1988) A 3-year study of continuous mixed grazing of cattle and sheep: Parasitism of offspring. *International Journal for Parasitology* 18, 779–784.

Kemp, P.D., Kenyon, P.R. and Morris, S.T. (2010) The use of legume and herb forage species to create high performance pastures for sheep and cattle grazing systems. *Revista Brasileira de Zootecnia* 39, 169–174.

Knox, M.R., Torres-Acosta, J.F. and Aguilar-Caballero, A.J. (2006) Exploiting the effect of dietary supplementation of small ruminants on resilience and resistance against gastrointestinal nematodes. *Veterinary Parasitology* 139, 385–393.

Koch, D.W., Kercher, C. and Jones, R. (2002) Fall and winter grazing of brassicas – A value-added opportunity for lamb producers. *Sheep and Goat Research Journal* 17, 1–13.

Kruidhof, H.M., Bastiaans, L. and Kropff, M.J. (2008) Ecological weed management by cover cropping: Effects on weed growth in autumn and weed establishment in spring. *Weed Research* 48, 492–502.

Lange, K.C., Olcott, D.D., Miller, J.E., Mosjidis, J., Terrill, T. *et al.* (2006) Effect of sericea lespedeza (*Lespedeza cuneata*) fed as hay, on natural and experimental *Haemonchus contortus* infections in lambs. *Veterinary Parasitology* 141, 273–278.

Lassoued, N., Rekik, M., Mahouachi, M. and Ben Hamouda, M. (2004) The effect of nutrition prior to and during mating on ovulation rate, reproductive wastage, and lambing rate in three sheep breeds. *Small Ruminant Research* 52, 117–125.

Leng, R.A. (1991) Optimising herbivore nutrition. In: Ho, Y.W., Wong, H.K., Abdullah, N. and TAJUDDIN, Z.A. (eds) *Recent advances on the nutrition of herbivores. Proceedings of the 3rd International Symposium on the Nutrition of Herbivores*, Serdang, Malaysia.

Li, F., Sørensen, P., Li, X. and Olesen, J.E. (2020) Carbon and nitrogen mineralization differ between incorporated shoots and roots of legume versus non-legume based cover crops. *Plant and Soil* 446, 243–257.

Liu, S., Masters, D. and Adams, N. (2003) Potential impact of nematode parasitism on nutrient partitioning for wool production, growth and reproduction in sheep. *Australian Journal of Experimental Agriculture* 43, 1409–1417.

Liu, X., Wei, R., Tian, M., Liu, J., Ruan, Y. *et al.* (2022) Combined transcriptome and metabolome profiling provide insights into cold responses in rapeseed (*Brassica napus* L.) genotypes with contrasting cold-stress sensitivity. *International Journal of Molecular Sciences* 23, 13546.

Lonngren, K.J., Barone, C.D., Zajac, A.M., Brown, R., Reed, J. *et al.* (2020) Effect of birdsfoot trefoil cultivars on exsheathment of *Haemonchus contortus* in fistulated sheep. *Veterinary Parasitology* 287, 109271.

Luginbuhl, J.M., Green, J.T., Poore, M.H. and Conrad, A. (2000) Use of goats to manage vegetation in cattle pastures in the Appalachian region of North Carolina. *Sheep and Goat Research Journal* 16, 124–135.

Macaluso, C. (2021) Evaluation of growth performance carcass and meat quality of lambs reared on cover crop and grain finishing systems. Master's thesis, Michigan State University, East Lansing, Michigan.

Mahieu, M. and Aumont, G. (2009) Effects of sheep and cattle alternate grazing on sheep parasitism and production. *Tropical Animal Health and Production* 41, 229–239.

Mahieu, M., Archimede, T., Fleur, J. and Mandonnet, M. (2008) Intensive grazing system for small ruminants in the tropics: The French West Indies experience and perspectives. *Small Ruminant Research* 77, 195–207.

Marley, C.L., Cook, R., Keatinge, R., Barrett, J. and Lampkin, N. (2003) The effect of birdsfoot trefoil (*Lotus corniculatus*) and chicory (*Cichorium intybus*) on parasite intensities and performance of lambs naturally infected with helminth parasites. *Veterinary Parasitology* 112, 147–155.

Marley, C.L., Cook, R., Barrett, J., Keatinge, R. and Lampkin, N. (2006) The effects of birdsfoot trefoil (*Lotus corniculatus*) and chicory (*Cichorium intybus*) when compared with perennial ryegrass (*Lolium perenne*) on ovine gastrointestinal parasite development, survival and migration. *Veterinary Parasitology* 138, 280–290.

Mechineni, A., Kommuru, D.S., Gujja, S., Mosjidis, J., Miller, J. *et al.* (2014) Effect of fall-grazed sericea lespedeza (*Lespedeza cuneata*) on gastrointestinal nematode infections of growing goats. *Veterinary Parasitology* 204, 221–228.

Michel, J.F. (1985) Strategies for the use of anthelmintics in livestock and their implications for the development of drug resistance. *Parasitology* 90, 621–628.

Min, B.R., Barry, T.N., Attwood, G.T. and McNabb, W. (2003) The effect of condensed tannins on the nutrition and health of ruminants fed fresh temperate forages: A review. *Animal Feed Science and Technology* 106, 3–19.

Min, B.R., Pomroy, W., Hart, S. and Sahlu, T. (2004) The effect of short-term consumption of a forage containing condensed tannins on gastro-intestinal nematode parasite infections in grazing wether goats. *Small Ruminant Research* 51, 279–283.

Min, B.R., Solaiman, S., Gurung, N., Behrends, J., Eun, J.-S. *et al.* (2012) Effects of pine bark supplementation on performance, rumen fermentation, and carcass characteristics of Kiko crossbred male goats. *Journal of Animal Science* 90, 3556–3567.

Molan, A.L., Duncan, A.J., Barry, T.N. and McNabb, W. (2003) Effects of condensed tannins and crude sesquiterpene lactones extracted from chicory on the motility and larvae of deer lungworm and gastrointestinal nematodes. *Parasitology International* 52, 209–218.

Moss, R. and Vlassoff, A. (1993) Effect of herbage species on gastro-intestinal roundworm populations and their distribution. *New Zealand Journal of Agricultural Research* 36, 371–375.

Niezen, J.H., Robertson, H.A., Waghorn, G.C. and Charleston, W. (1998) Production, faecal egg counts and worm burdens of ewe lambs which grazed six contrasting forages. *Veterinary Parasitology* 80, 15–27.

NRC (2007) *Nutrient Requirements of Small Ruminants*. National Academies Press, Washington, DC, USA.

Oates, L.G., Undersander, D.J., Gratton, C. and Bell, M. (2011) Management-intensive rotational grazing enhances forage production and quality of subhumid cool-season pastures. *Crop Science* 51, 892–901.

O'Connor, L.J., Walkden-Brown, S.W. and Kahn, L. (2006) Ecology of the free-living stages of major trichostrongylid parasites of sheep. *Veterinary Parasitology* 142, 1–15.

Pain, S., Corkran, J., Kenyon, P., Morris, S. and Kemp, P. (2014) The influence of season on lambs' feeding preference for plantain, chicory and red clover. *Animal Production Science* 55, 1241–1249.

Paolini, V., Farge, F., Prevot, F., Dorchies, P. and Hoste, H. (2005) Effects of the repeated distribution of Sainfoin hay on the resistance and the resilience of goats naturally infected with gastrointestinal nematodes. *Veterinary Parasitology* 127, 277–283.

Pardo, G. and Del Prado, A. (2020) Guidelines for small ruminant production systems under climate emergency in Europe. *Small Ruminant Research* 193, 106261.

Pembleton, K.G., Tozer, K.N., Edwards, G.R. and Jacobs, J. (2008) Simple versus diverse pastures: Opportunities and challenges in dairy systems. *Agricultural Systems* 97, 126–138.

Peña-Espinoza, M., Valente, A.H., Thamsborg, S.M., Simonsen, H., Boas, U. *et al.* (2018) Antiparasitic activity of chicory (*Cichorium intybus*) and its natural bioactive compounds in livestock: A review. *Parasites & Vectors* 11, 1–14.

Planisich, A., Utsumi, S.A., Larripa, M. and Galli, J. (2021) Grazing of cover crops in integrated crop-livestock systems. *Animal* 15, 100054.

Quinn, J.C., Kessel, A. and Weston, L.A. (2014) Secondary plant products causing photosensitization in grazing herbivores: Their structure, activity and regulation. *International Journal of Molecular Sciences* 15, 1441–1465.

Rao, P.S., Deshpande, S., Blümmel, M., Reddy, B. and Hash, T. (2012) Characterization of brown midrib mutants of sorghum (*Sorghum bicolor* (L.) Moench). *European Journal of Plant Science and Biotechnology* 6, 71–75.

Recktenwald, E.B. and Ehrhardt, R.A. (2024) Greenhouse gas emissions from a diversity of sheep production systems in the United States. *Agricultural Systems* 217, 103915.

Reed, K. and Morrissey, E.M. (2022) Bridging ecology and agronomy to foster diverse pastures and healthy soils. *Agronomy* 12, 1893.

Ridler, A., Hytten, K., Gray, D. and Reid, J. (2024) Reduced anthelmintic use on 13 New Zealand sheep farms: Farmer motivations and practical implementation. *New Zealand Veterinary Journal* 73, 29–40.

Rocha, R.A., Bresciani, K.D.S. and Barros, T.F.M. (2008) Sheep and cattle grazing alternately: Nematode parasitism and pasture decontamination. *Small Ruminant Research* 75, 135–143.

Satou, T., Koga, M., Matsuhashi, R., Koike, K., Tada, I. *et al.* (2002) Assay of nematocidal activity of isoquinoline alkaloids using third-stage larvae of *Strongyloides ratti* and *S. venezuelensis*. *Veterinary Parasitology* 104, 131–138.

Schipanski, M.E., Barbercheck, M., Douglas, M.R. and Finney, D. (2014) A framework for evaluating ecosystem services provided by cover crops in agroecosystems. *Agricultural Systems* 125, 12–22.

Smith, L.A., Marion, G., Swain, D.L., White, P. and Hutchings, M. (2009) The effect of grazing management on livestock exposure to parasites via the faecal-oral route. *Preventive Veterinary Medicine* 91,
95–106.

Sun, X., Waghorn, G., Hoskin, S. and Harrison, S. (2012) Methane emissions from sheep fed fresh brassicas (*Brassica* spp.) compared to perennial ryegrass (*Lolium perenne*). *Animal Feed Science and
Technology* 176, 107–116.

Teague, W. (2018) Forages and pastures symposium: Cover crops in livestock production: Whole-system
approach: Managing grazing to restore soil health and farm livelihoods. *Journal of Animal Science*
96, 1519–1530.

Thamsborg, S.M., Roepstorff, A. and Larsen, M. (1999) Integrated and biological control of parasites in
organic and conventional production systems. *Veterinary Parasitology* 84, 169–186.

Thomas, G.A., Dalal, R.C., Weston, E.J., Lehane, K., King, A. *et al*. (2009) Pasture-crop rotations for
sustainable production in a wheat and sheep-based farming system in Vertosol in South-West
Queensland, Australia. *Animal Production Science* 49, 682–695.

Tontini, J.F., Poli, C.H.E.C., Bremm, C., de Castro, J., Fajardo, M. *et al*. (2015) Distribution of infective
gastrointestinal helminth larvae in tropical erect grass under different feeding systems for lambs.
Tropical Animal Health and Production 47, 1145–1152.

Torres-Acosta, J.F. and Hoste, H. (2008) Alternative or improved methods to limit gastro-intestinal parasitism in grazing sheep and goats. *Small Ruminant Research* 77, 159–173.

Torres-Fajardo, R., González-Pech, P., Sandoval-Castro, C., Ventura-Cordero, J. and Torres-Acosta, J.
(2019a) Criollo goats limit their grass intake in the early morning suggesting a prophylactic self-
medication behaviour in a heterogeneous vegetation. *Tropical Animal Health and Production* 51,
2473–2479.

Torres-Fajardo, R.A., Navarro-Alberto, J.A., Ventura-Cordero, J., Gonzalez-Pech, P., Sandoval-Castro, C.
et al. (2019b) Intake and selection of goats grazing heterogeneous vegetation: Effect of gastrointestinal nematodes and condensed tannins. *Rangeland Ecology & Management* 72, 946–953.

Torres-Fajardo, R.A., González-Pech, P.G., Sandoval-Castro, C.A. and Torres-Acosta, J. (2020) Small
ruminant production based on rangelands to optimize animal nutrition and health: Building an interdisciplinary approach to evaluate nutraceutical plants. *Animals* 10, 1799.

Torres-Fajardo, R.A., Ortiz-Dominguez, G., González-Pech, P.G., Sandoval-Castro, C.A. and Torres-
Acosta, J. (2024) The complexity of goats' feeding behaviour: An overview of the research in the
tropical low deciduous forest. *Small Ruminant Research* 231, 107199.

Villalba, J.J., Beauchemin, K.A., Gregorini, P. and MacAdam, J. (2019) Pasture chemoscapes and their
ecological services. *Translational Animal Science* 3, 829–841.

Vlassoff, A., Leathwick, D. and Heath, A. (2001) The epidemiology of nematode infections of sheep. *New
Zealand Veterinary Journal* 49, 213–221.

Waghorn, G. (2008) Beneficial and detrimental effects of dietary condensed tannins for sustainable sheep
and goat production—progress and challenges. *Animal Feed Science and Technology* 147, 116–139.

Wang, Y., McAllister, T.M. and Archarya, S. (2015) Condensed tannins in Sainfoin: Composition, concentration, and effects on nutritive and feeding value of sainfoin forage. *Crop Science* 55, 13–22.

Warren, S.D., Nevill, M.B., Blackburn, W.H. and Garza, N. (1986) Soil response to trampling under intensive rotation grazing. *Soil Science Society of American Journal* 50, 1336–1341.

Warwick, S.I. (2011) *Brassicaceae* in agriculture. In: Schmidt, R. and Bancroft, I. (eds) *Genetics and
Genomics of the Brassicaceae. Plant Genetics and Genomics: Crops and Models*. Springer, New
York, pp. 33–65.

Westwood, C. and Mulcock, H. (2012) Nutritional evaluation of five species of forage brassica. *Proceedings
of the New Zealand Grassland Association* 31–37.

Yıldırır, M., Çakır, D.Ü. and Yurtman, İ.Y. (2022) Effects of restricted nutrition and flushing on reproductive
performance and metabolic profiles in sheep. *Livestock Science* 104870.

7 Bioactive Forages for the Control of Gastrointestinal Nematodes of Small Ruminants

Thomas H. Terrill[1]*, Juan Felipe de J. Torres-Acosta[2] and Hervé Hoste[3]

[1]*Department of Agricultural Sciences, Agricultural Research Station, Fort Valley State University, Fort Valley, Georgia, USA;* [2]*Facultad de Medicina Veterinaria y Zootecnia, Universidad Autónoma de Yucatán, Mérida, Yucatán, México;* [3]*Université de Toulouse, UMR 1225 IHAP INRAE/ENVT (retired), Toulouse, France*

Abstract

Infection with gastrointestinal nematode (GIN) parasites is a primary constraint to sustainable small ruminant production worldwide, and increased prevalence of GIN resistance to anthelmintic drugs has exacerbated the problem for producers. As an alternative to exclusive dependence on drugs, interest has been growing in the use of bioactive (antiparasitic) plants and plant products as a component of sustainable parasite management systems in livestock. This review is focused on the bioactive effectiveness of tannin-containing forages and plant by-products against GIN of small ruminants in tropical (Mexico – Yucatan), subtropical (southeastern USA – Georgia), and temperate (Europe – France) climatic environments. Supporting *in vitro* and *in vivo* data from experiments with tannin-rich cool-season and warm-season vegetative legumes, tropical legume trees, and plant by-products will be described, as well as possible antiparasitic mechanisms of action, and incorporation of bioactive plants as nutraceuticals into livestock farming systems.

Introduction

Gastrointestinal nematodes (GINs) remain a major threat in different small ruminant production systems based on outdoor grazing worldwide. Since the early 1960s, the control of these parasitic worms has relied on the systematic, regular use of three main families of broad-spectrum chemical anthelmintics (AH) with different mechanisms of action against the worms. More recently, monepantel, a derivate of aminoacetonitril (ADD), represents a fourth AH family that is currently available in some parts of the world. The quasi-exclusive reliance on chemical treatments to control GINs has led to the regular, exponential development and diffusion of AH-resistant parasites in sheep and goat farms (Rose Vineer *et al.*, 2020). This phenomenon of AH resistance seems to depend on the main characteristics of the breeding systems.

In North America, favorable climatic conditions for growth of the free-living life stages of GINs (eggs and larvae) on pasture led farmers to rely on the frequent use of AH dewormers in their small ruminant flocks and herds, inevitably leading to the current crisis of multiple AH-resistant GIN (Kaplan, 2004; Howell *et al.*, 2008). The exponential worldwide expansion/

*Corresponding author: terrillt@fvsu.edu

© CAB International 2026. *Management Practices for Controlling Nematode Parasites of Small Ruminants* (eds James E. Miller and Joan M. Burke)
DOI: 10.1079/9781800623767.0007

diffusion of AH-resistant GIN populations in small ruminant farms in temperate and tropical areas of the world has given a strong impetus to promote the concept of integrated management of GIN based on the combination of alternative approaches to chemical molecules corresponding to different principles of control (Torres-Acosta and Hoste, 2008).

One of these innovative approaches targeting GIN populations is aimed at exploring the potential antiparasitic effects of plants and their bioactive compounds to disturb GIN biology and the dynamics of infection on farm. The use of bioactive forages to assist in controlling gastrointestinal parasites in livestock is not a new concept but has been an important part of animal health management for millennia throughout the world (Athanasiadou et al., 2007). Many antiparasitic plants have been identified and utilized as a part of ethno-veterinary practices in Africa (Githiori et al., 2005, 2006), Asia (Badar et al., 2017), Europe (Manolaraki et al., 2010; Rodríguez-Hernández et al., 2023), and North and South America (Borges et al., 2020).

Tannin-containing Plants

The first impetus for using plants containing condensed tannins (CT) to control GINs in sheep and goats came from early empirical results obtained in a series of studies in New Zealand (NZ) (Niezen et al., 1995, 1998a). The main objective of these studies was to examine the potential effects on greenhouse gas (GHG) emissions of three CT-containing forages—sulla (Hedysarum coronarium), birdsfoot trefoil (Lotus corniculatus), and/or big trefoil (Lotus pedunculatus)—vs three control fodders with no tannins—perennial ryegrass (Lolium perenne), plantain (Plantago lanceolata), and alfalfa (Medicago sativa). Concomitant measurements of fecal egg counts (FEC) showed that the grazing of CT-containing legumes, particularly sulla, led to significant decreases in egg excretion.

These early results with cool-season legumes led to further explorations of a potential AH role of CT and other polyphenols contained in a wide range of plants, including warm-season and tropical legume forages. The special interest in legume (Fabaceae) plants in

early studies relates to the nutritional values of this family, the possibility to grow and select them in temperate countries, the wide distribution of legume trees under tropical conditions, and also the beneficial environmental effects, in particular by fixing N in the soils, thus reducing the need for chemical N2 fertilizers.

After the early results from NZ, further studies were performed worldwide to confirm that the ingestion of CT-containing legumes contributed to disturbing the biology of GINs, and that represented a new window of opportunities to improve the control of GIN infections as well as other positive consequences for the hosts and the environment.

Research on sainfoin (*Onobrychis viciifolia*) in France (National Veterinary School of Toulouse; INRA-ENVT)

Traditionally, sainfoin was present in Europe, especially in areas with chalky soils of high pH. The value of this legume has been recognized since the 16th century. The sanitary interest of this plant is briefly illustrated by its French name 'sain-foin,' which means 'healthy hay' in English.

The renewed interest in sainfoin has been associated with the novel objectives defined, at the end of the 1990s, to promote more sustainable agriculture and animal breeding in the European Union (EU), aiming at maintaining high levels of production while reducing chemical inputs, preserving the environment, and preparing for adaptation to climatic change.

Within this general framework, the renewed interest in sainfoin as a model for cool-season CT-containing legumes has been explored in two EU projects, coordinated by Professor Irene Mueller-Harvey, namely:

- Healthy Hay (https://cordis.europa.eu/ project/id/35805/reporting/fr)
- Legume Plus (https://cordis.europa.eu/ project/id/289377/reporting).

Within these two projects, several main tasks were defined to explore the potential AH properties of sainfoin. Some main objectives of specific tasks within these two projects concerned questions on both basic and applied research to define the on-farm use of sainfoin to control GIN infections. Some of these main tasks were as follows.

- To develop and/or validate *in vitro* methodologies to confirm the AH activiy of sainfoin and to explore the variability depending on different factors.
- To describe the *in vivo* effect of sainfoin consumption on the different key stages of the GIN biological life cycle in infected sheep and goats.
- To explore the mechanisms of action of CT and related polyphenols on GIN.
- To define the concept of nutraceuticals based on tannin-containing bioactive plants.
- To define the optimal conditions for use of sainfoin on farms.

The results obtained to address these different tasks with sainfoin are summarized in further sections of this chapter.

Many of these studies have been performed in a long-term collaboration between INRA/ ENVT and the Autonomous University of Yucatán (UADY), Mexico. In addition, many conclusions on the different items obtained with sainfoin have been confirmed with other models of tannin-containing bioactive legumes, namely the warm-season legume sericea lespedeza (SL; *Lespedeza cuneata*), and many plants of the tropical deciduous forest (TDF), as will be discussed below.

Research in the USA (Fort Valley State University [FVSU] and the American Consortium for Small Ruminant Parasite Control [ACSRPC])

Research at FVSU and the ACSRPC on the use of antiparasitic tannin-containing plants has focused primarily on SL, a warm-season perennial legume well adapted to the southeastern USA and other parts of the world with similar climates, such as in southern Africa (Terrill and Mosjidis, 2015).

The initial project was completed with ground SL hay because there were no established SL pastures at FVSU at the time. Despite reduced extractable tannin concentrations

in sun-dried SL forage (Terrill *et al.*, 1990), it reduced the FEC of goats, with significant reductions compared to a bermudagrass (*Cynodon dactylon*) hay control diet by the third and fourth weeks of a 28 day trial (Shaik *et al.*, 2004). In a longer (11 week) follow-up study, goats on an SL hay diet had an 80% reduction in FEC compared to controls a week after starting the treatment feeds, and these differences remained until the end of the experiment (Shaik *et al.*, 2006). The SL-fed goats also had increased blood packed cell volume (PCV) values and reduced development of GIN eggs to infective larvae. Numbers of adult female *Haemonchus contortus*, *Teladorsagia circumcincta*, and *Trichostrongylus colubriformis* were 76%, 36%, and 50% lower, respectively, in the SL group compared to controls (Shaik *et al.*, 2006). Despite skepticism that similar results would be observed in feeding an SL hay diet to a different species (sheep) in a different location (Louisiana State University), in a study with 4-month-old naturally and artificially infected ewe lambs fed SL or bermudagrass hays, FEC was reduced (67–78%) in both groups due to SL feeding, while worm burdens in the naturally infected lambs fed SL hay were 67% lower than for control animals (Lange *et al.*, 2006).

The research performed in the USA included several grazing studies with SL showing positive antiparasitic effects against small ruminant GIN in different regions, including Georgia (Mechineni *et al.*, 2014), North Carolina (Luginbuhl *et al.*, 2013), and Arkansas (Burke *et al.*, 2012a, b), and in an on-farm SL study completed in South Africa (Botha, 2015). While this gives farmers in these regions a natural (nonchemical) tool for parasite management in their herds or flocks, what about those farmers in regions where SL is not well adapted? To address this question, the USA group started research to determine the effect of pelleting SL on its bioactivity against GINs and coccidia (*Eimeria* spp.) in both goats (Terrill *et al.*, 2007; Kommuru *et al.*, 2014) and sheep (Burke *et al.*, 2013). These steps were seen as essential to determine whether farmers could grow and market SL as a nutraceutical feed for livestock (Hoste *et al.*, 2015).

Another important area of study was the effect of the pelleting process, which includes grinding and then pushing the feed through a die to form the pellets. It was unknown whether the heat used in such a process would reduce tannin bioactivity by altering its structure or increasing the amount of tannin bound to protein. However, an *in vivo* study with young goats showed that the FEC and adult abomasal worm number reductions relative to control were actually greater in SL pellet-fed kids than in those on the ground SL diet (Terrill *et al.*, 2007). Possible explanations for this result were: (i) pelleting improved overall intake of the ration in the goats, leading to greater intake of total tannins, (ii) tannin structure (prodelphinidin to procyanidin ratio and mean degree of polymerization, or molecule size) may be more important than tannin level in the plant, or (iii) tannin bound to protein may be released in the acid environment of the abomasum (Terrill *et al.*, 2007; Kommuru *et al.*, 2014). Regardless of the exact reason for these results, pelleting SL hay can add value to its use as a nutraceutical forage by increasing flexibility for feeding, storage, and shipping.

Additional SL pellet experiments with small ruminants were subsequently completed, both as the primary diet (Kommuru *et al.*, 2014) and as a supplement to animals grazing grass pasture (Gujja *et al.*, 2013; Burke *et al.*, 2014; Hamilton *et al.*, 2017). Furthermore, efficacy of pelleted SL against coccidia (*Eimeria* spp.) of goats was tested in a study where the authors created many conditions conducive to a coccidial outbreak by using recently weaned kids, transporting them for 2 hours in a stock trailer, holding them for 72 hours on pasture, and then placing them into covered pens with either SL leaf-meal pellets or a commercially available goat pellet as the sole diet for a 28-day trial (Kommuru *et al.*, 2014). A second set of kids (20-week-old Spanish bucks) were allowed to graze for 21 days and then moved to the covered pens with the same feeds for a 28-day trial. In Experiment 1, the fecal oocyst count (oocysts per gram, OPG) of control animals increased from 1200 to over 7000 within a week, while the SL pellet-fed goats' OPG decreased (96.9% reduction compared to control) and remained low for the duration of the trial (Kommuru *et al.*, 2014). GIN FEC were reduced by 78.7% in the SL-fed goats after 7 days. In the second experiment, both groups averaged 24,000 OPG at the start of the trial, and the kids fed the SL pellets had a 92.2% lower coccidial OPG after a week, suggesting that feeding SL pellets had both a preventive (Experiment 1) and a therapeutic (Experiment 2) effect against coccidial infection in goats.

In addition to studies with SL grazing, hay, leaf-meal, or pellets, the antiparasitic potential of ensiled SL was tested in naturally parasitized goats with treatment diets of ensiled SL, chopped SL hay, and ground bermudagrass hay at 70% of the diet, with the remainder of the feed consisting of a grain mixture formulated to balance dietary protein and energy. Despite some initial reluctance of the goats to consume the ensiled SL, after a few days, both SL groups were eating at a similar level, and both had significantly lower counts of nematode eggs and coccidial oocysts than goats on the bermudagrass diet during the 28-day trial (Whitley *et al.*, 2018).

To determine the chemical structure of CT tannins in SL, freeze-dried, ground SL leaf and stem material and SL leaf pellets were sent to the laboratory of Professor Irene Mueller-Harvey at the University of Reading, Great Britain. Their analyses revealed much higher tannin content in SL leaves than stems (16.0 g vs 3.3 g/100 g dry weight), larger CT molecules in leaves (42 mean degree of polymerization, mDP) than in stems (18 mDP), and a predominance of prodelphnidin (PD) tannin subunits in both SL leaf and stem CT (98% and 94%, respectively; Mechineni *et al.*, 2014). The concentration of CT in SL leaf-meal pellets was also high (13.2%), with nearly pure PD (97.4%) and high molecular weight compounds (26,316 da or 86 mDP; Kommuru *et al.*, 2014). This work suggested that this unique structure of SL CT was at least partially responsible for its antiparasitic effectiveness against both GIN and coccidia in small ruminants (Kommuru *et al.*, 2014).

To further investigate the potential mechanism of action of SL CT against internal parasites, adult females of *H. contortus* were recovered directly from the abomasum of goats fed SL pellets in a pen study or as a supplement in a bermudagrass grazing study and fixed for scanning electron microscopy examination (Kommuru *et al.*, 2015). Eight of ten worms (3 of 5 in pen study, 5 of 5 in grazing supplement study) from the SL treatment animals showed cuticular damage compared with no damage for the worms recovered from control animals, suggesting a direct effect of SL CT on the cuticle of adult female *H. contortus* in goats (Kommuru *et al.*, 2015).

Additional research is needed to elucidate the antiparasitic mechanism of action in SL, including whether it is due principally to the unique structure of its CT or to the many other secondary compounds in this plant (Baek *et al.*, 2018; Kang *et al.*, 2021), or a combination of both. Application of next-generation analytical techniques, including metabolomics and metagenomics, will likely be useful in determining the role of SL secondary compounds in enhancing the nutraceutical properties of SL (Pannell *et al.*, 2022).

Recent work with SL has focused on expanding the use of this bioactive forage to larger numbers of farmers and a wider geographic area worldwide. Forage quality and yield data for SL grown in small plots in North Carolina, Georgia, Alabama, Louisiana, and Texas (Muir *et al.*, 2014, 2017, 2018) were used, along with soil and weather data from each site, to develop a prediction model for optimal conditions for establishment and production of SL plants (Panda *et al.*, 2020). The model was applied to the entire country of Eswatini in southern Africa, most of which was predicted to be highly suitable for SL production (Panda *et al.*, 2020). Data from on-farm SL production sites in the USA and Africa will be used to validate and improve the prediction models over the next few years.

Research in Mexico on tropical legume trees

The heterogeneous vegetation of the Yucatan Peninsula, known as tropical deciduous forest (TDF), is characterized by its diversity of legume species. This vegetation has been used as food for domestic ruminants since these animals arrived in Mexico with the Spaniards in the 16th century. Despite their importance as animal feed, the contribution of TDF plants in terms of nutritional quality was unknown until recently. Researchers at UADY in Mexico spent four decades describing how sheep and goats consume more than 60 plant species when grazing and browsing in the TDF, as well as identifying the nutritional quality of the plants

and the diet consumed (Torres-Fajardo *et al.*, 2024). The presence of plant secondary compounds (PSC) that were generally considered to be antinutritional was also reported, including saponins, terpenes, and CTs (Sandoval-Castro *et al.*, 2012). When researchers from INRA-ENVT, France, demonstrated that CTs from some temperate Fabaceae species have AH properties (Hoste *et al.*, 2005), the research group at UADY decided to collaborate with the French to investigate the AH activity of CT-rich plants from the TDF of Mexico. In 2000, communication was established between both groups, resulting in several collaborative projects to investigate the AH activity of tropical plants with different PSC, particularly CT-rich plants.

The first plant species evaluated were those for which there was evidence of a high content of phenolic compounds (Armendariz-Yañez and Rivera-Lorca, 2006). The first *in vitro* evaluations of acetone:water extracts (70:30) from the leaves of TDF forage trees (*Acacia pennatula*, *Lysiloma latisiliquum*, *Leucaena leucocephala*, and *Piscidia piscipula*) were carried out at the INRA-ENVT laboratory in Toulouse, France, because the techniques were not available in Mexico. The larval motility inhibition test (LMIT) and larval exsheathment inhibition test (LEIT) were used to demonstrate the AH activity of tropical plant extracts against French isolates of *H. contortus* and *T. colubriformis* (Alonso-Díaz *et al.*, 2008a, b). These studies showed that the activity was associated with the polyphenol content in each extract. The first evaluation carried out in Mexico with *H. contortus* isolated in a temperate zone of Mexico demonstrated the *in vitro* AH activity of the acetone:water extract (70:30) of *Havardia albicans*, a plant species known for its high polyphenol content (Hernández-Orduño *et al.*, 2008).

More recently, research has focused on plant materials normally consumed by sheep and goats in the TDF, including some evaluated previously and others that had not been evaluated: *Acacia collinsi*, *Bunchosia swartziana*, *Gymnopodium floribundum*, and *Mimosa bahamensis* (Castañeda-Ramírez *et al.*, 2017a, 2018). These evaluations confirmed the plants' AH activity against *H. contortus* egg hatching and larval (L3) exsheathment. Pure compounds that were detected in some TDF plant extracts, such as cinnamic acid and its analogues, have also been evaluated (Castañeda-Ramírez *et al.*, 2019; Mancilla-Montelongo *et al.*, 2019). In addition, scanning electron microscopy was used to describe the damage caused to different stages of the GIN life cycle (Martínez-Ortíz-de-Montellano *et al.*, 2013), and transmission microscopy was used to describe damage to the ultrastructure of parasites exposed to extracts (Martínez-Ortiz-de-Montellano *et al.*, 2019; Mancilla-Montelongo *et al.*, 2021a).

When evaluating the TDF plant extracts against *H. contortus* isolates from Mexico, it was evident that some isolates from tropical zones had lower *in vitro* sensitivity to the plant extracts. It was hypothesized that these parasites could be adapted to the polyphenols of plants that are consumed by their ruminant hosts (Chan-Pérez *et al.*, 2016, 2017). Thus, it was important to have bioactive options that are not present in the diet of small ruminants. The latter stimulated the search for other nutraceutical options. The search began by testing agro-industrial by-products, such as *Coffea arabica* spent coffee (Ortiz-Ocampo *et al.*, 2016), the leaves and husks of *Theobroma cacao* (Mancilla-Montelongo *et al.*, 2021a), different spent substrates from the production of edible mushrooms (Castañeda-Ramírez *et al.*, 2022), and leaves of tropical plants that are not present in the diet of ruminants (Castañeda-Ramírez *et al.*, 2020).

The collaboration between Mexico and France has provided innovations to the *in vitro* methodologies in aspects such as the use of the effective concentration 50% (EC50) as a standard methodology for comparison between extracts (Alonso-Díaz *et al.*, 2011). It also initiated the e.g.g hatching inhibition test (EHIT), which is currently used to evaluate extracts of different plants such as *Phytolaca icosandra* (Hernández-Villegas *et al.*, 2011) and other materials (Castañeda-Ramírez *et al.*, 2019Castañeda-Ramírez *et al.*, 2020). This test led to the discovery that tropical plant extracts can cause an ovicidal effect (embryo death) and blocking effect on the hatching of L1, which is the most common effect of PSC (Vargas-Magaña *et al.*, 2014; Chan-Pérez *et al.*, 2016; Castañeda-Ramírez *et al.*, 2017a).

The studies with tropical legumes led to several findings. For example, the AH activity of some CT-rich plant materials is associated with bioactive PSC other than CT (Vargas-Magaña *et al.*, 2014; Hernández-Bolio *et al.*, 2018). It also helped to discover the importance of the age of L3 larvae in the efficiency of the LEIT for *H. contortus* (Castañeda-Ramírez *et al.*, 2017b) and *T. colubriformis* (Mancilla-Montelongo *et al.*, 2020) under tropical conditions. More recently, the group adapted an *in vitro* rumen incubation method, conventionally used t3o evaluate feed digestibility, as a novel test to evaluate the effect of PSC on the exsheatment of L3. This test is based on the principle that *H. contortus* L3 normally exsheath in the rumen liquor of ruminants (Marin-Tun *et al.*, 2023), so the PSC activity inside the animal rumen should affect this process. The test allows evaluation of the bioactive extracts under the conditions of the rumen liquor in terms of pH, temperature, lack of oxygen, and the presence of live bacteria and protozoa (Marin-Tun *et al.*, 2024).

Based on the promising *in vitro* results, several *in vivo* studies were performed. The consumption of *L. latisiliquum* foliage reduced the establishment of *H. contortus* and *T. colubriformis* in goats, and this effect was associated with the polyphenol content in the plant, as confirmed by the addition of polyethylene glycol (PEG) (Brunet *et al.*, 2008a). It was also found that the short-term consumption of *L. latisiliquum* foliage in goats reduced fecal excretion of nematode eggs and the size and fecundity of adult female *H. contortus* (Martínez-Ortíz-de-Montellano *et al.*, 2010). The reduction in the size and fecundity of *H. contortus* females was also reported for sheep consuming the foliage of *H. albicans* (Galicia-Aguilar *et al.*, 2012; Méndez-Ortíz *et al.*, 2012), and more recently, the same activity was reported for sheep consuming *G. floribundum* foliage (Méndez-Ortiz *et al.*, 2019).

The collaboration between France and Mexico led to a series of review articles with suggestions for evaluation of the AH activity of plants under *in vitro* and *in vivo* conditions. Hoste *et al.* (2005) provided the first common document about the use of plants with a direct AH effect against GINs. This was followed by several articles reflecting on important aspects in which the use of plants with a direct effect against GINs was deepened, with special emphasis on plants rich in polyphenols and their use as nutraceuticals (Hoste *et al.*, 2008, 2011, 2012, 2015, 2016. These articles provided advice on the various ways of choosing the plant candidates to be evaluated, the difference between nutraceuticals and phytotherapeutic drugs, and methodological suggestions for *in vitro* and *in vivo* testing. In addition, the need to be aware of possible adverse effects and the importance of considering environmental, technical, economic, and social aspects to optimize the sustainability of the use of these materials were described.

Meanwhile, reviews by Torres-Acosta *et al.* (2008, 2016, 2021), Alonso-Díaz *et al.* (2010), Sandoval-Castro *et al.* (2012), and Torres-Fajardo *et al.* (2020, 2021, 2024) reflected on various issues that should be considered for including polyphenol-rich plants from the TDF as nutraceuticals to improve the nutrition and the health of small ruminants. These articles also reflected on factors that should be considered to favor the sustainability of the use of these materials and understand the aspects that may cause variability in results.

Research Techniques to Determine Antiparasitic Effectiveness of Bioactive Plants

In vitro data

A range of *in vitro* assays targeting different key stages of the life cycle have been applied with a range of sainfoin extracts. The pros and cons of the different *in vitro* assays have been summarized previously (Jackson and Hoste, 2010). These *in vitro* assays are powerful means to address two main objectives. First, they represent nonexpensive ways to screen the potential AH values of a wide range of plant species and/ or of varieties within the same plant species (Paolini *et al.*, 2004). Second, these *in vitro* assays are also a main way to explore potential mechanisms of action of the bioactive PSC, and particularly CT, on GINs.

In vivo results

Briefly, the main consequences of the consumption of CT-containing legume forages on the three key stages of the GIN life cycle have been described, namely adult worms, third-stage larvae L3, and eggs.

- For adult worms, the main effect found was a reduction of egg excretion, contributing to a reduced contamination of pastures. These decreases in egg output have been related to a reduced fertility of female worms and/or reductions in worm numbers.
- A reduced rate of establishment of the third-stage infective larvae (L3) in the host, which means a decrease in the success of animals' infections.
- A decreased rate of development of eggs to L3, which leads to a reduced infectivity and parasitic risk associated with grazing the pastures. Most of the results described have been illustrated with sainfoin, sericea lespedeza, and some models of plants from the TDF (e.g. *Lysiloma latissilicum*), suggesting that these results and conclusions have some generic value (Hoste *et al.*, 2016).
- Variability of results has been found depending on the studies and the model of tannin-containing plants. Different explaining factors have also been identified.
- Besides disturbing effects on worm populations, positive effects on the resilience of the infected animals have been repeatedly measured either by reductions of pathophysiological effects (i.e. anemia due to hemonchosis, diarrhea for other GIN species) and/or maintenance of production (growth and meat production, milk production) despite GIN infections (Hoste *et al.*, 2016).

The Concept of Nutraceuticals

The finding of feed resources combining nutritional and sanitary benefits lead to the concept of nutraceuticals (functional food) in veterinary and human medicine (Andlauer and Fürst, 2002; Hoste *et al.*, 2016). In the specific case of the AH properties of tannin-containing plants, several conditions have been identified to achieve some efficacy against the different stages of GIN (Torres-Fajardo *et al.*, 2021): (i) a plant resource containing tannin with nutritional value for ruminants; (ii) good palatability; (iii) a sufficient threshold of concentration of PSCs (tannins) in the diet; and (iv) adequate length of feed distribution. For CT-rich forages with infected ruminants, different studies suggest that at least 2 weeks' consumption of the diet is needed.

The principal effect of a synthetic AH is to eliminate adult worms, with consequences for the rest of the biological cycle. The expected efficiency in susceptible strains is close to 100%. The overall result is to break the GIN life cycle by eliminating the stages of the parasitic phase with consequences for egg excretion and then, the environmental phases. By comparison with synthetic chemical AHs, bioactive PSCs contained in nutraceutical materials should affect both the parasitic phase and the free-living stages on pastures. Although the expected effects in each of the stages are below 100%, the combination of each relative effect on the three key impacted stages (namely adult worms, eggs, and infective third-stage larvae) of the GIN life cycle contributes to slow the dynamics of infection and reduce the accumulation of worm populations in sheep or goats and, consequently, to reduce and/or delay reliance on synthetic chemical AHs.

Another key difference between the effects of synthetic AH in GIN vs nutraceuticals is the observed variations in results. When launched, the efficiency of a novel synthetic AH molecule is expected to approach 100% (before the rise of AH resistance). In comparison, such high levels of efficacy have never been observed with bioactive forages, whatever the biological stage. By using sainfoin as a model of tannin-containing legume forage, some factors explaining the variability of antiparasitic effects have been identified. Genetic, phenological, and environmental factors related to the plant have been mentioned (Mueller-Harvey et al., 2019). It is suspected that some technological factors used to prepare the forage for ruminant feeding can affect the bioactivity by possible degradation of the bioactive metabolites as mentioned above.

Moreover, some variations in the efficiency of tannins and polyphenols against the worms seem also to depend on the GIN species (see, for example, Paolini et al., 2003b, 2005a). Some results suggest that this is related to the location of worms in the digestive tract (abomasum or small intestine) due to differences in the local environmental conditions (e.g. pH), which could influence interactions between the polyphenols and the different parasitic stages. Another hypothesis is that some intrinsic characteristic of the GIN, such as the quality of some major proteins of the larval sheath, the adult cuticle, and intestinal cells of worms, could also explain the variability.

Suspected Mechanisms of Action

Two hypotheses have been proposed to explain the effects of bioactive plants and their PSCs against GINs. The first suggests some pharmacological-like effects, related to direct consequences of bioactive natural compounds on the different parasitic stages. The second hypothesis supposes some indirect effects by stimulation of the mucosal host response when fed with bioactive fodders. The first hypothesis is mainly supported by in vitro results, since there is no possible involvement of the host immune or inflammatory response in this type of study. Fewer studies have been designed and results obtained to explore the second hypothesis. Last, it is worth underlining that the two hypotheses are nonexclusive. The observed AH effects can be explained by a combination of the two main mechanisms (Hoste et al., 2012).

Besides being a screening tool to identify bioactive plants of interest, the different in vitro assays previously described have also allowed researchers to dissect the modes of action of PSCs against GIN. These studies provided evidence to confirm a role not only of CTs but also different families of flavonoids. Furthermore, besides the concentration of CT, the structure of these polyphenols also influences AH activity (Quijada et al., 2015; Mueller-Harvey et al., 2019). To summarize, synthetic AHs correspond usually to one pure, well-standardized molecule, while the bioactive PSCs are explained by a 'cocktail' of polyphenolics and other molecules with variability in concentrations and quality.

Both in vitro and in vivo studies provided information on the interactions of tannins and other flavonoids with the different parasitic stages (eggs, L3, and adult worms). Observations using scanning and transmission electron microscopy have illustrated changes in different external and internal structures, especially the egg, L3 sheath and digestive tract, or adult cuticle, and intestinal cells (Brunet *et al.*, 2011; Martínez-Ortiz-de-Montellano *et al.*, 2013, 2019). *In vitro* assays also confirmed functional disturbances in some key event of the parasitic life cycle, such as egg hatching, L3 exsheathment, and further penetration into the digestive mucosae (Brunet *et al.*, 2007, 2008b; Hoste *et al.*, 2012; Vargas-Magaña *et al.*, 2014).

How to Use Bioactive Plants as Nutraceuticals

Temperate bioactive legume forages

Sericea lespedeza and sainfoin have been used to compare different ways to exploit the AH effects of CT-containing legumes by comparing grazing vs different preservation forms (hay, silage, dehydrated pellets) (Paolini *et al.*, 2003a, 2005b; Heckendorn *et al.*, 2006; Shaik *et al.*, 2006; Terrill *et al.*, 2007; Werne *et al.*, 2013; Arroyo-Lopez *et al.*, 2014; Gaudin *et al.*, 2016; Whitley *et al.*, 2018). An important question related to these different modes of exploitation concerns the preservation of bioactive PSCs when submitted to different physical affects, namely temperature, fermentations, and pressure. Overall results obtained with these two

temperate legumes indicated that only limited losses in PSC are associated with hay, silage, and pellets, and these technological treatments maintain their AH activities provided that the initial concentration of bioactive compounds in the raw material is high enough. For the specific case of pellets, the commercialization of final products supposes an organization of a whole system of production, from the seeds to the dehydration plants.

The pros and cons of the different modes of exploitation are summarized in Table 7.1 according to diverse criteria. The main advantages of conserved forms are related to easier distribution even on a large scale (exportation in different countries or territories), better standardization of the products and the possibility to characterize the products before use by measuring the level of bioactive PSC. The main disadvantages are related to the economic and environmental costs. In contrast, direct grazing of sainfoin or sericea lespedeza by sheep or goats on pastures corresponds to a higher autonomy of the farm and lower external costs. On the other hand, direct grazing is associated with more factors responsible for variations in the potential AH effects due to a range of additional difficulties which can affect the growth of the forage (meteorological and soil conditions) and the exploitation by infected small ruminants. A recent 4-year survey in France illustrated these

Table 7.1. Pros and cons of the different modes of exploitation of tannin-containing legume forage (sericea lespedeza, sainfoin) according to different criteria.

	Direct grazing	Hay	Silage	Dehydrated pellets
Farm autonomy	+++	+++	+++	+
Agronomical conditions/ technology	Variable	Variable	Variable	+++
Technological treatment of the raw material	Nil	Low	Medium	High
Conservation	+/-	+	+	+++
Measurement of plant secondary metabolites before use	+/-	++	++	+++
Standardization of the products	-	+/-	+/-	+++
Possible exportation	-	+/-	+/-	+++
Economic cost	+	+	++	+++
CO_2 balance	+	+	++	+++

+++ Very likely; ++ likely; + moderate; +/- variable; - not likely.

difficulties of grazing based on three bioactive forages: chicory (*Cichorium intybus*), plantain, and sainfoin (Reccueil_fastoche-2023.pdf (innovin.fr),

Nutraceutical plants from the TDF (Mexico)

The use of PSC-rich plants with AH activity can be designed in different ways depending on each farmer's resources. We can distinguish at least five ways of taking advantage of this type of plant (Alonso-Díaz *et al.*, 2010).

- Use of naturally available bioactive plants from the TDF. The simplest way to take advantage of these resources is to let animals consume the foliage of those bioactive plants that grow naturally in the TDF. Animals can help themselves directly during their grazing/browsing. Feeding behavior studies performed in the TDF showed that animals consume different bioactive plant species daily during the dry and rainy seasons (Torres-Fajardo *et al.*, 2024). Such behavior results in high consumption of PSCs, such as the CT. However, the heterogeneous nature of TDF results in a great variability in the availability of bioactive plants. In addition, sheep and goats show marked preferences for several plant species, and this preference depends on the grazing area and the time of year (Torres-Fajardo *et al.*, 2024). On the other hand, the AH bioactivity of PSC from plant species such as *G. floribundum* varies throughout the year, being higher in the rainy season (when there is a greater possibility of reinfection with GIN) and lower in the dry season when reinfection by GIN is lower (Ortíz-Ocampo *et al.*, 2021). Therefore, it is to be expected that the effect of bioactive plants against GIN varies throughout the year. A disadvantage of using direct grazing is that animals fed under such systems show a protein:energy dietary imbalance since there are often few available pastures and herbaceous plants, so energy supplementation with maize or soghum meal will be required (Torres-Acosta *et al.*, 2021).

- Bioactive trees/shrubs in rows within tropical grass paddocks. Tropical grasses are characterized by their low crude protein content (<7% CP). To improve the nutritional quality of the diet consumed in these paddocks, CP-rich legume trees/shrubs can be planted or allowed to grow inside the grass paddocks. In some cases, these have been placed along pasture paddocks forming rows that should be well planned to prevent their shade from affecting the growth of grasses. The foliage obtained can also be used to supplement the animals in the pen as a 'cut and carry' system. Rows of trees/shrubs allow animals to alternate consumption of grasses and legumes (Sarabia *et al.*, 2023).

- Trees/shrubs in living fences delimiting tropical grass paddocks. Thorny trees such as *H. albicans* could be selected to help prevent the passage of people or animals between the paddocks. The consumption of grasses and foliage of forage legumes should also be favored to obtain a more balanced diet in terms of energy and protein. In this case, trees and shrubs should also be maintained at a height that allows consumption of foliage by animals, but some trees can be left to grow to provide shade in some areas of the paddock, which helps with thermoregulation of animals in these tropical paddocks (Sarabia *et al.*, 2023).

- Establish protein banks for 'cut and carry' or grazing. Bioactive plants can be used as 'forage banks' (Alonso-Díaz *et al.*, 2010). This involves planting large numbers of plants of one or more bioactive species in a small area of a farm. Forage banks are planted as a monoculture with a high density of plants. Using the foliage of the protein banks by 'cut and carry' will include additional daily activity to cut the foliage and deliver it to the animals in their pens. Another way to use the foliage of the protein bank would be to let the animals enter this plantation to consume the foliage for a short period (one or more hours per day). The amount of time that animals should remain inside the protein bank depends on their need for protein-rich foliage, and this depends on the other dietary inputs on the farm. Thus, this will need to be finetuned by the farmers and their advisors to avoid animals destroying the bank but also to avoid negative effects to the animals' health.

- In recent years, agro-industrial by-products with nutraceutical potential have been suggested as part of the animals' diet (Hoste *et al.*, 2022) in temperate and tropical regions. A possible interaction has been proposed between cocoa farmers and sheep and goat farmers, where cocoa farmers could use sheep manure to fertilize their plants while sheep farmers could use the leaves as nutraceutical materials (Mancilla Montelongo *et al.*, 2021b).

Present and Future Issues in Implementing Nutraceutical Materials on Farms

Temperate regions

Although seeds of bioactive (antiparasitic) forages can be sold to individual farmers for use as a grazing crop, sun-drying bioactive forages for hay or processing into ground leaf-meal or pellets will allow commercialization and distribution of nutraceutical materials to a much wider geographic area. This is already under way to a certain degree with sainfoin in Europe and sericea lespedeza in the USA. Farmers in several states in the southern USA are marketing square bales of sericea lespedeza as a nutraceutical hay (R. Edwards, pers. comm.), while leaf-meal pellets are currently being manufactured and marketed throughout the country by a seed company in Alabama (Sims Brothers, Inc., Union Springs, AL). In Europe, the company which has developed sainfoin pellets is Sainfolia Ltd (Viapres le Petit, France).

Tropical forests

Many questions still need to be solved before the commercialization/implementation of TDF plant foliage as natural dewormers. However, it is possible to make more accurate suggestions if one considers the nutritional value *per se* of many of these plants.

- Promote the introduction of trees/shrubs into silvopastoral systems. Most low-income farmers use the TDF vegetation to feed their animals. In these systems, it will be important to optimize the protein intake from the vegetation by implementing an area of tropical grasses in their farms, either for grazing or 'cut and carry.' On the other hand, some farmers have created grass monoculture paddocks, fighting hard for decades to eliminate trees/shrubs from their pastures. These farmers should consider the advantages of having some forage trees/shrubs in their paddocks. Each farmer will need to find the optimal way to transform their grass monocultures into silvopastoral systems in a sustainable manner.

- Implementation of forage banks with bioactive trees/shrubs. There is ample opportunity to implement tree nurseries that could sell plants to farmers who want to 'build' silvopastoral paddocks. Another business option might be to create protein banks large enough to sell nutraceutical foliage. This option could be important in those regions of the world with long periods of drought. During the rainy season, this type of fodder can be sold for selective use in those animals showing signs of GIN infection.

- Optimize the number of bioactive forage/tree/shrub species and the number of individuals of each species. Those farms deciding to keep bioactive forages/trees/shrubs or include these plants in silvopastoral paddock will need advice on the optimal number and species required. It will be necessary to work hand in hand with agronomists and animal nutritionists with experience in the development of silvopastoral systems.

Other Positive Aspects/Benefits of Nutraceutical Fodders

As mentioned previously in this review, the consumption of nutraceutical foliage can help in controlling GIN infections in sheep and goats.

However, recent studies support the hypothesis that there are many other positive effects that can be obtained when CT-rich foliages are included in small ruminant production systems.

Legumes such as sainfoin and sericea lespedeza, and the tropical tree legumes, can fix N2 in the soil, which can help reduce the need for industrial chemical fertilizers in agriculture. Legume trees can help restore degraded soils (Sarabia *et al.*, 2023). Furthermore, sainfoin and legume trees are important sources of nectar and pollen for many species of bees and other pollinators, so these plants can help in providing vital ecosystem services as well as generating valuable products, such as honey.

The consumption of CT-rich legumes can help in reducing the environmental impacts of ruminant production by lowering greenhouse gas emissions (including ruminal methane) and shifting N2 excretion from urine to feces (Niderkorn *et al.*, 2020; Sarabia *et al.*, 2023).

Animals consuming CT-rich fodder and some CT-rich agricultural by-products show positive effects on the organoleptic quality of their products. For example, the meat of lambs and the milk of goats may increase in terms of omega-3 fatty acids (Girard *et al.*, 2016; Menci *et al.*, 2023).

In the TDF, sheep and goats consume the foliage of CT-rich trees and shrubs mainly seeking to obtain macronutrients to cover their maintenance and production requirements (Torres-Fajardo *et al.*, 2024). However, the diet harvested from TDF vegetation can be too high in protein content. Thus, sheep and goats select CT-rich plants as a strategy to block excess dietary protein. In this manner, animals avoid wasting energy to eliminate N in the urine and reduce the possibility of suffering from tympanism due to excess N (Torres-Acosta *et al.*, 2021).

Furthermore, when animals have access to fodder from legume trees/shrubs > 1 m tall, such fodder should usually have a negligible amount of L3 larvae. In this way, much of the tree/shrub foliage can be considered GIN free. This makes it possible to dilute infectivity in a silvopastoral paddock compared to grass monoculture paddocks (Torres-Fajardo *et al.*, 2024).

Future Research

It is essential to deepen our understanding of the mechanisms of action of PSCs in different GIN life stages in order to achieve optimal use of temperate and tropical nutraceutical resources. It is necessary to identify which PSC can be active, as well as the synergies and antagonisms between these compounds in a single plant species or in plant mixtures. This work should be carried out with different methodologies targeting different stages of the GIN life cycle. It is also important to explore the pharmacology of CT and other polyphenols in the hosts (Quijada *et al.*, 2018).

More research should be directed to understand the changes in quantity and quality of PSCs and how they affect bioactivity against GINs. It is also important to understand the potential negative and positive impacts of processing and storage on the biological activity of nutraceutical plant materials. Farmers require clear information about the environmental and plant factors that can cause variability in plant AH activity (Ortíz-Ocampo *et al.*, 2021). This complex task requires the development of low-cost, standardized methods to measure the bioactive compounds and their AH activity, such as near infrared spectroscopy.

The information on quality and quantity of bioactive compounds in plants can be used to develop AI modeling, which could help to predict different scenarios affecting the bioactivity of CT-rich plants. These interactions must then be confronted with the AI models describing and predicting parasite epidemiology. In this manner, we can develop our understanding of the important plant–animal–parasite interactions which can vary from day to day.

Another important interaction deserving further investigation is that between the PSCs in feed and the GIN populations inside the host, including the hosts' immune responses and their digestive metabiome (Correa *et al.*, 2020).

Up to now, most research has mainly been directed to ruminant GINs. However, some studies have shown that these bioactive forages might also represent an alternative to control other digestive parasitic infections (i.e. coccidiosis) in ruminants and other monogastric livestock species (Sandoval-Castro *et al.*, 2012). In this same sense, it is important to use CT bioactive forages as a model to explore therapeutic and prophylactic self-medication in GIN-infected ruminants, as proposed by Lisonbee *et al.* (2009) for temperate légumes and Torres-Fajardo *et al.* (2024) for tropical legumes.

Conclusion

Thirty years after the early results obtained in New Zealand on the potential AH activity of bioactive plants (Niezen *et al.*, 1995, 1998b), a large body of data has been generated worldwide. Over this time, the concept of CT-rich plants has changed from antinutritional or antibloating agents to a richer concept which involves their nutritional value, AH activity, and other positive effects on animal production and the environment. The complexity of this research field required an interdisciplinary approach that involved scientists with a high degree of specialization in a wide range of disciplines (i.e. parasitology, nutrition, animal production, phytochemistry, chemistry, etc.) (Torres-Fajardo

et al., 2020). These researchers have been able to identify the nutraceutical value of CT-rich plants.It will be important to define the required optimal conditions for the use of CT-containing plants to control GIN infections in small ruminants, and that implies even greater research efforts that can harness use of the bioactive materials to affect different key stages in the GIN biological life cycle.

Integrating the use of bioactive forages, trees, and shrubs as nutraceuticals to control GIN parasites of small ruminants into flock and herd management exemplifies the 'One Health' concept. This approach considers animal health, human health (by reducing chemical drug residues in the food and environment), economic sustainability for farmers, and the positive environmental impacts. Incorporating agro-industrial by-products into this strategy presents an opportunity to utilize materials currently considered waste, providing added value while limiting environmental pollution and promoting a circular economy.

References

Alonso-Díaz, M.A., Torres-Acosta, J.F.J., Sandoval-Castro, C.A., Capitello-Leal, C., Brunet, S. *et al.* (2008a) Effects of four tropical tanniniferous plant extracts on the inhibition of larval migration and the exsheathment process of *Trichostrongylus colubriformis* infective stage. *Veterinary Parasitology* 153, 187–192.

Alonso-Díaz, M.A., Torres-Acosta, J.F.J., Sandoval-Castro, C.A., Hervé, H., Aguilar-Caballero, A.J. *et al.* (2011) Comparing the sensitivity of two *in vitro* assays to evaluate the anthelmintic activity of tropical tannin rich plant extracts against *Haemonchus contortus*. *Veterinary Parasitology* 181, 360–364.

Alonso-Díaz, M.A., Torres-Acosta, J.F.J., Sandoval-Castro, C.A., Aguilar-Caballero, A. and Hoste, H. (2008b) *In vitro* larval migration and kinetics of exsheathment of *Haemonchus contortus* larvae exposed to four tropical tanniniferous plant extracts. *Veterinary Parasitology* 153, 313–319. DOI: 10.1016/j.vetpar.2008.01.042.

Alonso-Díaz, M.A., Torres-Acosta, J.F.J., Sandoval-Castro, C.A. and Hoste, H. (2010) Tannins in tropical tree fodders fed to small ruminants: A friendly foe? *Small Ruminant Research* 89, 164–173. DOI: 10.1016/j.smallrumres.2009.12.040.

Andlauer, W. and Fürst, P. (2002) Nutraceuticals: A piece of history, present status and outlook. *Food Research International* 35, 171–176.

Armendariz-Yañez, I.R. and Rivera-Lorca, J.A. (2006) Content of secondary metabolites of some indigenous browse legumes from the Yucatan Peninsula, with particular reference to phenolic compounds. In: Sandoval-Castro, C.A., Howell, F.D., Torres-Acosta, J.F.J. and Ayala-Burgos, A.J. (eds) *Herbivores: Assessment of Intake, Digestibility, and The Roles of Secondary Compounds*. Nottingham University Press, Nottingham, UK.

Arroyo-Lopez, C., Hoste, H., Manolaraki, F., Saratsi, K., Stefanakis, A. *et al.* (2014) Compared effects of two tannin rich resources carob (*Ceratonia siliqua*) and sainfoin (*Onobrychis viciifolia*) on the experimental trickle infections of lambs with *Haemonchus contortus* and *Trichostrongylus colubriformis*. *Parasite* 21, 71–80.

Athanasiadou, S., Githiori, J. and Kyriazakis, I. (2007) Medicinal plants for helminth parasite control: Facts and fiction. *Animal* 1, 1392–1400.

Badar, N., Iqbal, Z., Sajid, M.S. and Rizwan, H. (2017) Documentation of ethnoveterinary practices in district Jhang, Pakistan. *Journal of Animal & Plant Sciences* 27, 398–406.

Baek, K., Lee, T.K., Song, J.H., Choi, E., Ko, H.J. *et al.* (2018) Lignan glycosides and flavonoid glycosides from the aerial portion of *Lespedeza cuneata* and their biological evaluations. *Molecules* 23, 1920.

Borges, A.K.M., Barboza, R.R.D., Souto, W.M.S. and Alves, R. (2020) Natural remedies for animal health in Latin America. In: McGaw, L.J. and Abdalla, M.A. (eds) *Ethnoveterinary Medicine: Present and Future Concepts*. Springer International, Cham, Switzerland, pp. 311–344.

Botha, H. (2015) The use of sericea lespedeza (smart man's Lucerne) in South Africa. In: *Proceedings of the WWWW 2015 International Congress Sustainable Parasitic Controli*, Pretoria, South Africa, pp. 1–2.

Brunet, S., Martínez-Ortiz-de-Montellano, C., Torres-Acosta, J.F.J., Sandoval-Castro, C., Aguilar-Caballero, A. *et al.* (2008b) Effect of the consumption of *Lysiloma latisiliquum* on the larval establishment of parasitic gastrointestinal nematodes in goats. *Veterinary Parasitology* 157, 81–88.

Brunet, S., Aufrere, J., El Babili, F., Fouraste, I. and Hoste, H. (2007) The kinetics of exsheathment of infective nematode larvae is disturbed in the presence of a tannin-rich plant extract (sainfoin) both *in vitro* and *in vivo*. *Parasitology* 134, 1253–1262.

Brunet, S., Jackson, F. and Hoste, H. (2008a) Effects of sainfoin (*Onobrychis viciifolia*) extract and monomers of condensed tannins on the association of abomasal nematode larvae with fundic explants. *International Journal for Parasitology* 38, 783–790.

Brunet, S., Fourquaux, I. and Hoste, H. (2011) Ultrastructural changes in the third-stage, infective larvae of ruminant nematodes treated with sainfoin (*Onobrychis viciifolia*) extract. *Parasitology International* 60, 419–424.

Burke, J.M., Miller, J.E., Mosjidis, J.A. and Terrill, T. (2012a) Grazing sericea lespedeza for control of gastrointestinal nematodes in lambs. *Veterinary Parasitology* 186, 507–512.

Burke, J.M., Miller, J.E., Mosjidis, J.A. and Terrill, T. (2012b) Use of a mixed sericea lespedeza and grass pasture system for control of gastrointestinal nematodes in lambs and kids. *Veterinary Parasitology* 186, 328–336.

Burke, J.M., Miller, J.E., Terrill, T.H., Orlik, S., Acharya, M. *et al.* (2013) Sericea lespedeza as an aid in the control of *Emeria* spp. in lambs. *Veterinary Parasitology* 193, 39–46. DOI: 10.1016/j.vetpar.2012.11.046.

Burke, J.M., Miller, J.E., Terrill, T.H. and Mosjidis, J. (2014) The effects of supplemental sericea lespedeza pellets in lambs and kids on growth rate. *Livestock Science* 159, 29–36.

Castañeda-Ramírez, G.S., Torres-Acosta, J.F.J., Sandoval-Castro, C.A., Gonzalez-Pech, P., Parra-Tabla, V. *et al.* (2017a) Is there a negative association between the content of condensed tannins, total phenols, and total tannins of tropical plant extracts and *in vitro* anthelmintic activity against *Haemonchus contortus* eggs? *Parasitology Research* 116, 3341–3348.

Castañeda-Ramírez, G.S., Mathieu, C., Vilarem, G., Hoste, H., Mendoza-de-Gives, P. *et al.* (2017b) Age of *Haemonchus contortus* third stage infective larvae is a factor influencing the *in vitro* assessment of anthelmintic properties of tannin containing plant extracts. *Veterinary Parasitology* 243, 130–134.

Castañeda-Ramírez, G.S., Rodríguez-Labastida, M., Ortiz-Ocampo, G.I., Gonzalez-Pech, P., Ventura-Cordero, J. *et al.* (2018) An *in vitro* approach to evaluate the nutraceutical value of plant foliage against *Haemonchus contortus*. *Parasitology Research* 117, 3979–3991. DOI: 10.1007/s00436-018-6107-0.

Castañeda-Ramírez, G.S., Torres-Acosta, J.F.J., Sandoval-Castro, C.A., Borges-Argaez, R., Caceres-Farfan, M. *et al.* (2019). Bio-guided fractionation to identify *Senegalia gaumeri* leaf extract compounds with anthelmintic activity against *Haemonchus contortus* eggs and larvae. *Veterinary Parasitology* 270, 13–19.

Castañeda-Ramírez, G.S., Torres-Acosta, J.F.J., Mendoza-de-Gives, P., Tun-Garrido, J., Rosado-Aguilar, J. *et al.* (2020) Effects of different extracts of three *Annona* species on egg-hatching processes of *Haemonchus contortus*. *Journal of Helminthology* 94, e77,1–8.

Castañeda-Ramírez, G.S., Lara-Vergara, I.Y., Torres-Acosta, J.F.J., Sandoval-Castro, C., Sanchez, J. *et al.* (2022) *In vitro* anthelmintic activity of extracts from coffee pulp waste, maize comb waste and *Digitaria eriantha* S. hay alone or mixed, against *Haemonchus contortus*. *Waste and Biomass Valorization* 13, 3523–3533.

Chan-Pérez, J.I., Torres-Acosta, J.F.J., Sandoval-Castro, C.A., Hoste, H., Castaneda-Ramirez, G. *et al.* (2016) *In vitro* susceptibility of ten *Haemonchus contortus* isolates from different geographical origins towards acetone: Water extracts of two tannin rich plants. *Veterinary Parasitology* 217, 53–60.

Chan-Pérez, J.I., Torres-Acosta, J.F.J., Sandoval-Castro, C.A., Castaneda-Ramirez, G., Vilarem, G. *et al.* (2017) Susceptibility of ten *Haemonchus contortus* isolates from different geographical origins towards acetone: Water extracts of polyphenol-rich plants. Part 2: Infective L3 larvae. *Veterinary Parasitology* 240, 11–16.

Correa, P.S., Mendes, L.W., Lemos, L.N., Crouzoulon, P., Niderkorn, V. *et al.* (2020) Tannin supplementation modulates the composition and function of ruminal microbiome in lambs infected with gastrointestinal nematodes. *FEMS Microbiology Ecology* 96, fiaa024.

Galicia-Aguilar, H.H., Rodríguez-González, L.A., Capetillo-Leal, C.M., Camara-Sarmiento, R., Aguilar-Caballero, A. *et al.* (2012) Effect of *Havardia albicans* supplementation on feed consumption and dry matter digestibility of sheep and the biology of *Haemonchus contortus*. *Animal Feed Science and Technology* 176, 178–184.

Gaudin, E., Simon, M., Quijada, J., Schelcher, F., Sutra, J. *et al.* (2016) Efficacy of sainfoin (*Onobrychis viciifolia*) pellets against multi resistant *Haemonchus contortus* and interaction with oral ivermectin: Implications for on-farm control. *Veterinary Parasitology* 227, 122–129.

Girard, M., Dohme-Meier, F., Wechsler, D., Goy, D., Kreuzer, M. *et al.* (2016) Ability of 3 tanniferous forage legumes to modify quality of milk and Gruyère-type cheese. *Journal of Dairy Science* 99, 205–220.

Githiori, J.B., Höglund, J. and Waller, P.J. (2005) Ethnoveterinary plant preparations as livestock dewormers: Practices, popular beliefs, pitfalls and prospects for the future. *Animal Health Research Reviews* 6, 91–103.

Githiori, J.B., Athanasiadou, S. and Thamsborg, S.M. (2006) Use of plants in novel approaches for control of gastrointestinal helminths in livestock with emphasis on small ruminants. *Veterinary Parasitology* 139, 308–320.

Gujja, S., Terrill, T.H., Mosjidis, J.A., Miller, J., Mechineni, A. *et al.* (2013) Effect of supplemental sericea lespedeza leaf meal pellets on gastrointestinal nematode infection in grazing goats. *Veterinary Parasitology* 191, 51–58.

Hamilton, T., Terrill, T., Kommuru, D. and Rivers, A. (2017) Effect of supplemental sericea lespedeza pellets on internal parasite infection and nutritional status of grazing goats. *Journal of Agricultural Science and Technology A* 7, 334–344.

Heckendorn, F., Häring, D.A., Maurer, V., Zinsstag, J., Langhans, W. *et al.* (2006) Effect of sainfoin (*Onobrychis viciifolia*) silage and hay on established populations of *Haemonchus contortus* and *Cooperia curticei* in lambs. *Veterinary Parasitology* 142, 293–300.

Hernández-Bolio, G.I., García-Sosa, K., Escalante-Erosa, F., Castaneda-Ramirez, G., Sauri-Duch, E. *et al.* (2018) Effects of polyphenol removal methods on the *in vitro* exsheathment inhibitory activity of *Lysiloma latisiliquum* extracts against *Haemonchus contortus* larvae. *Natural Product Research* 32, 508–513.

Hernández-Orduño, G., Torres-Acosta, J.F.J., Sandoval-Castro, C., Aguilar-Caballero, A., Reyes Ramirez, R. *et al.* (2008) *In vitro* anthelmintic effect of *Acacia gaumeri*, *Havardia albicans* and Quebracho tannin extracts on a Mexican strain of *Haemonchus contortus* L_3 larvae. *Tropical and Subtropical Agroecosystems* 8, 191–197.

Hernández-Villegas, M.M., Borges-Argaez, R., Rodriguez-Vivas, R.I., Torres-Acosta, J., Mendez-Gonzalez, M. *et al.* (2011) Ovicidal and larvicidal activity of crude extracts of *Phytolacca icosandra* against *Haemonchus contortus*. *Veterinary Parasitology* 179, 100–106.

Hoste, H., Torres-Acosta, J.F., Paolini, V., Aguilar-Caballero, A., Etter, E. *et al.* (2005) Interactions between nutrition and gastrointestinal infections with parasitic nematodes in goats. *Small Ruminant Research* 60, 141–151.

Hoste, H. and Torres-Acosta, J.F.J. (2011) Non-chemical control of helminths in ruminants: Adapting solutions for changing worms in a changing world. *Veterinary Parasitology* 180, 144–154.

Hoste, H., Torres-Acosta, J.F.J., Alonso-Díaz, M.A., Brunet, S., Sandoval-Castro, C. *et al.* (2008) Identification and validation of bioactive plants for the control of gastrointestinal nematodes in small ruminants. *Tropical Biomedicine* 25, 56–72.

Hoste, H., Martinez-Ortiz-De-Montellano, C., Manolaraki, F., Brunet, S., Ojeda-Robertos, N. *et al.* (2012) Direct and indirect effects of bioactive tannin-rich tropical and temperate legumes against nematode infections. *Veterinary Parasitology* 186, 18–27.

Hoste, H., Torres-Acosta, J.F.J., Sandoval-Castro, C.A., Mueller-Harvey, I., Sotiraki, S. *et al.* (2015) Tannin containing legumes as a model for nutraceuticals against digestive parasites in livestock. *Veterinary Parasitology* 212, 5–17.

Hoste, H., Meza-Ocampos, G., Marchand, S., Sotiraki, S., Sarasti, K. *et al.* (2022) Use of agro-industrial by-products containing tannins for the integrated control of gastrointestinal nematodes in ruminants. *Parasite* 29, article number 10.

Hoste, H., Torres-Acosta, J.F.J., Quijada, J., Chan-Perez, I., Dakheel, M. *et al.* (2016) Interactions between nutrition and infections with *Haemonchus contortus* and related gastrointestinal nematodes in small ruminants. *Advances in Parasitology* 93, 239–251.

Howell, S.B., Burke, J.M., Miller, J.E., Terrill, T., Valencia, E. *et al.* (2008) Prevalence of anthelmintic resistance on sheep and goat farms in the southeastern United States. *Journal of the American Veterinary Medical Association* 233, 1913–1919.

Jackson, F. and Hoste, H. (2010) *In vitro* methods for the primary screening of plant products for direct activity against ruminant gastrointestinal nematodes. In: Vercoe, P., Maklar, H. and Schlink, A. (eds) *In Vitro Screening of Plant Resources for Extra-Nutritional Attributes in Ruminants: Nuclear and Related Methodologies*. Springer, Dordrecht, The Netherlands, pp. 25–45.

Kang, H., Yoo, M.J., Yi, S.A., Kim, T.W., Ha, J.W. *et al.* (2021) Phytochemical constituents identified from the aerial parts of *Lespedeza cuneata* and their effects on lipid metabolism during adipocyte maturation. *Separations* 8, 203.

Kaplan, R.M. (2004) Drug resistance in nematodes of veterinary importance: A status report. *Trends in Parasitology* 20, 477–481.

Kommuru, D.S., Barker, T., Desai, S., Burke, J., Ramsay, A. *et al.* (2014) Use of pelleted sericea lespedeza (*Lespedeza cuneata*) for natural control of coccidia and gastrointestinal nematodes in weaned goats. *Veterinary Parasitology* 204, 191–198.

Kommuru, D.S., Whitley, N.C., Miller, J.E., Mosjidis, J., Burke, J. *et al.* (2015) Effect of sericea lespedeza leaf meal pellets on adult female *Haemonchus contortus* in goats. *Veterinary Parasitology* 207, 170–175.

Lange, K.C., Olcott, D.D., Miller, J.E., Mosjidis, J., Terrill, T. *et al.* (2006) Effect of sericea lespedeza (*Lespedeza cuneata*) fed as hay, on natural and experimental *Haemonchus contortus* infections in lambs. *Veterinary Parasitology* 141, 273–278.

Lisonbee, L.D., Villalba, J.J., Provenza, F.D. and Hall, J. (2009) Tannins and self-medication: Implications for sustainable parasite control in herbivores. *Behavioural Processes* 82, 184–189.

Luginbuhl, J.-M., Glennon, H.M., Miller, J.E. and Terrill, T. (2013) Grazing and pasture management. In: *Proceedings of the American Consortium for Small Ruminant Parasite Control 10th Anniversary Conference*, May 20–22, Fort Valley, GA, pp. 63–67.

Mancilla-Montelongo, M.G., Gaudin-Barbier, E., Castañeda-Ramírez, G.S., Canul-Velasco, M., Chan-Perez, J. *et al.* (2021a) *In vitro* evaluation of the nutraceutical potential of *Theobroma cacao* pod husk and leaf extracts for small ruminants. *Acta Parasitológica* 66, 1122–1136.

Mancilla Montelongo, M.G., Sandoval Castro, C.A., Torres-Acosta, F. and García Ceballos, C.A. (2021b) Subproductos agroindustriales: Alimentos nutracéuticos para cabras y borregos. *Bioagrociencias* 14, 32–40.

Mancilla-Montelongo, G., Castañeda-Ramírez, G.S., Torres-Acosta, J.F.J., Sandoval-Castro, C. and Borges-Argaez, R. (2019) Evaluation of cinnamic acid and six analogues against eggs and larvae of *Haemonchus contortus*. *Veterinary Parasitology* 270, 25–30.

Mancilla-Montelongo, M., Castañeda-Ramírez, G.S., Can-Celis, A., Chan-Perez, J., Sandoval-Castro, C. *et al.* (2020) Optimal age of *Trichostrongylus colubriformis* larvae (L3) for the *in vitro* larval exsheathment inhibition test under tropical conditions. *Veterinary Parasitology* 278, 109027.

Manolaraki, F., Sotiraki, S., Stefanakis, A., Skampardonis, V., Volanis, M. *et al.* (2010) Anthelmintic activity of some mediterranean browse plants against parasitic nematodes. *Parasitology* 137, 685–696. DOI: 10.1017/S0031182009991399.

Marin-Tun, C.G., Mancilla-Montelongo, M.G., Torres-Acosta, J.F.J., Capitello-Leal, C., Sandoval-Castro, C. *et al.* (2023) An *in vitro* rumen incubation method to study exsheathment kinetics of *Haemonchus contortus* third-stage infective larvae. *Parasitology Research* 122, 833–845. DOI: 10.1007/s00436-023-07780-z.

Marin-Tun, C.G., Mancilla-Montelongo, M.G., Capetillo-Leal, C.M., Sandoval-Castro, C., Hoste, H. *et al.* (2024) Adapting the *in vitro* rumen incubation method to evaluate the effect of a plant extract on the exsheathment inhibition of *Haemonchus contortus* infective larvae. *Veterinary Parasitology* 327, 110135.

Martínez-Ortíz-de-Montellano, C., Vargas-Magaña, J.J., Canul-Ku, H.L., Miranda-Soberanis, R., Capetillo-Leal, C.M. *et al.* (2010) Effect of a tropical tannin-rich plant *Lysiloma latisiliquum* on adult populations of *Haemonchus contortus* in sheep. *Veterinary Parasitology* 172, 283–290. DOI: 10.1016/j.vetpar.2010.04.040.

Martínez-Ortíz-de-Montellano, C., Arroyo-López, C., Fourquaux, I., Torres-Acosta, J., Sandoval-Castro, C. *et al.* (2013) Scanning electron microscopy of *Haemonchus contortus* exposed to tannin-rich plants under *in vivo* and *in vitro* conditions. *Experimental Parasitology* 133, 281–286.

Martínez-Ortíz-de-Montellano, C., Torres-Acosta, J.F., Fourquaux, I., Sandoval-Castro, C. and Hoste, H. (2019) Ultrastructural study of adult *Haemonchus contortus* exposed to polyphenol-rich materials under *in vivo* conditions in goats. *Parasite* 26, 65.

Mechineni, A., Kommuru, D.S., Gujja, S., Mosjidis, J., Miller, J. *et al.* (2014) Effect of fall-grazed sericea lespedeza (*Lespedeza cuneata*) on gastrointestinal nematode infections of growing goats. *Veterinary Parasitology* 204, 221–228.

Menci, R., Natalello, A., Stamilla, A., Mangano, F., Torrent, A. *et al.* (2023) Chestnut shells in the diet of lamb: Effects on growth performance, fatty acid metabolism, and meat quality. *Small Ruminant Research* 228, 107105.

Méndez-Ortiz, F.A., Sandoval-Castro, C.A., Ventura-Cordero, J., Sarmiento-Franco, L., Santos-Ricalde, R. *et al.* (2019) *Gymnopodium floribundum* fodder as a model for the *in vivo* evaluation of nutraceutical value against *Haemonchus contortus*. *Tropical Animal Health and Production* 51, 1591–1599.

Méndez-Ortíz, F.A., Sandoval-Castro, C.A. and Torres-Acosta, J.F.J. (2012) Short term consumption of *Havardia albicans* tannin rich fodder by sheep: Effects on feed intake, diet digestibility and excretion of *Haemonchus contortus* eggs. *Animal Feed Science and Technology* 176, 185–191.

Mueller-Harvey, I., Bee, G., Dohme-Meier, F., Hoste, H., Karonen, M. *et al.* (2019) Benefits of condensed tannins in forage legumes fed to ruminants: Importance of structure, concentration, and diet composition. *Crop Science* 59, 861–885.

Muir, J.P., Terrill, T.H., Kamisetti, N.R. and Bow, J. (2014) Environment, harvest regimen, and ontogeny change *Lespedeza cuneata* condensed tannin and nitrogen. *Crop Science* 54, 2903–2909.

Muir, J.P., Terrill, T.H., Mosjidis, J.A., Luginbuhl, J., Miller, J. *et al.* (2018) Harvest regimen changes sericea lespedeza condensed tannin, fiber and protein concentrations. *Grassland Science* 64, 137–144. DOI: 10.1111/grs.12186.

Muir, J.P., Terrill, T.H., Mosjidis, J.A., Luginbuhl, J., Miller, J. *et al.* (2017) Season progression, ontogenesis, and environment affect *Lespedeza cuneata* herbage condensed tannin, fiber, and crude protein concentrations. *Crop Science* 57, 515–524.

Niderkorn, V., Barbier, E., Macheboeuf, D., Torrent, A., Mueller-Harvey, I. *et al.* (2020) *In vitro* rumen fermentation of diets with different types of condensed tannins derived from sainfoin (*Onobrychis viciifolia* Scop.) pellets and hazelnut (*Corylus avellana* L.) pericarps. *Animal Feed Science and Technology* 259, 114357.

Niezen, J.H., Waghorn, T.S., Charleston, W.A.G. and Waghorn, G. (1995) Growth and gastrointestinal nematode parasitism in lambs grazing either lucerne (*Medicago sativa*) or sulla (*Hedysarum coronarium*) which contains condensed tannins. *Journal of Agricultural Science* 125, 281–289.

Niezen, J.H., Waghorn, G.C. and Charleston, W.A.G. (1998a) Establishment and fecundity of *Ostertagia circumcincta* and *Trichostrongylus colubriformis* in lambs fed lotus (*Lotus pedunculatus*) or perennial ryegrass (*Lolium perenne*). *Veterinary Parasitology* 78, 13–21.

Niezen, J.H., Robertson, H.A., Waghorn, G.C. and Charleston, W.A.G. (1998b) Production, faecal egg counts and worm burdens of ewe lambs which grazed six contrasting forages. *Veterinary Parasitology* 80, 15–27.

Ortiz-Ocampo, G., Chan-Pérez, J.I., Covarrubias-Cárdenas, A.G. and Santos-Ricalde, R. (2016) Efecto antihelmíntico *in vitro* e *in vivo* de residuos de *Coffea arabica* sobre un aislado de *Haemonchus contortus* con baja susceptibilidad a taninos. *Tropical and Subtropical Agroecosystems* 19, 41–50.

Ortíz-Ocampo, G.I., Sandoval-Castro, C.A., Mancilla-Montelongo, G., Castaneda-Ramirez, G., Chan-Perez, J. *et al.* (2021) Variabilidad en el contenido de polifenoles, actividad biológica y antihelmíntica de extractos metanol:agua de las hojas de *Gymnopodium floribundum* Rolfe. *Revista Mexicana de Ciencias Pecuarias* 12, 1168–1187.

Panda, S.S., Terrill, T.H., Mahapatra, A.K., Kelly, B., Morgan, E. *et al.* (2020) Site-specific forage management of sericea lespedeza: Geospatial technology-based forage quality and yield enhancement model development. *Agriculture* 10, 419.

Pannell, D., Kouakou, B., Terrill, T.H., Ogunade, I., Estrada-Reyes, Z. *et al.* (2022) Adding dried distillers grains with solubles influences the rumen microbiome of meat goats fed lespedeza or alfalfa-based diets. *Small Ruminant Research* 214, 106747.

Paolini, V., Dorchies, P. and Hoste, H. (2003a) Effects of sainfoin hay on gastrointestinal infection with nematodes in goats. *Veterinary Record* 152, 600–601.

Paolini, V., Frayssines, A., De La Farge, F., Dorchies, P. and Hoste, H. (2003b) Effects of condensed tannins on established populations and on incoming larvae of *Trichostrongylus colubriformis* and *Teladorsagia circumcincta* in goats. *Veterinary Research* 34, 331–339.

Paolini, V., Fouraste, I. and Hoste, H. (2004) *In vitro* effects of three woody plant and sainfoin extracts on 3rd-stage larvae and adult worms of three gastrointestinal nematodes. *Parasitology* 129, 69–77. DOI: 10.1017/S0031182004005268.

Paolini, V., Prevot, F., Dorchies, P. and Hoste, H. (2005a) Lack of effects of quebracho and sainfoin hay on incoming third-stage larvae of *Haemonchus contortus* in goats. *Veterinary Journal* 170, 260–263.

Paolini, V., De La Farge, F., Prevot, F., Dorchies, P. and Hoste, H. (2005b) Effects of the repeated distribution of sainfoin hay on the resistance and the resilience of goats naturally infected with gastrointestinal nematodes. *Veterinary Parasitology* 127, 277–283. DOI: 10.1016/j.vetpar.2004.10.015.

Quijada, J., Fryganas, C., Ropiak, H.M., Ramsay, A., Mueller-Harvey, I. *et al.* (2015) Anthelmintic activities against *Haemonchus contortus* or *Trichostrongylus colubriformis* from small ruminants are influenced by structural features of condensed tannins. *Journal of Agricultural and Food Chemistry* 63, 6346–6354.

Quijada, J., Drake, C., Gaudin, E., El-Korso, R., Hoste, H. *et al.* (2018) Condensed tannin changes along the digestive tract in lambs fed with sainfoin pellets or hazelnut skins. *Journal of Agricultural Food Chemistry* 66, 2136–2142.

Rodríguez-Hernández, P., Reyes-Palomo, C., Sanz-Fernández, S., Rufino-Moya, P., Zafra, R. *et al.* (2023) Antiparasitic tannin-rich plants from the south of Europe for grazing livestock: A review. *Animals* 13, 201.

Rose Vineer, H., Morgan, E.R., Hertzberg, H., Bartley, D., Bosco, A. *et al.* (2020) Increasing importance of anthelmintic resistance in European livestock: Creation and meta-analysis of an open database. *Parasite* 27, 69.

Sandoval-Castro, C.A., Torres-Acosta, J.F.J., Hoste, H., Salem, A. and Chan-Perez, J. (2012) Using plant bioactive materials to control gastrointestinal tract helminths in livestock. *Animal Feed Science and Technology* 176, 192–201.

Sarabia, L., Solorio, F., Galindo, F., Rojas-Hernández, S., Sánchez, R. *et al.* (2023) Tropical trees and shrubs for healthy agroecosystems, including animal health and welfare. In: Fiebrig, I.N. (ed.) *Medicinal Agroecology: Review, Case Studies, and Research Methodologies*. CRC Press, Boca Raton, Florida, pp. 155–174.

Shaik, S.A., Terrill, T.H., Miller, J.E. and Kouakou, B. (2004) Effects of feeding sericea lespedeza hay to goats infected with *Haemonchus contortus*. *South African Journal of Animal Science* 34(Suppl. 1), 248–250.

Shaik, S.A., Terrill, T.H., Miller, J.E., Kouakou, B., Kannan, G. *et al.* (2006) Sericea lespedeza hay as a natural deworming agent against gastrointestinal nematode infection in goats. *Veterinary Parasitology* 139, 150–157.

Terrill, T.H. and Mosjidis, J.A. (2015) Smart man's lucerne and worm control. In: *Proceedings of the WWWW 2015 International Congress Sustainable Parasitic Control*, Pretoria, South Africa, pp. 25–26.

Terrill, T.H., Windham, W.R., Evans, J.J. and Hoveland, C. (1990) Condensed tannin concentraton in sericea lespedeza as influenced by preservation method. *Crop Science* 30, 219–224. DOI: 10.2135/cropsci1990.0011183X003000010047x.

Terrill, T.H., Mosjidis, J.A., Moore, D.A., Shaik, S., Miller, J. *et al.* (2007) Effect of pelleting on efficacy of sericea lespedeza hay as a natural dewormer in goats. *Veterinary Parasitology* 146, 117–122. DOI: 10.1016/j.vetpar.2007.02.005.

Torres-Acosta, J.F.J. and Hoste, H. (2008) Alternative or improved methods to limit gastro-intestinal parasitism in grazing sheep and goats. *Small Ruminant Research* 77, 159–173.

Torres-Acosta, J.F.J., Alonso-Díaz, M.A., Hoste, H. and Sandoval-Castro, C. (2008) Efectos negativos y positivos del consumo de forrajes ricos en taninos en la producción de caprinos. *Tropical and Subtropical Agroecosystems* 9, 83–90.

Torres-Acosta, J.F.J., Gonzalez-Pech, P.G., Ortiz-Ocampo, G.I., Rodriguez-Vivas, I., Tun-Garrido, J. *et al.* (2016) Revalorizando el uso de la selva baja caducifolia para la reproducción de rumiantes. *Tropical and Subtropical Agroecosystems* 19, 73–80.

Torres-Acosta, J.F.J., Sandoval-Castro, C.A., González-Pech, P.G. and Mancilla-Montelongo, G. (2021) Interacción entre la nutrición y los nematodos gastrointestinales en pequeños rumiantes pastoreando la selva baja caducifolia – contribuciones de la FMVZ-UADY. *Tropical and Subtropical Agroecosystems* 24, 1–18.

Torres-Fajardo, R.A., González-Pech, P.G., Sandoval-Castro, C.A. and Torres-Acosta, J. (2020) Small ruminant production based on rangelands to optimize animal nutrition and health: Building an interdisciplinary approach to evaluate nutraceutical plants. *Animals* 10, 11–32.

Torres-Fajardo, R.A., González-Pech, P.G., Torres-Acosta, J.F.J. and Sandoval-Castro, C. (2021) Nutraceutical potential of the low deciduous forest to improve small ruminant nutrition and health: A systematic review. *Agronomy* 11, 1403.

Torres-Fajardo, R.A., Ortíz-Domínguez, G.A., González-Pech, P.G. and Sandoval-Castro, C. (2024) The complexity of goat feeding behaviour: A historical overview from decades of research in the tropical low deciduous forest. *Small Ruminant Research* 231, 107199.

Vargas-Magaña, J.J., Torres-Acosta, J.F.J., Aguilar-Caballero, A.J., Sandoval-Castro, C., Hoste, H. *et al.* (2014) Anthelmintic activity of acetone–water extracts against *Haemonchus contortus* eggs: Interactions between tannins and other plant secondary compounds. *Veterinary Parasitology* 206, 322–327.

Werne, S., Perler, E., Maurer, V., Probst, J., Hoste, H. *et al.* (2013) Effect of sainfoin and faba bean on gastrointestinal nematodes in periparturient ewes. *Small Ruminant Research* 113, 454–460.

Whitley, N., Terrill, T., Griffin, E. and Greer-Mapson, L. (2018) Effect of ensiling on efficacy of sericea lespedeza against gastrointestinal nematodes and coccidia in goats. *Journal of Agricultural Science and Technology A* 8, 377–387.

8 Diagnostics for the Management of Gastrointestinal Nematode Infections in Small Ruminants

Adriano F. Vatta*

Department of Pathobiological Sciences, Louisiana State University School of Veterinary Medicine, Baton Rouge, Louisiana, USA

Abstract

In wishing to manage gastrointestinal nematode parasites, it is important that a diagnosis of parasitism is made and, insofar as is possible, the species of parasites and their relative abundance should be determined. This chapter focuses on the diagnosis of gastrointestinal nematode parasites in small ruminants and provides information on collecting, storing, and shipping fecal samples, quantitative fecal egg counts (including the McMaster, Mini-FLOTAC, centrifugal fecal flotation, and automated fecal egg counting methods), and parasite identification (including the fluorescein-labeled peanut agglutinin method, coproculture, and molecular-based approaches to parasite identification). Tests for liver flukes, lungworms, and tapeworms are described and measuring packed cell volume, evaluating pasture contamination with infective larvae, and the use of necropsy are also discussed. A review of the methods available for testing for anthelmintic resistance (including the use of the fecal egg count reduction test, egg hatch and larval development assays, and sequencing to determine the frequency of resistance-conferring genetic mutations) concludes the chapter.

Introduction

This chapter is intended to provide the readership of this book, including university researchers and instructors, practicing veterinarians, extension specialists, and animal science and veterinary science students (at both undergraduate and graduate levels), with a summary of the parasitology diagnostic procedures currently available or likely to become available for routine diagnosis in small ruminants in the near future. The chapter will provide a brief description of the diagnostic methods most applicable to sheep and goats, when the methods might be used, and what their advantages and limitations are. Our aim is to provide some guidance on how the various diagnostic techniques may be used as part of a parasite management plan. This chapter is not intended to provide standard operating procedures or to outline the procedures in detail, but brief descriptions of the methods will be provided together with further references that the reader may then consult when necessary. In this regard, one useful reference is Veterinary Clinical Parasitology by Zajac *et al.* (2021).

In sheep or goat farming, we are most often concerned with the effects of parasites in the herd or flock, rather than the individual animal. However, many people keep sheep, goats, or camelids as pets and are distinctly interested in

*Corresponding author: avatta2@lsu.edu

© CAB International 2026. *Management Practices for Controlling Nematode Parasites of Small Ruminants* (eds James E. Miller and Joan M. Burke)
DOI: 10.1079/9781800623767.0008

the health and wellbeing of specific individual animals. When one of these individuals becomes sick and we suspect gastrointestinal nematode parasitism to be the cause of the illness, a thorough physical examination is required. We would like to know the degree to which the host is infected and the species of parasites infecting the host. In such cases, identification of the parasite species may not always be possible, and we may have to use past experience to help us, such as knowledge that *Haemonchus contortus* or barber pole worm is the predominant parasite in our small ruminants at this time of year. Nevertheless, to estimate the degree to which the animal is infected, use of a quantitative diagnostic method, such as a fecal egg count, is required. The results of the test, the egg count in our case, will then be evaluated together with any abnormal findings on physical examination, such as pale mucous membranes, to decide whether a diagnosis of parasitism is warranted.

In the more common situation where we are concerned with parasitism in the herd or flock as a whole, which is likely of more relevance to the readership of this book, quantitative diagnostic methods, of which fecal egg counts are the most commonly used, are also needed. Fecal egg counts for a herd or flock will indicate which individual animals are shedding parasite eggs heavily on pasture and are contributing to a significant build-up of infective larvae, which in turn poses the threat of heavy infection to other members of the group, if the heavy-shedding individuals are not treated. Fecal egg counts may therefore be used to identify individuals to be treated.

While it is never our aim (and indeed, it is impossible) to eliminate parasites from the herd or flock completely, it may occasionally be necessary to treat a large proportion of the herd or flock and fecal egg counts may then be used to estimate when to intervene at the herd basis to prevent clinical disease. Please note that the correlation between egg count and actual worm burden in ruminants is, at best, nematode species specific, and is influenced by such factors as the ages of the animals and their reproductive status. This makes it difficult to define what constitutes a 'heavily shedding' individual. Nonetheless, over time, veterinarians and producers do develop their own cut-offs for treatment based on egg count. It should also be

noted, at least for barber pole worm infection, that the use of the FAMACHA© system, rather than egg count, is recommended to identify individuals that are clinically affected by parasitism and require treatment.

With the widespread occurrence of anthelmintic (dewormer) resistance, diagnostics are used not only for assessing the severity of a gastrointestinal parasite infection in a herd or flock, but also to assess the resistance status of the parasites on a farm. Fecal egg counts, for example, are used in the fecal egg count reduction test to estimate the level of anthelmintic resistance on a farm (Kaplan *et al.*, 2023).

Collecting, Storing, and Shipping Fecal Samples

Fecal samples should be collected directly from the rectum whenever possible. Samples picked up from the ground may be contaminated with soil and bedding, as well as nonparasitic free-living nematodes which, if the feces are cultured, will contaminate the cultures. It is advisable that an experienced person train others attempting to collect feces from the rectum for the first time. The sheep or goat should be properly restrained, and the feces carefully extracted from the rectum using the fingers. Disposable gloves should be worn and changed between animals and lubricant should be used. Fecal samples should be collected individually in suitable containers (such as small cups with lids or Ziploc® bags).

As recommended by Dunn (1969), the container should be filled as full as possible and the container sealed with the lid, to exclude as much air as possible. Nematode eggs require oxygen to develop, so excluding air will stop any eggs present from hatching in the feces. This is especially relevant where the samples are to be shipped to a laboratory.

Fecal samples should be transported in a cooler box with ice. The samples should be stored in a refrigerator overnight or when not in use in the laboratory. Fecal samples for fecal egg count or coproculture should never be frozen, to preserve egg viability and morphology (Van Wyk and Van Wyk, 2002). In this regard, when samples are placed in a cooler, they should not be in direct contact with the ice, as direct contact with icepacks can cause the feces to freeze. Feces intended for culture should not be refrigerated for more than 1 day before delivery to the lab, because this could interfere with the hatching of the eggs and development of the larvae. Although egg counts conducted on fecal samples that have been properly refrigerated for 2–3 weeks may still give valid results, a good rule of thumb is to complete the egg counts within 7 days.

Sometimes, for reason of cost or time, fecal egg counts may be conducted on pooled fecal samples. In such cases, samples from individual animals should be submitted and the feces pooled in the laboratory, where the personnel can weigh the same amount of feces from each animal prior to pooling the weighed feces and conducting the count.

Quantitative Fecal Egg Counts

Fecal egg counts are the most commonly used method to diagnose gastrointestinal nematode infections. In many cases, a fecal egg count will be performed to confirm a diagnosis of parasitism when an animal or group of animals is showing signs indicative of worm infection, such as pale mucous membranes, bottlejaw, diarrhea, or poor body condition. In other cases, fecal egg counts will be used as a surveillance or monitoring tool to track the infection level in a herd or flock or the levels of egg shedding on pasture. Fecal egg counts are one of the best tools we have on hand to monitor gastrointestinal nematode infections, but they are not without their own limitations. Before we discuss some of the commonly used fecal egg count methods, it is useful to consider some of these limitations.

We can start with a consideration of the technical limitations of the actual tests. For a full discussion of certain concepts as they apply to fecal egg counts, including sensitivity, accuracy, precision, and detection limit, we refer the reader to Nielsen (2021). Nielsen (2021) defines diagnostic accuracy as 'a measure of how close a test measures to the true value of a given sample,' which, in the case of fecal egg counts, is 'a measure of how close a determined egg count is to the true count of the sample.' Recognizing that some loss of eggs should always be expected during the preparation of a fecal sample for egg counting, accuracy may be defined 'by the egg

loss occurring during processing and flotation' (Nielsen, 2021). The problem with trying to measure accuracy of fecal egg counts is that the true count of the sample is never known. Precision, on the other hand, is 'a measure of variation between repeated measures on the same sample and is synonymous with repeatability' (Nielsen, 2021). In contrast with accuracy, the precision of a technique may be estimated and has important implications for fecal egg counting. For example, poor precision will increase data variability, which will mask statistically significant differences between pre- and posttreatment counts when performing a fecal egg count reduction test. (The fecal egg count reduction test is discussed below.)

We should also consider the biological sources of variation in egg counts. A fecal nematode egg count is simply a measure of the concentration of nematode eggs in the feces. However, nematode eggs are not distributed evenly throughout the feces, which can contribute to variation between egg counts performed on separate subsamples of the same fecal sample. Any factors that affect the consistency of the feces will also affect the final egg count. For example, the number of eggs per gram of feces may be vastly underestimated in diarrheic feces compared with what the egg count would have been in normally formed feces, because the eggs are diluted by the extra fluid in the fecal material. In such cases, it is important to realize that a low egg count, by itself, may not be a good measure of whether the animal is suffering from gastrointestinal parasitism. The different species of nematodes also shed eggs at dramatically different levels. For example, *H. contortus* is a prolific egg layer while *Trichostrongylus* spp. produce many fewer eggs. Therefore, theoretically speaking, since pure infections seldom occur, a fecal egg count of 2000 eggs per gram of feces (epg) of a pure *Trichostrongylus colubriformis* infection in a sheep may be significant while a fecal egg count of 2000 epg of a pure *H. contortus* infection in a sheep may not be of concern (see Hansen and Perry, 1994, p.79, for a proposed interpretation of level of infection based on fecal egg count).

As alluded to previously, fecal egg counts are a poor measurement of actual worm burden. We can expect all grazing animals to be infected with gastrointestinal nematodes, but some individuals may have levels that are too low to detect with a fecal egg count. This may be for several reasons. First, eggs are only laid by mature female nematodes. A fecal egg count will tell us nothing about the presence or absence of adult male and immature nematodes in the animal, which may be affecting its health. A positive fecal egg count will tell us that the animal is infected, but failure to demonstrate eggs (or larvae) in a fecal sample does not definitively mean that the animal is worm free, as adult males and immatures of both sexes may be present. Indeed, as far as immature worms are concerned, grazing animals are likely to be ingesting infective larvae on a constant basis, at least during times when conditions for the survival of the larvae on pasture are favorable. In turn, a proportion of these larvae will be developing towards maturity in the animal. If the adult worm burden has been removed through anthelmintic treatment or host immune responses, at the time of sampling, few or no eggs will be seen because the majority of the worm population in the host will be immature.

Sometimes when we treat animals that harbor resistant worms, resistant female worms will survive but not lay eggs. This occurs with resistance to the benzimidazoles and moxidectin. When the drug does not kill the worms, it suppresses the females' egg-laying ability, making fecal egg counts unreliable in detecting the presence of worms. Egg-laying may resume after some time but if egg counts are conducted too soon after treatment, the presence of the worms will be missed.

Fecal egg counts are a better indication of worm burden in young animals which are still developing an immunity to the parasites than in older animals, but the degree to which immunity develops to the various parasite species and the age of onset of such immunity vary greatly in individual young animals too. Host immune mechanisms act on nematodes in several ways, for example by limiting the establishment of nematode infections, by expelling worms that have established, or by limiting the number of eggs laid by females (Dobson *et al.*, 1992). The ability of the host to use these mechanisms for its own protection will depend on the nematode species involved. Factors such as the age, sex, breed, nutritional status, and reproductive status of the host will also play important roles in the expression of these immune mechanisms. As such, the numbers of parasites present in

an animal and in particular, as far as fecal egg counts are concerned, the numbers of eggs laid by the females of that worm population will be affected by the host immunity–parasite interactions.

Parasites are said to be overdispersed within a population of host animals, which means that a small proportion of the herd or flock (~20–30%) will be infected with most of the parasites (~70–80%). If we do not examine a representative number of animals in the flock or herd, we run the risk of either severely underestimating or overestimating the worm burden in the host population. When trying to understand the infection status of the herd or flock as a whole, rather than that of an individual animal, it is better to sample more animals than fewer. For example, Hansen and Perry (1994) recommend that where there are 1–10 animals, all animals should be sampled; where there are 11–25, at least 10 animals; and where there are 26–100 animals, at least 30 animals. Whenever possible, include in the sampling those individual animals which are in poor body condition or showing signs typically associated with clinical parasitism such as pale mucous membranes (anemia), bottle jaw (hypoproteinemia), or diarrhea.

Fecal egg counts will most often be a composite of eggs from different nematode species, even if one species predominates at a certain time of the year. Whether a fecal egg count is considered low, moderate, or high will depend on the host (sheep or goat), but also on the species composition of the nematodes in the gastrointestinal tract at the time the egg count is conducted. Certain nematode species such as *H. contortus*, the barber pole worm, are prolific egg layers while others such as *Teladorsagia circumcincta* and *Trichostrongylus* spp. are considerably less prolific than *H. contortus*. Producers who have farmed, and veterinarians who have practiced, in a particular area for many years will be useful sources of information regarding the local parasite epidemiology, including the parasite species that predominate during different seasons of the year. Nonetheless, nematode species composition will also vary greatly from farm to farm and across seasons. As will be discussed below, laboratory techniques may (and should) be used to determine the species composition of the nematode population present in the herd or flock at different times of the year. This is important to know because different worms differ in their pathogenicity and cause different clinical signs.

Different fecal egg counting techniques are better suited to quantify the egg count at lower or higher egg counts. This is related to the so-called multiplication factor that is used and will be discussed in the following sections. Here we consider the McMaster method, the Mini-FLOTAC method, centrifugal fecal flotation methods, and automated methods. We will discuss the strengths and important limitations of each method and consider when they each might best be used in the diagnosis of gastrointestinal nematode parasitism.

McMaster method

The McMaster method (Gordon and Whitlock, 1939) is the most widely used and recommended method for fecal examination in sheep and goats. In fact, when we speak about fecal egg counts in small ruminants, we tend to assume that fecal egg counts by the McMaster method are being discussed!

In brief, to perform a McMaster fecal egg count (Fig. 8.1.), a small amount of feces (for example, 2 g) is weighed and mixed with a measured quantity of flotation solution (for example, 28 ml salt solution). The suspension is strained (for example, through a tea strainer or cheese cloth). The strained suspension is mixed and the chambers of a McMaster slide are filled (there may be two or three chambers, depending on the design). After allowing any eggs present in the sample to float in the chambers, all the eggs within the scored grid on each chamber of the slide are counted. The eggs counted are then multiplied by a factor to derive the number of eggs per gram of feces in the sample. In our example, using 2g feces, 28 ml salt solution, and a McMaster slide with two chambers, each with a volume of 0.15 ml, the multiplication factor is calculated as $(30\,ml/2\,g)/0.30\,ml = 50$. The method is easily learned and, in that sense, can

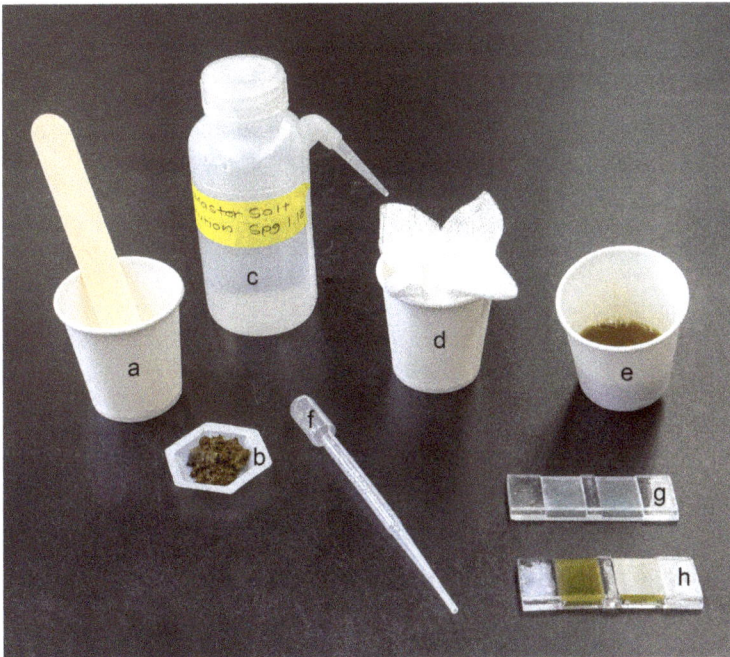

Fig. 8.1. Items required to perform a McMaster fecal egg count, in various stages of preparation: (a) cup and tongue depressor (for mixing); (b) feces; (c) flotation solution; (d) cup with gauze for straining the fecal suspension; (e) cup containing strained fecal suspension; (f) pipette; (g) clean McMaster slide; and (h) McMaster slide with filled chambers. Photo credit: Christopher Jones, Louisiana State University.

be used by anyone with an interest in performing fecal egg counts, including veterinarians, animal scientists, veterinary technicians, and producers. However, it does require that those performing the egg counts be trained. There is also some capital outlay for the purchase of a standard compound microscope and the McMaster slides, as well as flotation solutions (or the ingredients to produce these in house) and ancillary items.

The McMaster method is used to determine the number of strongylid eggs per gram in a fecal sample. As such, the test is quantitative and most often used because it allows for easy quantification of the nematode eggs in a sample when moderate and high infections are present. Commonly, as in our example above, the multiplication factor used is 50 epg, which makes the method less useful for detecting eggs when light infections are present.

Strongylid eggs are those produced by nematodes in the taxonomic order Strongylida, which includes nematodes in the superfamilies Strongyloidea and Trichostrongyloidea. These include the common nematodes *H. contortus*, *Trichostrongylus* spp., *T. circumcincta*, *Oesophagostomum* spp., *Chabertia ovina*, and others. The eggs of these nematodes cannot easily and reliably be differentiated from each other and are therefore not differentiated during fecal egg counts. This is the reason why laboratories will report strongyle-type or, more commonly, trichostrongyle-type eggs. That said, eggs of the nematodes *Nematodirus*, *Trichuris*, and *Strongyloides* may also be noted when carrying out a McMaster count. These eggs have characteristics that allow them to be easily identified and differentiated from other eggs. Similarly, eggs of tapeworms (cestodes), for example, *Moniezia expansa*, and oocysts of coccidia (*Eimeria* spp.) may be detected.

Tapeworm eggs are never quantitatively evaluated using the McMaster method. Tapeworms shed segments (proglottids) which contain the eggs, and the segments are mostly passed out intact. Tapeworm eggs are only detected in the feces if the eggs have been expelled from the segments while inside the digestive tract of the host or if the segments have ruptured. All parasite eggs, including tapeworm eggs, are not evenly distributed throughout the feces and given the erratic presence of tapeworm

eggs in the feces, attempting to determine whether an animal is infected with tapeworms through fecal examination for the eggs is not a reliable or useful method. Therefore, while finding tapeworm eggs during a fecal examination will indicate infection, their absence does not confirm that the animal is not infected. The producer would do better to look for the presence of the tapeworm segments on the fecal pellets or to note whether any tapeworms are protruding from the anus rather than relying on egg counts to detect infection.

Oocysts of coccidia (*Eimeria* spp.) may be enumerated and an oocyst per gram (opg) count determined, though this is rarely done for diagnostic purposes. Based on a visual estimate of the number of oocysts noted in each chamber of the McMaster slide, the presence of oocysts may be subjectively scored (for example, on a scale of 1+ to 4+, where 0 would indicate no oocysts seen, a score of 1+ would indicate a few oocysts seen, and a score of 4+ would indicate many oocysts, too numerous to count). There is, however, no correlation between oocyst count and severity of disease, and disease may occur before infections become patent. Rather, the presence of clinical signs consistent with coccidiosis together with finding oocysts on fecal examination suggest coccidiosis as a diagnosis. One cannot diagnose coccidiosis based on the presence of oocysts alone.

One drawback of the McMaster method is that it has a relatively high multiplication factor. As discussed above, the multiplication factor, or conversion factor, is the value by which the number of actual eggs counted is multiplied to derive the number of eggs per gram of feces (Nielsen, 2021). This means, for example, that if the multiplication factor is 50, detecting a single egg using the McMaster method will give a result of 50 epg. Conversely, not detecting the single egg will result in the sample being recorded as having no parasite eggs detected. If fecal egg counts are <50 epg, the McMaster is likely to yield a negative result, but it does not mean that there are no eggs present. Also, as noted previously, the eggs of most parasitic strongylid nematodes cannot be accurately differentiated from each other during a McMaster fecal egg count (or indeed, any method of direct fecal examination for eggs). To identify *H. contortus* or barber pole worm eggs in feces, a fluorescein-labeled peanut agglutinin test (Palmer and McCombe, 1996) may be requested from a laboratory that offers the test.[1] Alternatively, a fecal coproculture needs to be prepared or one of the new molecular-based methods needs to be used (see below).

Aside from the limitations of the McMaster method, it is still the most practical method for gastrointestinal parasite monitoring in sheep and goats.

Take-home message: Use the McMaster method as your first choice for routine monitoring of fecal egg counts in sheep and goats. Choose the McMaster method especially when the egg counts are expected to be moderate to high.

Mini-FLOTAC

The Mini-FLOTAC system (Cringoli *et al.*, 2017) is sold as a kit consisting of a Fill-FLOTAC apparatus, a Mini-FLOTAC counting chamber, and an adaptor for a standard compound microscope stage to facilitate the reading of the counting chamber (Fig. 8.2).[2] The Fill-FLOTAC apparatus consists of a plastic cup with a screw-on lid, through which a conical collector passes. The lid also contains a built-in sieve and a capped outlet port. The opening of the conical collector is such that when the screw-on lid is held upside down in your hand, it resembles a miniature martini glass, which, for the ruminant version of the system, is designed to hold 5 g feces.

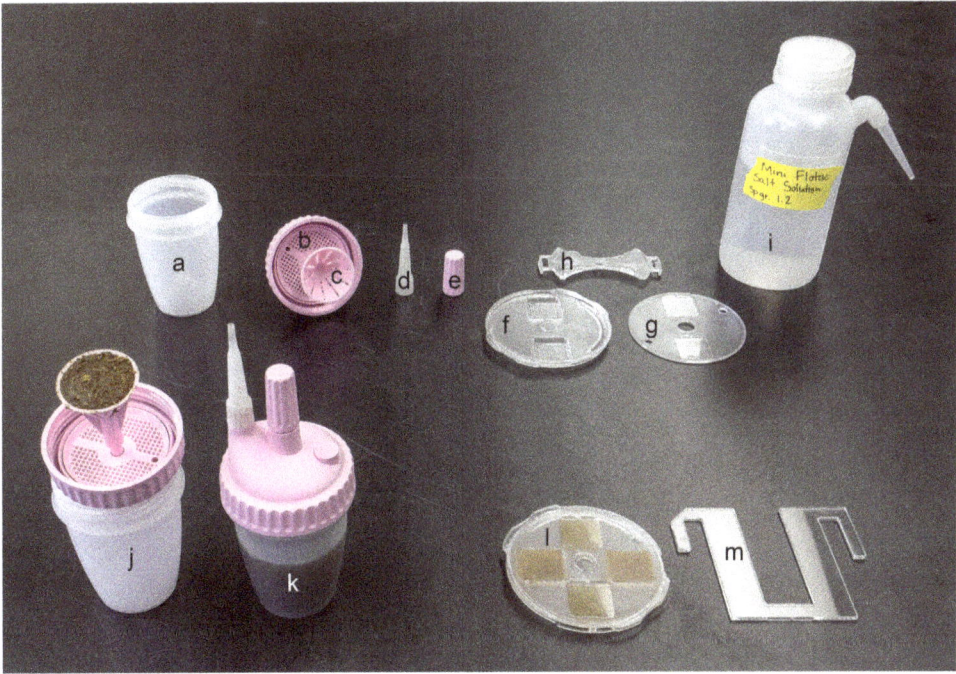

Fig. 8.2. Items required to perform a Mini-FLOTAC fecal egg count, in various stages of preparation: (a) Fill-FLOTAC cup; (b) Fill-FLOTAC built-in sieve in Fill-FLOTAC cap; (c) Fill-FLOTAC conical collector; (d) Fill-FLOTAC pipette for connecting to outlet (side) port; (e) Fill-FLOTAC cap for central port; (f) Mini-FLOTAC base with flotation chambers; (g) Mini-FLOTAC reading disc; (h) Mini-FLOTAC key used to turn reading disc into position for reading egg count; (i) flotation solution; (j) Fill-FLOTAC with conical collector filled with feces; (k) Fill-FLOTAC containing feces mixed with flotation solution and pipette in place on outlet port for filling Mini-FLOTAC flotation chambers; (l) Mini-FLOTAC filled with fecal suspension and reading disc turned in preparation for reading egg count; and (m) microscope adaptor to hold Mini-FLOTAC in place on microscope stage. Photo credit: Christopher Jones, Louisiana State University.

The conical collector is filled with feces and the surface leveled. The cup is filled with 45 ml of flotation solution. The lid is then screwed on to the cup, causing the feces to be dispersed into the flotation fluid in the cup, and the feces are mixed with the fluid using an up-and-down pumping action on the collector. Once mixed, the cup is inverted, the cap removed from the outlet port and the suspension is poured through the built-in sieve and, using a pipette connected to the outlet port, is used to fill the flotation chambers in the Mini-FLOTAC apparatus. A reading disc is attached to the apparatus and, using the microscope adaptor, the eggs are counted within the chambers using a standard compound microscope. A useful video demonstrating the technique is available on YouTube at www.youtube.com/watch?v= HahNA8yayuo.

The Mini-FLOTAC system has a smaller multiplication factor than the McMaster method. For our ruminant example, the multiplication factor is calculated as $(50\,\text{ml}/5\,\text{g})/2\,\text{ml} = 5$. Compare this value with the multiplication value for the McMaster method of 50 in our example above. The Mini-FLOTAC is useful for evaluating samples where the egg counts are expected to be low. As such, the method has greater application for cattle, where the egg counts are typically much lower than those of sheep and goats.

Because the conical collector of the Fill-FLOTAC is designed to accommodate a known weight of feces and because the sieve is built in to the apparatus, using the system does not require the use of a scale and there is less mess than with the McMaster method. The multiplication factor is close to that of a centrifugal fecal flotation (see next section) but does not require the use of a centrifuge.

Take-home message: Use the Mini-FLOTAC method when you expect the egg counts to be low in sheep and goats. Choose this method when you want a low multiplication factor similar to that of a centrifugal fecal flotation, but do not have access to a centrifuge.

Centrifugal fecal flotation methods

Several methods which use centrifugation and flotation, including the modified Stoll test method, the Wisconsin method,

the Cornell–Wisconsin method, and other methods that are simply referred to as 'centrifugation-flotation' methods, have been developed that essentially employ the same basic technique—a certain amount of feces is mixed with a flotation solution followed by centrifugation of the suspension in a test tube to concentrate the larger debris in the base of the tube (Fig. 8.3). The centrifugation also promotes the flotation of parasite eggs, oocysts, cysts, larvae, or other parasitic structures of interest present in the sample to float to the top of the tube where they are collected on a cover slip. The cover slip is transferred to a microscope slide and examined under a standard compound microscope.

These techniques are useful for screening for certain nematodes, such as *Trichuris* spp., and for screening protozoan parasites, such as *Giardia* and *Cryptosporidium* spp., where flotation solutions of the specific gravity most suitable for the recovery of these parasites may be substituted for the salt or sugar solutions standardly used in the laboratory for the McMaster or Mini-FLOTAC methods. See Zajac *et al.* (2021), for example, for details.

If the feces used in the procedure are weighed, a centrifugal fecal flotation method may be used to quantitate eggs or other parasitic structures. Several studies comparing centrifugal fecal flotation methods to the McMaster (Cain *et al.*, 2020) or to the McMaster and Mini-FLOTAC methods (Bosco *et al.*, 2018; Paras *et al.*, 2018) have demonstrated that the centrifugal fecal flotation method is less accurate and less precise than the other methods used to determine the fecal egg count. From a practical perspective, when attempting to perform a fecal egg count using a centrifugal fecal flotation method and the concentration of eggs in the feces is high, the eggs will be very close to each other or even overlap under the cover slip, making it difficult for the operator to distinguish between the eggs in order to count them. In these cases, the ability to count the eggs accurately is greatly diminished, especially when several hundreds or even thousands of eggs are concentrated on the microscope slide. Repeating the test using a smaller amount of feces (for example, 1g instead of 3 g) may make it easier to count the eggs on the microscope slide.

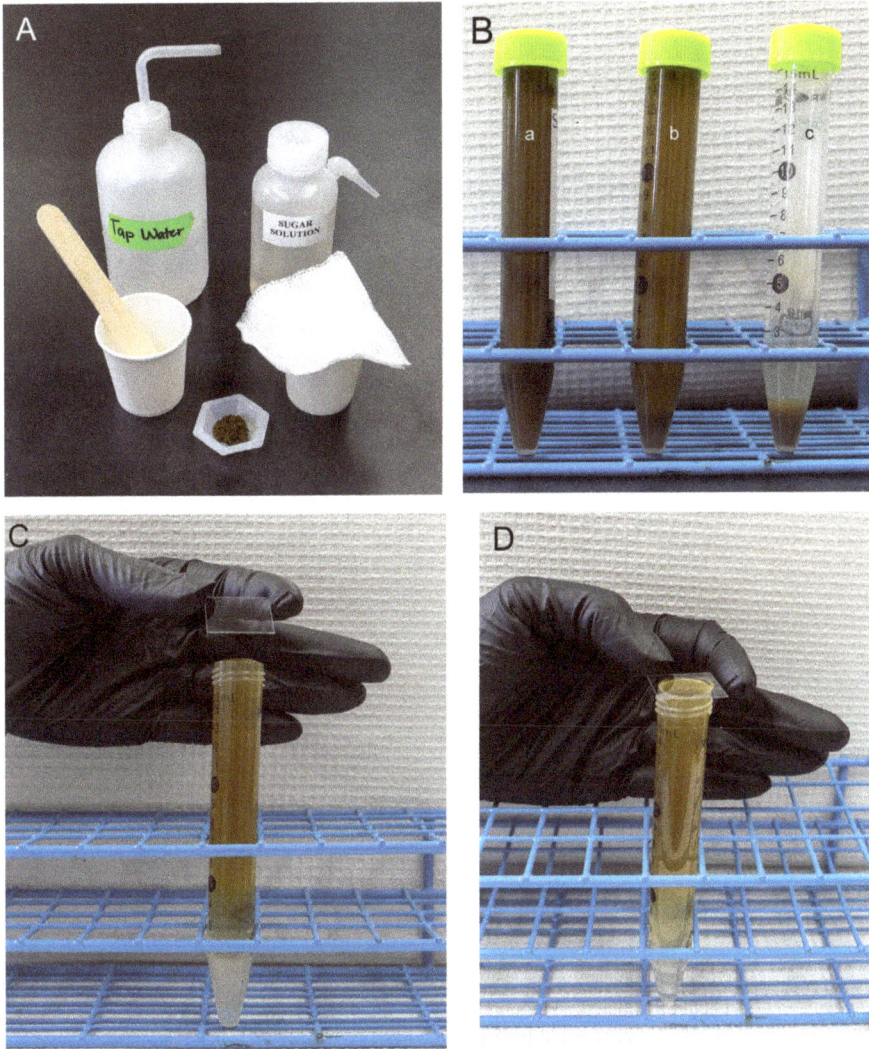

Fig. 8.3. (A) Items required to perform a centrifugal fecal flotation. (B) (a) Feces mixed with water; (b) after centrifugation; and (c) after decanting of the supernatant. (C) Placing a cover slip on the positive meniscus of a suspension of feces and flotation solution. (D) Centrifuge tube with cover slip in place. Photo credit: Christopher Jones, Louisiana State University.

One final point to note is that passive flotation of eggs is not recommended, even though the kits to perform such flotations are commonly available. Aside from the fact that they are not quantitative, it has been shown that use of centrifugation consistently recovers more eggs than passive flotation (Dryden *et al.*, 2005).

Take-home message: Use a centrifugal fecal flotation method for fecal egg count when other methods with lower multiplication factors than the McMaster method, such as the Mini-FLOTAC method, are unavailable or cannot be performed. Choose a centrifugal fecal flotation method when screening for protozoan parasites and use a fecal solution of the appropriate specific gravity.

Automated methods

In the past decade, automated fecal egg counting systems have become commercially available for use in companion animals (see, for example, Nagamori *et al.*, 2020) and horses (Slusarewicz *et al.*, 2016). These systems allow for the rapid processing of large batches of samples by operators who do not have the technical skills to identify and count nematode eggs. Most of the current automated fecal egg counting methods work by utilizing high-magnification visible light imaging systems which are coupled to automated moving stages (Britton *et al.*, 2024). Large, high-resolution files are generated for subsequent computational analysis. On the other hand, one automated system, developed by Parasight System Inc., utilizes fluorescence imaging following labeling of nematode ova with a recombinant chitin-binding protein that attaches to the surface of the eggs (Slusarewicz *et al.*, 2016). Originally developed for fecal egg counts in horses, this system has since been modified for use in sheep and goats (Slusarewicz *et al.*, 2021). More recently, Parasight System Inc. has adapted its method further to identify and count eggs of *H. contortus* using a fluorescein-labeled lectin, specifically a peanut agglutinin (Cain *et al.*, 2024). For those using the automated system, the ability to provide a count of the *H. contortus* eggs within a sample adds significant value.

Take-home message: An automated fecal egg counting system may be useful for veterinarians offering a high-throughput diagnostic service to small ruminant producers as part of their clinical practice. Large commercial producers, or producer cooperatives, may also find investment in such a system to be worthwhile.

Parasite Identification

When recommendations on parasite management are made in the United States, especially in the south-eastern region, most of these are geared towards the control of *H. contortus*. While this assumption will be true in the majority of cases, especially during the summer, good practice is always to identify the parasite species in question responsible for the clinical signs or production losses. Such confirmation may take the form of a history of the parasite in question being the cause of the problem. *Haemonchus contortus*, for example, may have been previously diagnosed on the farm when animals died and were subjected to necropsy. In subsequent years, when anemic animals are noted, the weather is warm, there has been good rainfall, and the pastures are lush such that hemonchosis would be expected, the producer can assume with relative safety that the cause of the anemia is the barber pole worm. The FAMACHA© system may be used to identify anemic animals for treatment and is therefore in and of itself a diagnostic tool (Malan *et al.*, 2001; Vatta *et al.*, 2001).

In cases where sheep or goats are showing signs other than anemia, such as diarrhea, poor body condition, and weight loss, or they are anemic and are also showing other signs, we cannot know which species of nematodes are causing the signs, or indeed whether worms are the major problem. In such cases, fecal egg counts and methods for identifying the parasites will need to be employed to make or rule out a definitive diagnosis of parasitism. Identification of species is also recommended when testing for anthelmintic resistance and the techniques discussed in this section may be used to provide valuable information regarding the resistance status of the various nematode populations on the farm.

In the live animal, we are forced to base our identification of any gastrointestinal nematodes present on the collection and testing of a fecal sample. However, as discussed earlier, identification of the strongylid (trichostrongyle and strongyle) eggs noted on fecal examination by one of the egg-counting methods is difficult, if not impossible, to do with certainty. The exception here is *Nematodirus* which, while being a strongylid, has an egg 2–3 times the size of the other common strongylid eggs. (The eggs of the nonstrongylid nematodes, *Trichuris*, *Strongyloides*, and *Moniezia* may, of course, be identified.)

Here we discuss some of the specialized laboratory techniques that may be used to identify the strongylid species or genera present in a fecal sample. Fecal samples will need to be submitted to a laboratory that offers the desired test—the identification to species or genus level requires specialized expertise in identification or in the execution and interpretation of the laboratory techniques to be used for the identification. These techniques include a fluorescein-labeled peanut agglutinin to identify *H. contortus* eggs, fecal coproculture with larval identification, and molecular-based approaches. It should be noted that there are very few laboratories that offer these methods of identification of strongylid eggs in fecal samples, and to the author's knowledge, there is no lab that offers all three techniques discussed here.

Fluorescein-labeled peanut agglutinin method

As mentioned earlier, an automated system is available that can provide a count of *H. contortus* eggs within a sample. The specific lectin used in the automated system, a peanut agglutinin, was originally discovered by Palmer and McCombe (1996) who observed that it binds selectively to *H. contortus* eggs. When the lectin is conjugated to fluorescein isothiocyanate, the *H. contortus* eggs can be visualized under ultraviolet illumination. An automated system may therefore provide a value for the *H. contortus* fecal egg count. However, it should be noted that certain diagnostic laboratories do conduct a peanut lectin assay manually to differentiate *H. contortus* eggs from other strongylid eggs and submitting fecal samples to such laboratories may be an option for some to consider.

Coproculture

Various methods of coproculture, or fecal culture, have been described and each laboratory will have its own variation on the method. However, the basic principle behind the culture method is to mimic in the laboratory the environment in which strongylid eggs develop on pasture. This invariably involves mixing the feces with a substrate such as vermiculite and adding sufficient water to the sample to ensure that the sample remains moist but not too wet during the incubation process. (Note that some prefer to incubate the sample without the substrate.) The culture is incubated at a constant temperature of approximately 25–26°C for 7–10 days, to allow the eggs to

hatch and the larvae to develop through to the third stage. The larvae are then recovered for identification using a Baermann apparatus or a modification of that technique. One method of larval recovery is illustrated in Fig. 8.4.

A number of larval identification keys have been published, but the identification remains difficult, requires a great deal of experience, and is best left to trained personnel. The results for the larval identification are expressed as percentages of the various genera of strongylid larvae identified—most larvae can only be identified to genus and not species. If desired, the relative percentages of larvae present in the sample may be used to apportion the egg counts to the genera or species of larvae identified.

Coprocultures may also be performed in a quantitative manner if the feces are weighed prior to culture, the egg count for the feces is known, and the numbers of larvae recovered are counted. The results are expressed as larvae per gram or as a percentage development based on the original egg count. This approach is generally only ever used for research purposes, such as to quantify the effects on larval development in fecal samples containing the spores of nematophagous fungi.

Molecular-based approaches to parasite identification

Aside from the drawback of the time required for eggs to develop to the third larval stage, and the specialist knowledge needed to identify the larvae, various factors may affect the actual development of larvae in culture, including temperature of incubation, moisture content of the culture (Kassai, 1999), and duration of incubation (Van Wyk and Mayhew, 2013), and variations in these factors may promote the development of certain nematode species over others. This may skew the final percentages of larvae identified in favor of those nematodes which show better development under the specific conditions of incubation.

On the other hand, certain molecular-based approaches have been developed that overcome some or all of these limitations. Molecular-based approaches include real-time multiplex PCR

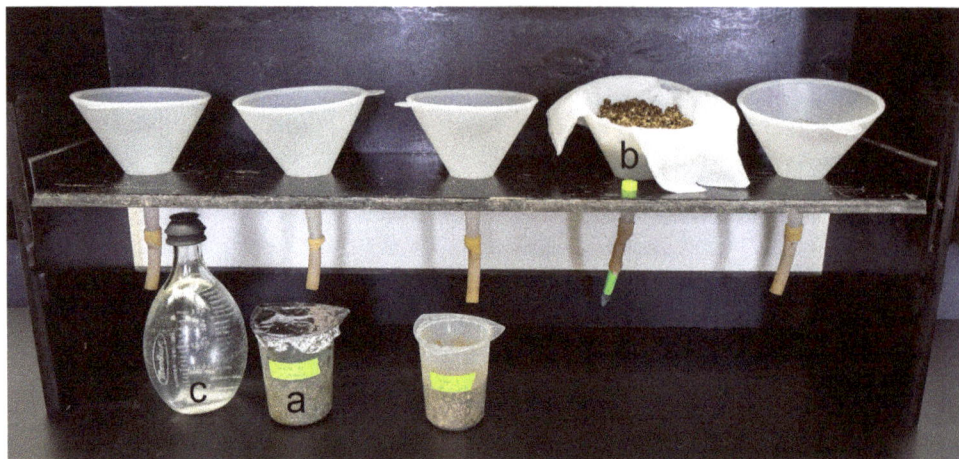

Fig. 8.4. Items required to perform a coproculture and larval recovery: (a) beaker containing feces mixed with vermiculite and water and covered with aluminum foil for incubation; (b) Baermann apparatus consisting of a funnel holding a metal mesh (not shown) and feces contained within cheesecloth; and (c) water to add to the funnel to submerge the feces. The stem of the funnel containing the feces (b) is attached to a rubber tube that is closed off with a 15 ml centrifuge tube. Photo credit: Christopher Jones, Louisiana State University.

(qPCR; Roeber *et al.*, 2017) and nemabiome metabarcoding (Avramenko *et al.*, 2015) which can both be potentially integrated with the fecal egg count reduction test to add species-specific information (Kaplan *et al.*, 2023) (see later in this chapter). Once standardized in the molecular biology laboratory, these tests do not require the specialized diagnostic skill that nematode larval identification demands.

The molecular-based techniques may be used for both strongylid eggs and larvae. While for the most part larvae may be identified morphologically only to the genus level, and strongylid eggs of small ruminants, with the few exceptions noted previously, cannot easily and reliably be differentiated, multiplex PCR and nemabiome metabarcoding can be used to identify eggs or larvae to the species level. Both multiplex PCR and nemabiome metabarcoding also provide quantitation of species present in a sample. Further details of the nemabiome sequencing-based approach are available at nemabiome.ca.[3] Though nemabiome metabarcoding is not available for routine, quick-turnaround diagnostic purposes at the time of writing, multiplex PCR tests are offered by a laboratory in Canada.[4] By arrangement,

samples may also be submitted from the United States to the laboratory in Canada.

The nemabiome metabarcoding approach, which employs deep amplicon sequencing, was originally developed using the Illumina platform. However, the method may be shifted to other sequencing platforms. One such platform is that provided by Oxford Nanopore. Indeed, Oxford Nanopore sequencing devices have already been applied in nemabiome metabarcoding and have the potential to provide greater speed and flexibility, and ultimately greater affordability, than the original Illumina sequencing platform (Charrier, 2024; John S. Gilleard, University of Calgary, personal communication, 2024).

Tests for Parasites Other than Gastrointestinal Nematodes

Liver flukes

Sheep and goats infected with liver flukes, specifically *Fasciola hepatica* and less commonly *Fasciola gigantica*, may develop anemia and when they are coinfected with *H. contortus*, the anemia may be exacerbated. This is something to bear in mind when using the FAMACHA© system on the farm, because while using a FAMACHA© card will help you identify anemic animals, it will not identify the cause of the anemia. In cases where liver fluke infection is suspected, a sedimentation test should be performed on, say, 6–10 animals from the flock or herd. If fluke eggs are found in the feces, it would be proper to conclude that liver flukes are contributing to the anemia seen. Because the eggs of *Fasciola* spp. are relatively dense, they do not float in the commonly used flotation solutions. Instead, they are allowed to sediment out during the laboratory test, hence the name, sedimentation test.

Several methods have been used to perform a sedimentation test. In all these methods, a fecal suspension is first sieved to remove the largest particulate matter before the filtrate is cleaned by being subjected to repeated sedimentation steps. In each step, the particulate matter is allowed to sediment out and the supernatant is discarded, before the sediment is resuspended in water and the process repeated until the supernatant is relatively clear. At that stage, the remaining sediment is stained with methylene blue and examined for fluke eggs. One commercially available system, the FLUKEFINDER® (Soda Springs, Idaho; Fig. 8.5), is commonly used as it makes the procedure easier to perform than some of the other methods.

Although not available in the United States, a copro-antigen ELISA (BIO K 201 – Monoscreen AbELISA *Fasciola hepatica*, Bio-X Diagnostics

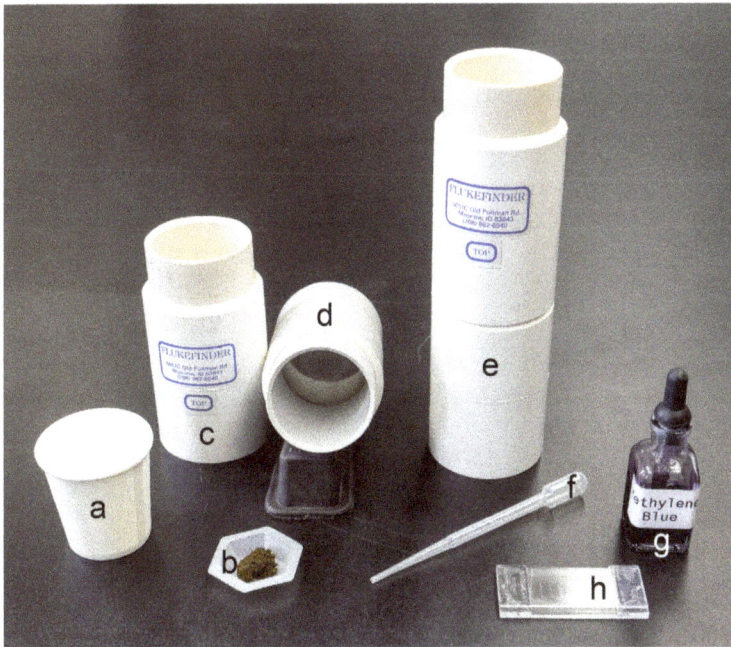

Fig. 8.5. Items required to perform a fecal sedimentation examination using the FLUKEFINDER® apparatus: (a) cup; (b) feces; (c) top portion of FLUKEFINDER apparatus; (d) bottom portion of FLUKEFINDER apparatus; (e) assembled FLUKEFINDER apparatus; (f) pipette; (g) methylene blue; and (h) trematode egg counting chamber. Once the fecal material has been sieved through the FLUKEFINDER apparatus, the sediment remaining on the bottom sieve (d) is washed into a 50 ml centrifuge tube (not shown) and the material is allowed to sediment for a determined period of time, whereafter the supernatant is discarded and the sediment is resuspended in water. The process is continued until the supernatant which is discarded is relatively clean. At that stage, a few drops of methylene blue (g) are added to the sediment and the suspension is transferred to the counting chamber (h) for examination under a microscope. Photo credit: Christopher Jones, Louisiana State University.

S.A., Rochefort, Belgium) has been developed for the diagnosis of *F. hepatica* infections in fecal samples and is available in several other countries. The copro-antigen ELISA is mentioned here as a placeholder in case the assay or other serological tests become available in the future for the diagnosis of *F. hepatica* in the United States.[5] The ELISA is an indirect sandwich test for feces. It uses 96-well microplates which have been sensitized with a specific antibody to copro-antigens of *F. hepatica*, which are antigens of the parasite present in the feces. Diluted fecal material is incubated in the wells of the microplate and if the copro-antigens are present, they are captured on the microplate. The plate is then washed and conjugate is added to the plate; this is an antibody coupled to biotin and it binds to the copro-antigens already captured on the plate. Following further incubation and washing, a second conjugate, a peroxidase-coupled avidine specific to biotin, is added. After incubation, the plate is washed again and a chromogen is added. If the *F. hepatica* copro-antigens are present, the conjugates remain bound and the peroxidase catalyzes the transformation of the colorless chromogen into a pigmented compound (blue). The intensity of the resulting color will be in proportion to the copro-antigen titer of the sample. The enzymatic reaction is stopped and the optical density of the sample is read using a photometer.

For practical purposes, diagnostics for liver flukes are normally always conducted by submitting fecal samples to state or private commercial laboratories. In this regard, we need to note that there are no laboratory diagnostic tests available to test for the deer fluke, *Fascioloides magna*. As the common name implies, this is a liver fluke of white-tailed deer (*Odocoileus virginianus*). In deer, the adult flukes are found in cysts in the liver and the cysts communicate with the bile ducts, allowing eggs to move via the bile into the gastrointestinal tract and to pass out in the feces. In sheep and goats, the flukes are not encapsulated in the liver and the young flukes wander aimlessly and destructively in the liver tissue. Sheep and goats will die from the infections before the flukes mature and reach adulthood. As such, eggs of *F. magna* will not be seen in the feces of sheep and goats. A definitive diagnosis of *F. magna* is made on necropsy.

Lungworms

Occasionally, larvae of the lungworms *Muellerius capillaris* or *Dictyocaulus filaria* will be noted on fecal examination, particularly if a centrifugal fecal flotation method is used. If lungworms are suspected to be the cause of a respiratory problem, fresh feces from affected individuals should be submitted to the laboratory. First-stage larvae will be collected using a Baermann apparatus, in the same way that third-stage larvae are recovered following coproculture. Identification of lungworm larvae requires a trained diagnostic parasitologist; there are many things, including free nematodes, that look like lungworm larvae to the untrained eye.

Tapeworms (cestodes)

The most common tapeworms found in sheep and goats are *Moniezia* spp. Tapeworms are much more commonly found in lambs and kids than in adult sheep and goats. As noted earlier, tapeworm infections are best diagnosed by noting the segments of the tapeworms as they exit the anus or attach to the wool or hair on the hindquarters of the animal. Alternatively, segments may be noted on freshly passed fecal samples. Though almost never required, if a specific diagnosis is desired, the segments may be submitted in alcohol or formalin to a diagnostic laboratory for identification. Tapeworm eggs will also be noted from time to time during fecal examination, but as previously discussed, fecal examination is not a reliable test or method of choice for the diagnosis of tapeworm infections.

Complementary Diagnostic Tests and Evaluations

Packed cell volume or hematocrit

Although mainly used for research purposes or as part of a diagnostic work-up to determine whether a sheep or goat requires a blood transfusion, the hematocrit or packed cell volume measurement may be used to confirm the anemic status of a sheep when the FAMACHA© score is equivocal or in cases where a new operator is being trained in the scoring system. Normally the packed cell volume, or percentage red blood cells, is determined by the microhematocrit method, which measures the relative amount of red blood cells in the blood. The normal range for the packed cell volume for goats is narrower and the high end of the normal range lower than for sheep. In both species, however, animals with a packed cell volume less than 15% should be treated for the cause of the anemia and should be provided with adequate nursing care. An individual with a packed cell volume of 10% or less may require a blood transfusion to prevent it from dying from anemia.

Evaluating pasture contamination with infective larvae

Thus far we have only considered diagnostics to assess the presence and degree of infection with parasites within the host itself. However, methods also exist to estimate the level of pasture contamination with infective larvae. Although truly only a research tool, the use of tracer animals probably provides the most accurate indication of the levels and species of nematodes that small ruminants on the pasture are ingesting. In brief, preferably parasite-naïve sheep or goats are dewormed and their egg counts assessed following deworming to ensure, as far as possible, that any infections present have been cleared. The animals are then allowed to graze on a pasture for a defined period of time, after which they are removed, generally maintained on a dry lot to allow any immature larvae to develop to adulthood, and then humanely euthanized. Parasites are recovered from the gastrointestinal tract during necropsy, counted, and identified to species using established procedures.

Another method which does not require the sacrifice of animals involves sampling herbage within the pasture on which sheep or goats are grazing. Samples of the grass are clipped at predetermined intervals while crisscrossing the pasture in such a manner as to be representative of the herbage in the pasture (Hansen and Perry, 1994). Several methods have been published, and all involve washing the grass and recovering any larvae from the grass samples. Any larvae so collected are identified and counted. The herbage is dried and the number of larvae per kilogram biomass is calculated. Isolating infective larvae from herbage is very labor intensive, requires specialized knowledge to identify the larvae, and is not sufficiently accurate to support a diagnosis in clinically infected animals, but it does have application in research when examining changes in pasture contamination with infective larvae over time.

Necropsy

Sheep and goats that die should, whenever possible, be subjected to necropsy by a veterinarian to determine the cause of death. However, this may be impractical (for example, if the animal is found in an advanced state of decomposition), the cause of death is obvious (for example, in the case of predation), or requesting a necropsy is cost-prohibitive.

Experienced veterinary pathologists who, based on the history provided, suspect that an animal has died of worm infection will examine for relevant signs, such as pallor of the carcass and bleeding in the abomasum, submit feces for a fecal egg count, and collect any worms that may be spotted and submit them to the laboratory. Finding worms in the gastrointestinal tract is unlikely, however, because of their small size. One exception is *H. contortus*, but even the barber pole worm may be hard to find when not present in the hundreds or thousands. Established procedures to recover worms, such as those employed by parasitology laboratories, are outside the normal scope of performing a necropsy. If a worm count is desired, this needs to be requested specifically of a parasitology laboratory, preferably before starting the necropsy itself. Consequently, a diagnosis of parasitism as the cause of death is normally made based on the history, postmortem signs, and fecal egg count.

We should note that an animal which has been recently dewormed may still die of the worm infection even though worms may not be found on necropsy. Such individuals succumb to the effects of the infection (for example, anemia) before their bodies are able to undergo the processes of repair and regeneration that are necessary following removal of the parasitic worms.

Diagnostic Tests for Anthelmintic Resistance

With the widespread occurrence of anthelmintic resistance to the products in the three anthelmintic classes available in the US, namely the benzimidazoles (for example, fenbendazole and albendazole), imidazothiazoles (for example, levamisole), and macrocyclic lactones (for example, ivermectin and moxidectin), it is essential to know the efficacy of the products, or combination of products, that are being used on a particular farm. Here we discuss three methods that may be used to test for anthelmintic resistance on a farm: the fecal egg count reduction test, *in vitro* methods including egg hatch and larval development assays, and the use of molecular biology methods.

Fecal egg count reduction test

Of the methods used to assess anthelmintic resistance, the fecal egg count reduction test requires the least technical experience and may be conducted by any producer in collaboration with a veterinarian or laboratory that performs fecal egg counts. Kaplan *et al.* (2023) have provided a comprehensive guideline for the conduct of a fecal egg count reduction test, and we will not repeat those details here. However, basing this discussion closely on the work by Kaplan *et al.* (2023), we will seek to explain the principles behind the test and to highlight certain conditions that must be met to obtain reliable results. As the name implies, the test aims to determine the reduction in fecal egg count following treatment with an anthelmintic, but the methodology now endorsed also permits the use of diagnostic criteria that provide greater statistical validity and clinical relevance than previously published recommendations.

In evaluating the data from a fecal egg count reduction test, several assumptions are made, including that the animals were treated with the minimum label dosage, they were administered the anthelmintic using a proper technique, and

the drugs had not expired and had been stored according to the label. The proper conduct of the test also relies on the ability of the operators to collect, label, store, and ship fecal samples correctly and that fecal egg counts be conducted using proper laboratory techniques.

A fecal egg count reduction test is performed by conducting pre- and posttreatment fecal egg counts for the same animals. This is referred to as a paired study design. Previous recommendations were to use separate treated animals and untreated control animals (an unpaired study design), but the use of pre- and posttreatment fecal egg counts from the same animals has been shown to provide more reliable results than when unpaired study designs are used.

Certain specific recommendations apply when conducting a fecal egg count reduction test.

- It is important that the same animals are sampled pre- and post treatment, which means that the animals have to be correctly identified (by means of ear tags, ear tattoos, RFID tags, or other methods).
- Young weaned animals are the preferred group to test if sufficient animals of that age are available, but sheep and goats of any age may be tested.
- The animals to be included in the test should be grazing on the same pastures.
- The animals should not have been dewormed in the previous 8–12 weeks with one or more of the most commonly used anthelmintic products.
- Animals should be weighed on the day of treatment and the doses of anthelmintic to be administered should be calculated based on those weights. If the animals cannot be weighed, an alternative is to use a weigh tape. Alternatively, although not recommended, the weight can be estimated, but the dose administered to each animal should be targeted to the heaviest animal of the group so that each animal gets the label dose as a minimum. Treating to average weight would mean that some animals would be underdosed.
- Fecal samples are collected prior to the treatment of the group, the animals are then treated, and fecal samples are collected again after an interval of 10–14

days, depending on the anthelmintic under evaluation. For short-acting drugs (benzimidazoles and levamisole), collecting samples 10–14 days post treatment is valid, while samples should be collected 14 days post treatment when the macrocyclic lactones are being tested or when a combination of short-acting drugs and a macrocyclic lactone is used.

For the test to be valid, a minimum total number of eggs has to be counted before treatment; that is, the sum of the raw counts of eggs (for all the animals included in the test before application of a multiplication factor) has to meet a certain minimum number. This means that one of the several different fecal egg count methods may be selected—the choice of method will be based on the mean fecal egg count of the group and the number of animals being tested. Note that Kaplan *et al.* (2023), citing Bosco *et al.* (2018), Paras *et al.* (2018), and Cain *et al.* (2020), do not recommend the use of centrifugal fecal flotation methods in fecal egg count reduction tests.

At a minimum, at least five animals are required to derive reliable results from a fecal egg count reduction test. However, Kaplan *et al.* (2023) provide three options for the required size of the treatment group depending on the total number of eggs counted before treatment. The required size, in turn, is determined by whether you wish to follow the so-called 'clinical protocol' or the so-called 'research protocol.' For on-farm purposes, the clinical protocol is sufficient, whereas the research protocol should be employed when experimental research is being conducted. The clinical protocol prescribes that when the minimum mean number of eggs counted (the total number of eggs counted before treatment divided by the total number of animals sampled) is 40, a minimum of eight animals is required; when the mean is 15, a minimum of 11 animals is required; and when the mean is 8, a minimum of 14 animals is required. Note that this mean value refers to the mean of the number of actual eggs counted in the samples, not the epg value. For example, if the multiplication factor for your fecal egg count technique is 50 (as may be used in a McMaster fecal egg count protocol), the minimum mean fecal egg count would need to be 2000 epg if you

wished to include only eight animals; it would need to be 750 epg if you wished to include only 11 animals; and it would need to be 400 epg if you wished to include 14 animals. If the fecal egg counts are lower than these values, the McMaster method should be adjusted so that a multiplication factor of 25 is used, or the Mini-FLOTAC system should be used.

A website (fecrt.com) has been created which will calculate the relevant required statistical outputs once the fecal egg count data have been entered. The data may, of course, be analyzed by a qualified statistician or another appropriate web-based analysis tool may be used. Two terms are of relevance here. The first is the target or expected efficacy, which is the efficacy of the drug when first introduced on the market or, differently, when applied to a population of susceptible parasites. The second term of relevance is the lower efficacy threshold, which is the smallest possible reduction in efficacy that can be reliably diagnosed as 'resistant.' The interval between the lower efficacy threshold and the expected efficacy is referred to as the 'gray zone.' By way of example, the guidelines for sheep have an expected efficacy of 99% and a lower efficacy threshold of 90% for the clinical protocol. The gray zone is then 90–99%. To conform with the guidelines of Kaplan *et al.* (2023), the analysis must yield values for an upper and lower 90% confidence interval (or provide results of separate hypothesis tests using a prespecified expected efficacy and a lower efficacy threshold). Based on these statistical outputs, the worm population is then classified as susceptible or resistant, or the results are considered inconclusive. The following interpretation of the results has been reproduced directly from Kaplan *et al.* (2023), pp. 5–6:

- "*Susceptible*: when the lower 90% confidence interval is greater than or equal to the lower efficacy threshold (corresponding to the lower limit of the gray zone) and the upper 90% confidence interval is greater than or equal to the expected efficacy (corresponding to the upper limit of the gray zone). *Simplified explanation*: the worst probable true efficacy is still within an acceptable margin of the expected efficacy, and the best probably true efficacy is equal to or greater than the expected efficacy.

- *Resistant*: when the upper 90% confidence interval (CI) is less than the expected efficacy (corresponding to the upper limit of the gray zone). This includes the subclassification of 'low resistant,' which meets the additional criteria of the lower 90% CI being greater than or equal to the lower efficacy threshold (lower limit of the gr–y zone). *Simplified explanation*: the best probable true efficacy is less than the expected efficacy of the drug.
- *Inconclusive*: if neither of these criteria is met. *Simplified explanation*: given the established gray zone, the data are not sufficient to make any positive conclusions regarding the true efficacy with respect to resistance or susceptibility."

If the outcome is inconclusive, repeating the fecal egg count reduction test using more animals and counting more eggs will increase the likelihood of obtaining a conclusive result.

When conducting a fecal egg count reduction test, additional valuable information may be obtained by identifying the nematode species present in the fecal samples before and after treatment. When species are present post treatment, we can infer that they are the nematodes contributing to any resistance noted. With due consideration given to the limitations of each method, any one of the methods discussed in the section above entitled 'Parasite Identification' may be used to provide the genus- or species-specific information.

Conversely, if there is no improvement or even a deterioration in the condition of the animal, you can assume that the treatment was ineffective or that the animal requires additional supportive care. Aside from rechecking the FAMACHA© score, if a fecal egg count is conducted before treatment, there is value in assessing whether there is any reduction in fecal egg count following treatment. The posttreatment sample should be collected at the same interval post treatment as recommended for that drug in the fecal egg count reduction test guidelines. The result will not give you a statistically valid determination of the resistance status of the worm population on the farm, but it may provide data that have clinical relevance to the animal in question. For example, if the treatment only results in a 50% reduction in the egg count, you may still see an improvement clinically, but the worms in the animal are highly resistant to the drug with which the animal was treated and it may be necessary to use an anthelmintic from a different class, or a combination of drugs from different anthelmintic classes going forward.

Another situation where checking the fecal egg counts post treatment is strongly advised is when animals have been recently introduced to the farm and are being kept in quarantine. Such animals should be dewormed with a combination of drugs from different classes and their egg counts checked with a method employing a low multiplication factor, to ensure that the worm burden is reduced to the extent that no eggs are detected on fecal examination.

Assessing effectiveness of treatment in individual animals

Where the current efficacy of the available anthelmintics is not known for the farm (for example, if a fecal egg count reduction test has never been conducted or has not been performed for several years), it is important to determine whether there is clinical improvement in the animal following treatment. If you used a FAMACHA© score to determine that the animal required treatment, examining the color of the conjunctival mucous membranes a week after treatment and finding that the color has improved (is pinker) will give you an indication that the treatment was clinically effective.

Egg hatch and larval development assays

The basic principle of the egg hatch and larval development assays is the incubation of parasite eggs in wells of tissue culture plates containing varying concentrations of the drug in question, from no drug up to a determined maximum concentration. From the data generated, various parameters are calculated, including the concentration at which the drug is able to inhibit either the hatching of the eggs by 50% or 95% (egg hatch assay) or the development of the larvae to the third stage (larval development assay).

One larval development assay that has been commercialized is the DrenchRite™ assay[6] which allows for the characterization of the resistant status on farm to the benzimidazoles, levamisole, ivermectin, and moxidectin. One advantage of the assay is that the producer can submit a single composite fecal sample rather than have to sample the herd or flock on two separate occasions, as would be required if performing a fecal egg count reduction test. The results of the assay allow the resistance status of the worm population on the farm to be characterized as resistant, suspected resistant, or susceptible. In other words, it is possible to relate the results of the assay with the level of clinical resistance (an expression of the phenotype) on the farm. Though results may be calculated for other species that develop in sufficient numbers on the plate, for example *Trichostrongylus* spp., the DrenchRite™ assay is best suited to characterizing resistance in *H. contortus* populations.

Egg hatch and larval development assays require specialized training and expertise and are not routinely conducted except for research purposes or as screening assays for compounds with potential anthelmintic activity. The assays require specialized laboratory equipment, employ labor-intensive procedures, and require a substantial turnaround time. In turn, these factors make the assays expensive to perform, unless subsidized by institutional or grant funding.

The DrenchRite™ assay is currently being used for research purposes at Louisiana State University, Baton Rouge, Louisiana, but the aim is to make the assay available to producers and veterinarians within the US in due course.[7] The assay is not currently available as a commercial diagnostic test in any other countries.

Deep amplicon sequencing

The use of nemabiome metabarcoding to determine the frequency of the different nematode species within a fecal sample has been discussed earlier. The deep amplicon sequencing approach on which nemabiome metabarcoding is based has been adapted to screen for genetic mutations that have been identified to confer resistance to the benzimidazoles in gastrointestinal nematode populations (Avramenko *et al.*, 2019). Deep amplicon sequencing can be used to determine the frequency of benzimidazole resistance mutations in gastrointestinal nematode populations as an alternative approach to fecal egg count reduction testing or *in vitro* egg hatch and larval development assays (Avramenko *et al.*, 2019). Recent work has extended this capability to screening for genetic mutations to levamisole based on the characterization of a major marker for levamisole resistance in *H. contortus* (Antonopoulos *et al.*, 2022). The genetic mechanisms that confer macrocyclic lactone resistance are still being studied and screening for genetic mutations in this class of anthelmintics is not yet available.

Deep amplicon sequencing allows us to determine the frequency of resistance-conferring genetic mutations by nematode species. Because anthelmintic resistance is species specific, this characteristic of the sequencing makes this tool a particularly powerful addition to the methodologies available to test for anthelmintic resistance.[8] The correlation of allele frequency for resistance mutations and phenotypic resistance (or the degree to which a drug will actually work in killing the nematodes in a worm population in a herd or flock on a farm) is not well worked out for benzimidazole (or levamisole) resistance, but future research is likely to provide further insights here. Deep amplicon sequencing has the ability, however, to detect the frequency of resistance-conferring alleles even though resistance may not yet be clinically evident on the farm.

While still very much a research tool at the moment, the progress made thus far with the deep amplicon sequencing approach bodes well for its use as a diagnostic tool in the future.

Conclusion

We have presented here the diagnostic methods and tests that are most commonly used to diagnose gastrointestinal parasite infections in sheep and goats, as well as some techniques that are not yet available, or not yet widely available, but should become more commonplace in the future. We hope that the information presented here may assist university researchers and instructors, practicing veterinarians, extension specialists, and animal science and veterinary science students to understand some of the advantages and limitations of the tests discussed so that informed decisions may be made not only for the initial diagnosis of a parasite problem but also for the ongoing monitoring of parasitic infections and anthelmintic resistance on farm.

Notes

[1] The Animal Health Diagnostic Center at Cornell University College of Veterinary Medicine offers a 'Haemonchus egg test' which is a fluorescein-labeled groundnut agglutinin test.

[2] At the time of going to press, the University of Georgia had indicated that limited numbers of the Fill-FLOTAC apparatus and Mini-FLOTAC counting chambers were available for purchase.

[3] Through prior agreement with the principal investigator, the Gilleard Laboratory, Faculty of Veterinary Medicine, University of Calgary (https://vet.ucalgary.ca/labs/jsgilleard/home) will provide nemabiome metabarcoding on a fee-for-service basis.

[4] Biovet, a Division of Antech, Mars Petcare Science & Diagnostics, has recently developed several real-time multiplex PCR tests that identify and provide an estimate of the parasitic burden that shows a strong correlation with nemabiome data of the main gastrointestinal nematodes of small ruminants, namely Haemonchus contortus, Teladorsagia spp., Cooperia spp., and Nematodirus spp. These tests are offered as a diagnostic service.

[5] The Bio-X Diagnostics copro-antigen ELISA has been used as part of a USDA-APHIS-funded research project (NAHMS Sheep 2024; www.aphis.usda.gov/livestock-poultry-disease/nahms/sheep) in the Parasitology Laboratory at Louisiana State University School of Veterinary Medicine, Department of Pathobiological Sciences. Please contact the author for further details (avatta2@lsu.edu).

[6] The intellectual property for the DrenchRite™ assay is held by Microbial Screening Technologies, Smithfield, New South Wales, Australia.

[7] Please contact the author (avatta2@lsu.edu) at Louisiana State University School of Veterinary Medicine, Department of Pathobiological Sciences, for further information regarding the availability of the assay.

[8] With prior agreement with the principal investigator, the Gilleard Laboratory, Faculty of Veterinary Medicine, University of Calgary (https://vet.ucalgary.ca/labs/jsgilleard/home) will provide deep amplicon sequencing for certain genetic mutations for anthelmintic resistance on a fee-for-service basis.

References

Antonopoulos, A., Doyle, S.R., Bartley, D.J., Morrison, A., Kaplan, R. et al. (2022) Allele specific PCR for a major marker of levamisole resistance in Haemonchus contortus. International Journal for Parasitology: Drugs and Drug Resistance 20, 17–26.

Avramenko, R.W., Redman, E.M., Lewis, R., Yazwinski, T., Wasmuth, J. et al. (2015) Exploring the gastro-intestinal "nemabiome": Deep amplicon sequencing to quantify the species composition of parasitic nematode communities. PLoS One 10, e0143559.

Avramenko, R.W., Redman, E.M., Melville, L., Bartley, Y., Wit, J. et al. (2019) Deep amplicon sequencing as a powerful new tool to screen for sequence polymorphisms associated with anthelmintic resistance in parasitic nematode populations. International Journal for Parasitology 49, 13–26.

Bosco, A., Maurelli, M.P., Ianniello, D., Morgoglione, M., Amadesi, A. et al. (2018) The recovery of added nematode eggs from horse and sheep faeces by three methods. BMC Veterinary Research 14, 7.

Britton, L., Ripley, B. and Slusarewicz, P. (2024) Relative egg extraction efficiencies of manual and auto-mated fecal egg count methids in equines. Helminthologia 61, 20–29.

Cain, J.L., Slusarewicz, P., Rutledge, M.H., McVey, M., Wielgus, K. et al. (2020) Diagnostic performance of McMaster, Wisconsin, and automated egg counting techniques for enumeration of equine strongyle eggs in fecal samples. Veterinary Parasitology 284, 109199.

Cain, J.L., Gianechini, L.S., Vetter, A.L., Davis, S., Britton, L. et al. (2024) Rapid, automated quantification of Haemonchus contortus ova in sheep faecal samples. International Journal for Parasitology 54, 47–53.

Charrier, E. (2024) Developing long-read Oxford Nanopore nemabiome metabarcoding for ovine gastrointestinal nematode community analysis and diagnostics. Doctoral thesis, University of Calgary, Alberta, Canada. Available at: https://prism.ucalgary.ca. https://hdl.handle.net/1880/118168

Cringoli, G., Maurelli, M.P., Levecke, B. and Utzinger, J. (2017) The mini-FLOTAC technique for the diagnosis of helminth and protozoan infections in human and animals. *Nature Protocols* 12, 1723–1732.

Dobson, R.J., Barnes, E.H. and Windon, R.G. (1992) Population dynamics of *Trichostrongylus colubriformis* and *Ostertagia circumcincta* in single and concurrent infections. *International Journal for Parasitology* 22, 997–1004.

Dryden, M.W., Payne, P.A., Ridley, R. and Smith, V. (2005) Comparison of common fecal flotation techniques for the recovery of parasite eggs and oocysts. *Veterinary Therapeutics* 6, 15–28.

Dunn, A.M. (1969) *Veterinary Helminthology*. Heinemann, London, UK.

Gordon, H.M. and Whitlock, H.V. (1939) A new technique for counting nematode eggs in sheep faeces. *Journal of the Council of Scientific and Industrial Research* 12, 50–52.

Hansen, J. and Perry, B. (1994) *The Epidemiology, Diagnosis and Control of Helminth Parasites of Ruminants*. International Livestock Center for Africa, Addis Ababa, Ethiopia.

Kaplan, R.M., Denwood, M.J., Nielsen, M.K., Thamsborg, S., Torgerson, P. *et al.* (2023) World Association for the Advancement of Veterinary Parasitology (W.A.A.V.P.) guideline for diagnosing anthelmintic resistance using the faecal egg count reduction test in ruminants, horses and swine. *Veterinary Parasitology* 318, 109936.

Kassai, T. (1999) Diagnostic helminthology. In: Kassai, T. (ed.) *Veterinary Helminthology*. Butterworth-Heinemann, Oxford, UK, pp. 192–193.

Malan, F.S., Van Wyk, J.A. and Wessels, C.D. (2001) Clinical evaluation of anaemia in sheep: Early trials. *Onderstepoort Journal of Veterinary Research* 68, 165–174.

Nagamori, Y., Hall Sedlak, R., DeRosa, A., Pullins, A., Cree, T. *et al.* (2020) Evaluation of the VETSCAN IMAGYST: An in-clinic canine and feline fecal parasite detection system integrated with a deep learning algorithm. *Parasites & Vectors* 13, 346.

Nielsen, M.K. (2021) What makes a good fecal egg count technique? *Veterinary Parasitology* 296, 109509.

Palmer, D.G. and McCombe, I.L. (1996) Lectin staining of trichostrongylid nematode eggs of sheep: Rapid identification of *Haemonchus contortus* eggs with peanut agglutinin. *International Journal for Parasitology* 26, 447–450.

Paras, K.L., George, M.M., Vidyashankar, A.N. and Kaplan, R. (2018) Comparison of fecal egg counting methods in four livestock species. *Veterinary Parasitology* 257, 21–27.

Roeber, F., Morrison, A., Casaert, S., Smith, L., Claerebout, E. *et al.* (2017) Multiplexed-tandem PCR for the specific diagnosis of gastrointestinal nematode infections in sheep: An European validation study. *Parasites & Vectors* 10, 226.

Slusarewicz, P., Pagano, S., Mills, C., Papa, G., Chow, K. *et al.* (2016) Automated parasite faecal egg counting using fluorescence labelling, smartphone image capture and computational image analysis. *International Journal for Parasitology* 46, 485–493.

Slusarewicz, P., Slusarewicz, J.H. and Nielsen, M.K. (2021) Development and performance of an automated fecal egg count system for small ruminant strongylids. *Veterinary Parasitology* 295, 109442.

Van Wyk, J.A. and Van Wyk, L. (2002) Freezing sheep faeces invalidates Haemonchus contortus faecal egg counts by the McMaster technique. *Onderstepoort Journal of Veterinary Research* 69, 299–304.

Van Wyk, J.A. and Mayhew, E. (2013) Morphological identification of parasitic nematode infective larvae of small ruminants and cattle: A practical lab guide. *Onderstepoort Journal of Veterinary Research* 80, 539.

Vatta, A.F., Letty, B.A., Linde, M.J., Wijk, E., Hansen, J. *et al.* (2001) Testing for clinical anaemia caused by *Haemonchus* spp. in goats farmed under resource-poor conditions in South Africa using an eye colour chart developed for sheep. *Veterinary Parasitology* 99, 1–14.

Zajac, A.M., Conboy, G.A., Little, S.E. and Reichard, M. (2021) *Veterinary Clinical Parasitology*, 9th edn. Wiley-Blackwell, Hoboken, USA.

9 Improving the Effectiveness and Sustainability of Gastrointestinal Nematode Control in Cattle: Applying Lessons Learned from Management of Small Ruminants to Forge a Brighter Future

Leonor Sicalo Gianechini[1]* and Ray M. Kaplan[1,2]

[1]*Department of Infectious Diseases, College of Veterinary Medicine, University of Georgia Athens, Georgia, USA;* [2]*School of Veterinary Medicine, St George's University, Grenada, West Indies*

Abstract

Gastrointestinal nematodes (GIN) pose a major challenge to the health and productivity of small ruminants and cattle. There is a considerable amount of published research on sustainable parasite control strategies for small ruminants, and the benefits of these approaches are well documented. However, comparable data for cattle remain limited due to the substantially higher costs and logistical challenges of performing similar studies in cattle. Consequently, sustainable parasite control strategies for cattle are extrapolated from small ruminant research. This chapter examines approaches to parasite control in cattle, incorporating lessons from small ruminants while emphasizing key differences in GIN biology and epidemiology between them. A central focus is placed on refugia-based strategies, which help maintain drug-susceptible alleles in parasite populations. By adopting refugia-based strategies and reducing reliance on whole-herd treatments, cattle producers can improve the sustainability of parasite control, preserve the efficacy of current treatments, and reduce losses due to drug resistance.

Introduction

Gastrointestinal nematodes (GIN) are one of the main constraints on the health and productivity of cattle and small ruminants (Gibbs, 1992; Sykes, 1994; Corwin, 1997; Sykes and Greer, 2003). Evidence-based recommendations constitute the foundations of sustainable parasite control programs for small ruminants. However, similar data demonstrating the benefits of sustainable parasite control programs for cattle are sparse. The primary reasons for this limited evidence are linked to the much higher costs and increased logistical complexity involved with performing long-term research studies in cattle. Thus, many of the recommendations for sustainable parasite control being made for cattle are based on research performed in small ruminants. Cattle, sheep, and goats are closely related members of the Bovidae family, and they

*Corresponding author: sicalo.leonor@uga.edu

© CAB International 2026. *Management Practices for Controlling Nematode Parasites of Small Ruminants* (eds James E. Miller and Joan M. Burke)
DOI: 10.1079/9781800623767.0009

share many similar biological features. This includes the common and important species of helminth parasites. Some helminth species infect both cattle and small ruminants, but most are host specific and do not crossinfect. However, these host-specific parasite species are extremely closely related, and have very similar life cycles and host–parasite dynamics.

Nevertheless, there are some key differences in the management practices used for raising cattle vs small ruminants, and these need to be considered when developing optimal parasite control programs. In this chapter, we will address two major areas (1) sustainable approaches for parasite control that work universally for ruminants, and (2) sustainable approaches developed for use in small ruminants that are applicable to cattle, and which can be practically implemented on cattle operations to improve long-term sustainability of parasite control.

Biology and Epidemiology of Important GIN in Cattle

In both cattle and small ruminants, the most pathogenic GIN species reside in the abomasum and intestine and belong to the superfamily Strongyloidea (Veglia, 1915; Fox, 1993; Stear *et al.*, 2003; Charlier *et al.*, 2020). Nematodes from other taxonomic orders such as whipworms (*Trichuris* spp.) will not be a focus in this chapter since they rarely are a health concern in cattle.

Gastrointestinal nematodes of livestock have a direct life cycle that involves an obligatory phase in the animal and free-living stages that develop within the feces in the environment. Weather and climatic conditions have a direct and profound impact on GIN biology and the epidemiology of parasitic infections. Given adequate moisture and temperature, larval contamination can rapidly increase in the environment, translating also into high worm burdens in the hosts. However, the timing and levels of development and survival of free-living stages will vary in different climatic regions. For instance, in the northern regions of the US, free-living stages will be exposed to prolonged freezing temperatures for a substantial part of the year. Worms will need to take advantage

of the short summer to infect the animals and build up their numbers in the grass. In contrast, in the southern states, transmission of GIN can occur during the entire year. However, the survival of cold-tolerant species will be limited during the warm season, while the survival of cold-intolerant species will be limited during the winter (Navarre, 2020).

Therefore, the prevalence, distribution, and seasonal patterns of GIN transmission will be different across the US. For example, *Ostertagia* spp., a cold-tolerant worm and the most pathogenic species of GIN in cattle, has a limited survival outside the animal during the hot summers of the south and in the cold winters of the north. However, this parasite can undergo arrested development in the host when climatic conditions are not optimal for its survival in the environment. Thus, in the south, it will arrest in the host during the summer, whereas in the north, this period of arrest occurs during the harsh winter (Myers and Taylor, 1989; Hildreth and McKenzie, 2020). The synchronous reactivation of *Ostertagia* larvae from the abomasal mucosa following this period of arrest can cause severe damage to the mucosa of this organ. This may result in clinical disease marked by significant weight loss, hypoproteinemia, diarrhea, anorexia, and even death (Fox, 1993). In the southern states, in addition to *Ostertagia*, *Cooperia* spp., *Haemonchus placei*, and *Haemonchus contortus* can also have an important impact on the health and productivity of cattle (Navarre, 2020). The two species of *Haemonchus* tend to mainly affect younger animals in their first grazing season. *Haemonchus* spp. feed on blood causing anemia, hypoproteinemia, and edema in affected animals. These effects are usually much less severe in cattle compared to the levels of disease observed in small ruminants. *Haemonchus* spp. can also undergo a period of arrested development, typically during cold winter conditions.

Cooperia spp. are found in the small intestine and although they are less pathogenic than *Ostertagia* and *Haemonchus*, they may produce significant negative effects in growing cattle (Stromberg *et al.*, 2012). Consequently, despite not causing clinical disease to the extent of *Ostertagia*, substantial production losses can result from high levels of infection with *Cooperia*. Over the past few decades, because of the heavy use of macrocyclic lactone drugs (e.g. ivermectin) and the propensity of this worm to become resistant, the relative intensity of *Cooperia* compared to other species has risen substantially. Considering these facts, *Cooperia* should be regarded as an important pathogen in cattle production systems both in the northern and southern regions.

Factors that affect pasture contamination with infective larvae play an important role in the epidemiology of infection with GIN in all ruminants. Levels of pasture contamination can vary greatly depending on a variety of factors including climate, season, weather, age of animals, and stocking rate. However, levels of larval contamination on pasture follow predictable seasonal patterns, with lowest levels tending to occur early and highest levels tending to occur late in the grazing season (Eysker *et al.*, 1998). As the grazing season progresses, young animals will recycle the worms on the pasture, yielding increases in their worm burdens and fecal egg counts (FEC), which then lead to increased levels of contamination. As this process continues, these first-year grazers begin to develop immunity, which then leads to reduced worm burdens and FEC (Charlier *et al.*, 2020). In this regard, sheep and cattle will develop immunity against certain species of worms by their second grazing season, whereas goats remain fairly susceptible even as adult animals (Michel, 1963; Vercruysse and Claerebout, 1997; Nisbet *et al.*, 2016). Another peculiarity is that ewes and does experience a periparturient rise in fecal egg counts, that spans the period from 2 weeks prior to lambing/kidding, until around 8 weeks postpartum (Taylor, 1935; O'Sullivan and Donald, 1970). This increased egg shedding occurs due to temporary immunosuppression, and nutrients being prioritized for fetal development, mammary development, and milk production. However, this phenomenon does not occur in cattle. Adult cows will typically shed few GIN eggs (<25 eggs per gram; epg) even when harboring moderate worm burdens (Armour, 1989).

Another issue is that fecal pats can act as a reservoir source of infective larvae for a long time. Even in harsh cold climates, larvae of some species of cold-tolerant worms can overwinter in fecal pats and survive in sufficient numbers to get the cycle started again in the spring (Wang *et al.*, 2020). Other cold-intolerant species like *Haemonchus* will survive the winter arrested

in the host, as opposed to inside the fecal pats (Waller *et al.*, 2004). So, depending on the species of worm, they will be able to survive severe environmental conditions in the host, in the pasture, or in both.

It is important to note that cattle and sheep can share several species of nematodes. The most common of these include *Trichostrongylus axei*, several species of *Cooperia* and *Nematodirus*, and *H. contortus* (Toledo *et al.*, 2019). This could potentially be of relevance when cograzing small and large ruminants, but only rarely leads to infections that are clinically significant.

Anthelmintic Resistance and Deworming Practices in Cattle and Small Ruminant Farms

For many decades, parasite control in ruminants has relied on the frequent and/or strategic use of anthelmintic drugs in order to maximize livestock health, productivity, and profitability. Although this approach was initially highly successful, we are now experiencing ever-increasing levels of anthelmintic (dewormer) resistance in all drug classes, involving virtually all of the most economically important parasites of livestock (Kaplan, 2004; Kaplan and Vidyashankar, 2012). Since the introduction of ivermectin in 1981, no new classes of anthelmintic have been marketed in the US for ruminants. Currently, there is no evidence that new anthelmintic drugs are in the late-phase pipeline, nor that the new drugs available elsewhere (monepantel and derquantel) will be commercialized in the US any time soon. Thus, it could be many years before a new anthelmintic drug class is introduced to the North American ruminant market. Consequently, the development and spread of anthelmintic resistance will almost certainly outpace the introduction of new anthelmintic classes, and in the future when a new anthelmintic is finally introduced for use in livestock, it will almost certainly be considerably more expensive than the most expensive of the current products. Thus, the cattle industry needs to change the way parasite control is practiced, bring back critical thinking to the process, and establish sustainable programs that help to preserve the efficacy of anthelmintics.

The development of anthelmintic resistance is a threat on every farm that uses anthelmintics, although the rate at which resistance develops is affected by a large number of variables including the host, the parasite species, the drug, the frequency of anthelmintic administration, and the amount of refugia present at the time treatments are performed (Prichard, 2005). On sheep and goat farms, anthelmintic resistance originally developed and spread considerably more rapidly than on cattle farms, and the problem is more severe on small ruminant farms. However, anthelmintic resistance is now an increasingly serious problem in cattle parasites, and is continually worsening. Therefore, it is important that the cattle industry make use of the lessons learned from the sheep and goat industry to slow the process of resistance in GIN infecting cattle.

Under natural conditions, the development of anthelmintic resistance usually requires numerous generations of worms to be under drug selection (Gilleard and Beech, 2007), taking many years to reach levels that cause a significant reduction in drug efficacy. However, anthelmintic resistance can appear very rapidly on a farm if new additions to the herd harbor drug-resistant parasites. Depending upon how many animals are purchased that harbor resistant worms, the worm burdens of those animals, and other management and pasture factors such as amount of refugia, treatment failure due to drug resistance can occur practically instantly or over a relatively short period. This is why appropriate quarantine periods and treatments, along with regular testing for drug resistance, should be implemented on all ruminant farms.

Studies performed in the southern states between 2002 and 2006,showed that *H. contortus* was resistant to all three classes of anthelmintics in 48% of sheep and goat farms. In the mid-Atlantic region (2007–2009), 82% of all farms tested had multiple resistance to at least two different drug classes, and the prevalence of moxidectin resistance was detected on 47% of the farms (Crook *et al.*, 2016). Other unpublished data (Kaplan *et al.*, 2023, personal communication) suggests that this problem has further worsened since these studies were conducted.

Resistance in parasites of cattle has developed at a slower pace than in the small ruminant and equine sectors, but over the past decade there has been a rapid increase in the levels and distribution of anthelmintic resistance in gastrointestinal worms of cattle worldwide (Waghorn *et al.*, 2006; Ramos *et al.*, 2016; Waghorn *et al.*, 2016; Cristel *et al.*, 2017; Rose Vineer *et al.*, 2020). In the US, there are some published case reports of resistance in parasites of cattle (Gasbarre *et al.*, 2009; Edmonds *et al.*, 2010) but no studies have been performed to establish the national prevalence of resistance. However, a study performed by the Kaplan Laboratory on 12 cow-calf farms in Georgia and on stocker cattle purchased at various stockyards in the southern region suggests that anthelmintic resistance to the macrocyclic lactone family (e.g. ivermectin) in cattle is both very common and widespread (Gianechini *et al.*, 2025). More than 90% of farms tested by our laboratory in the last 10 years show *Cooperia* spp. resistant to the macrocyclic lactone class. Resistance in *Cooperia* spp. and *Haemonchus* spp. was the most common, but resistance in *Ostertagia ostertagi* was also found. Other recent data (unpublished) indicates that macrocyclic lactone drugs have lost the ability to kill inhibited *Ostertagia* L4 in weaned beef calves in the southern US. Overall, in the southern US, it appears that resistance to macrocyclic lactone drugs is highly prevalent in *Cooperia* spp. and *Haemonchus* spp., and is in the emerging stages for *Ostertagia* (Gianechini *et al.* 2025).

Further supporting these observations, the United States Department of Agriculture (USDA) National Animal Health Monitoring System (NAHMS) conducted a study in 2008 to examine the efficacy of anthelmintic treatment on 72 beef cow-calf operations across 19 states (Gasbarre *et al.*, 2015). Notably, they found suboptimal fecal egg count reduction on 100% of the farms that had used a pour-on macrocyclic lactone as treatment 14–16 days prior. PCR analysis of the parasite populations surviving treatment indicated that the lack of efficacy was most likely due to anthelmintic resistance in *Cooperia* spp. and possibly *Haemonchus* spp. Therefore, even with limited information regarding the national prevalence of resistance in cattle nematodes, there is no evidence that would suggest that there are major differences in other regions in terms of anthelmintic resistance.

Other countries where data are available indicate the problem is even worse than in the

US. For instance, the problem of widespread anthelmintic resistance was confirmed in New Zealand in a survey conducted on 62 cattle farms in 2006 (Waghorn et al., 2006). At that time, resistance to ivermectin, albendazole, and levamisole was reported on 92%, 76%, and 6% of the farms, respectively, while only 7% of the farms showed susceptibility to all three drug classes. Furthermore, Cooperia spp. was resistant to ivermectin and albendazole on 74% of the farms. In contrast, the more pathogenic Ostertagia spp. was still susceptible to ivermectin and levamisole on 91% of the farms, whereas resistance to the benzimidazoles was observed in 35% of the farms. However, 10 years later, Waghorn conducted further testing on six commercial farms, showing macrocyclic

lactone failure to control Ostertagia spp. on all farms (Waghorn et al., 2016). In addition, inefficacy of albendazole and levamisole was also observed towards Ostertagia spp. in 50 and 100% of the farms, respectively. Similar results showing a high prevalence of resistance in multiple species of cattle nematodes including Ostertagia have been reported in multiple other countries (Suarez and Cristel, 2007; Soutello et al., 2007; Rendell, 2010). Consequently, evidence strongly suggests that resistance in Ostertagia is already a problem on some farms, and will continue to worsen and become a serious threat to cattle health and productivity in the US in the near future unless major changes in anthelmintic treatment strategies are implemented immediately.

Table 9.1. Available anthelmintics in the US market for use in cattle.

Drug class	Chemical name	Product name	Dose (mg/kg)	Route of administration
Benzimidazoles	Albendazole	Valbazen®	10	Oral
	Fenbendazole	Safe-Guard®, Panacur®	5–10	Oral (several different oral formulations exist)
	Oxfendazole	Synanthic®	4.5	Oral
Macrocyclic lactones	Ivermectin	Ivomec®, Ivermectin®, Bimectin®, Noromectin®, Ivermax®, Phoenectin®	0.2	s/c
		Privermectin®, Ivermectin®, Ivomec®, Bimectin®, Iver-On™, Phoenectin®	0.5	Pour-on
	Ivermectin + clorsulon	Ivomec® Plus, Noromectin® Plus	0.2 + 2	s/c
	Eprinomectin	Eprinex®, Eprizero™, LongRange®	0.5	Pour-on
			1	s/c
	Doramectin	Dectomax®	0.2	s/c
			0.5	Pour-on
	Moxidectin	Cydectin®	0.2	s/c
			0.5	Pour-on
		Tauramox™	0.2	s/c
Imidazothiazoles	Levamisole	Prohibit®, LevaMed™	8	Oral
Combination	Doramectin + levamisole	Valcor™	0.2 + 6	s/c

mg/kg, milligrams per kilogram; s/c, subcutaneous.

Table 9.1 provides a summary of all the anthelmintic drugs (dewormers) commercially available for cattle in the US (FDA, 2023), along with their recommended doses.

The Refugia-based Strategy

In sheep, several novel approaches have proven effective for reducing the development of resistance and managing resistant gastrointestinal nematodes. The common factor among these approaches is the preservation of refugia and the implementation of highly efficacious treatments (Greer *et al.*, 2020; Kaplan, 2020). By administering anthelmintics only to the animals that are suffering the consequences of parasitism at clinical and/or economically relevant levels, and thus will most likely benefit from treatment, herd-level parasite control can be achieved while allowing a proportion of worms to escape drug selection (Van Wyk, 2001). As this strategy is based on the principle of preserving and managing refugia, these are often referred to as refugia-based strategies.

Within the context of drug resistance, refugia represent the portion of the worm population that has escaped drug selection, either in animals that did not receive treatment or by being in the environment (on pasture) at the time of treatment (Van Wyk, 2001; Greer *et al.*, 2020). By escaping drug selection, this portion of the worm population will help maintain a pool of drug-susceptible alleles that will dilute the resistant worms that survived treatment. Furthermore, the fewer the number of surviving resistant worms, the greater the dilution effect from the refugia. By maximizing the efficacy of all anthelmintic treatments that are administered, the number of surviving resistant worms will be minimized. Achieving high efficacy therefore results in greater levels of dilution by existing refugia, thereby maximizing the benefits of refugia-based strategies. Given the reductions in efficacy that can be expected due to drug resistance, the only practical means available to increase the efficacy of treatments is to use anthelmintics in combination, whereby two or more different anthelmintics from different drug classes are administered at the same time. To illustrate

this point, data are presented in Table 9.2 that illustrate the impact of using combination treatments of more than one anthelmintic class to increase efficacy, and Table 9.3 shows the impact of treatment efficacy on the level of dilution achieved when a portion of the herd is left untreated.

To illustrate the relevance of the data presented in these tables, we present two scenarios. Scenario 1: if we administer an anthelmintic with 80% efficacy, 20% of the worms will survive (resistant worms). That 20% of worms surviving will have virtually no dilution (1.5-fold dilution), even when leaving 30% of our animals untreated. Scenario 2: achieving a treatment efficacy of 99%, and leaving 30% of the herd untreated, will achieve a 30-fold dilution. In general, the higher the efficacy, the lower the proportion of the herd that needs to be left untreated to achieve significant levels of dilution of the resistant phenotypes (see Table 9.3). However, to achieve high efficacy (>95%) in a scenario of widespread resistance, combining products that belong to different drug classes becomes a near necessity. It is important to note that from a purely clinical perspective, if the efficacy of an anthelmintic (used singly) is >80%, it is very possible that the farmer will not notice any difference in the clinical response of treatments when applied singly vs in combination (e.g. with a second drug also with 80% efficacy, which will then yield a 96% efficacy). However, the impact on the further development of resistance could be quite substantial, and that is why we need to monitor the efficacy of our drugs. The different mechanisms of action provided by different drug classes will act on worms that may be resistant to one drug class but are still susceptible to another dewormer in the combination.

As illustrated in Table 9.3, the success of refugia-based strategies is closely linked to the efficacy of the treatments. Consequently, every livestock farmer needs to know the efficacy of the anthelmintics being used on their farm. This is the only way in which evidence-based decisions can be made on drug choice, including which anthelmintics to include in a combination treatment. Having a good knowledge of the prevalence of resistance in your area is helpful but ultimately, this only tells you what can be expected across many farms; it does not provide any information of the situation on a particular farm. The reluctance of most

Table 9.2. Impact of using anthelmintics in combination on the efficacy of treatments. The increases in efficacy when using drug combinations are due to an additive effect as illustrated in the table. Calculations of efficacy are based on the following equations: where D1 = efficacy of drug 1, D2 = efficacy of drug 2, D3 = efficacy of drug 3, C2 = efficacy of D1 + D2, and C3 = efficacy of D1 + D2 + D3. C2% = D1% + (100-D1%) *D2% .C3% = C2% + (100 C2%) *D3%.

Drug 1 (%)	Drug 2 (%)	Drug 3 (%)	Combination (%)	High efficacy (>95%) achieved?
60	60	-	84	x
60	70	-	88	x
60	80	-	92	x
60	90	-	96	✓
60	95	-	98	✓
70	80	-	94	x
70	90	-	97	✓
70	95	-	98.5	✓
80	90	-	98	✓
80	95	-	99	✓
90	90	-	99	✓
90	95	-	99.5	✓
90	99	-	99.9	✓
60	60	70	95.2	✓
60	80	70	97.6	✓

Source: Adapted from Kaplan (2020).

Table 9.3. The level of dilution of resistant eggs (shed by treated animals) achieved at different levels of efficacy when leaving three different proportions of the herd untreated. The eggs shed from untreated animals dilute the eggs shed by treated animals, and the level of dilution increases as both the efficacy and the proportion left untreated increase.

	~ Fold dilution from refugia		
Efficacy	90% Treated	80% Treated	70% Treated
99.9	100	200	300
99.5	20	40	60
99	10	20	30
98	5	10	15
95	2	4	6
80	0.5	1	1.5

producers to test for anthelmintic resistance is not rational from an economic perspective since the evidence is strong that highly efficacious treatments are currently not achieved on most farms. Given the widespread levels of resistance that exist to some anthelmintics, in order to achieve the high efficacy desired on most farms it is necessary to use multiple drugs from different anthelmintic classes simultaneously. This is referred to as combination treatment, and research has demonstrated quite clearly that the use of anthelmintics in combination is a beneficial practice if used within the context of a refugia-based parasite control strategy (Bartram et al., 2012; Geary et al., 2012; Leathwick et al., 2012).

There are three major benefits to using drugs in combination. (i) There is an additive effect with each drug used (see Table 9.2), so the efficacy of the treatment increases with each additional drug given. (ii) There is a return to broad-spectrum efficacy; since resistance is species and drug specific, a second (or third) drug may kill any species resistant to the first (or second) drug. This will then return the broad-spectrum efficacy that one aims to achieve (and that is specified on the product label). (iii) By achieving a higher efficacy, there are fewer resistant survivors, thus there is a greater dilution of resistant worms by the susceptible portion of the population. However, for this strategy to achieve the desired goal, anthelmintics included in the combination need to have at least 60% efficacy or higher (Dobson *et al.*, 2011; Leathwick, 2012). If two anthelmintics each with 60% efficacy are included, then the treatment will yield an 84% overall efficacy. But if a third drug with a 70% efficacy is included, then the efficacy increases to 95% (see the examples in Table 9.2). It is important to note that the sooner a combination treatment strategy is implemented, the greater the benefits since the greatest difference in the percent of resistant survivors is seen when efficacy of anthelmintics is very high. Thus, this strategy should be implemented immediately on farms, and not just used as a last-ditch salvage approach once resistance becomes a severe problem.

At the time of this publication, there is only one FDA-approved product (Valcor™) on the US market that provides a combination of two actives belonging to different drug classes (see Table 9.1 for available products). For all the other available anthelmintics, each drug (dewormer) included in the combination needs to be administered separately. Just as when used singly, when used in combination drugs need to be administered at the full recommended dose for each individual dewormer. Additionally, different anthelmintics should not be mixed in the same container or syringe since they may not be chemically compatible. But they can be administered concurrently, meaning one after the other. Of important consideration is that unless combination treatments are done in tandem with practices that maintain/manage refugia, drug resistance to all the dewormers in the combination could escalate rapidly. Therefore, combination treatments should only be used in a parasite control program if efforts are made to manage refugia.

The optimal approach for instituting combination treatments is to first conduct a fecal egg count reduction test (FECRT) to gain knowledge of the efficacy of the dewormers individually. This will then permit the calculation for estimating the overall expected efficacy of the combination (see Table 9.2). Knowing this, producers can then determine the proportion of animals to leave untreated based on the level of dilution they wish to achieve (see Table 9.3) (Leathwick, 2007). Ideally, the efficacy of the combination will also be checked using a FECRT to confirm the expected efficacy was achieved.

Testing the efficacy of drugs with a FECRT is the best way for a farmer to make sure he/she is using effective drugs, and to decide which products to use in combination (Kaplan *et al.*, 2023). To optimally implement the FECRT, we recommend accessing (available free on open access) and following the new international guidelines published by the World Association for the Advancement of Veterinary Parasitology (WAAVP) (Kaplan *et al.*, 2023). These guidelines provide detailed explanation and instruction on how to perform a FECRT, and how to analyze and interpret the resulting data.

Transitioning from the "Old System" to More Sustainable Strategies

The latest beef study from NAHMS, conducted in 2017, collected information on common management and health practices, representing 78.9% of US cow-calf operations and 86.6% percent of US beef cows (USDA, 2020). Results of that study indicate that 89% of the operations that dewormed cattle at least occasionally did so on a regular schedule. Almost half (43.5%) of those operations rotated anthelmintic drug classes in an attempt "to prolong or improve the efficacy of dewormers." However, rotation of drugs and whole-herd treatments have long been associated with the development of resistance (Smith, 1990; Barnes *et al.*, 1995). Therefore, the cattle industry needs to move away from these practices and into evidence-based control strategies. However, a major problem that affects the awareness of drug resistance by producers is that unless they are carefully monitoring production parameters, the impact of anthelmintic resistance in cattle will most likely go unnoticed until late in the process. Change is difficult, however, especially when a new system requires more thought, time, and expense. Consequently, to achieve a shift in the way parasite control is practiced by the US cattle industry, new recommendations need to be both practical and cost-effective (McArthur and Reinemeyer, 2014).

Control programs that promote the sustainable use of anthelmintics and preservation of susceptible worms are rarely applied by cattle farmers, and changing these practices will require innovative approaches to the way parasite control is being applied (McArthur and Reinemeyer, 2014). In sheep, there are a number of successful and novel approaches (FAMACHA©, Five Point Check©, Happy Factor™ method, milk yield, body condition score, diarrhea score) (Table 9.4) that allow the identification of individual animals requiring treatment, leading to a reduction in the use of anthelmintics, preservation of susceptible worms in untreated animals, and increased

Table 9.4. Evidence-based targeted selective treatment (TST) options in sheep and their possible use in cattle.

TST indicator	Use in sheep	Possible use in cattle
FAMACHA© (anemia score)	For blood-sucking parasites, mainly *Haemonchus* spp.	Could work for *Haemonchus* and *Mecistocirrus* or *Bunostomum phlebotomum* but very impractical and potentially unsafe to perform in cattle
Happy Factor (weight gain)	For all nematodes; reduced weight gain as hallmark of clinical and subclinical PGE	Demonstrated as a reliable indicator for the first two grazing seasons in cattle. Need to improve practicality (e.g. remote automated scales)
Diarrhea score (DISCO)/ Dag score	For *Teladorsagia* and *Trichostrongylus* primarily; other causes of diarrhea (e.g. coccidiosis, *Strongyloides*, nutritional, etc.)	More difficult to implement in cattle since feces are naturally less solid than in small ruminants. With more research could possibly be applied for most nematodes in young calves, but only once parasites are causing clinical disease. Not practical for identifying cattle with subclinical PGE
FEC	For all nematodes but primarily *Haemonchus* spp. Impractical unless small flock; not a pen-side test	FEC is highly dependent on the predominant worm species, time of year, animal category, etc. Little evidence that FEC is correlated with production parameters. Not practical in cattle as it is not cost-effective
BCS	Used in the prelambing period, adult animals; also paired with FEC. For all nematodes	Practical but no evidence to date. Not sensitive enough for calves but might be useful for cows
Milk yield	On sheep/goat dairy farms for all nematodes	Could be used for *Ostertagia* spp., mainly. Practical. Some countries in Europe use bulk tank antibody levels for targeted treatment decisions of dairy cattle
Five Point Check (eye, nose, jaw, back, and tail)	For nasal bots and multiple species of GIN	No validation done in cattle. Unlikely to be useful or practical
Plasma pepsinogen concentration	Not used	Could potentially be useful for *Ostertagia* spp. Currently this is only a laboratory-based test, but a pen-side test would be needed to implement selective treatments

BCS, body condition score; FEC, fecal egg count; GIN, gastrointestinal nematodes; PGE, parasitic gastroenteritis.

overall farm sustainability (Van Wyk and Bath, 2002; Bath and Van Wyk, 2009; Gallidis *et al.*, 2009; Bentounsi *et al.*, 2012; Walker *et al.*, 2015; McBean *et al.*, 2016). However, most of these would be difficult and impractical to implement on cattle farms. In cattle, some studies have shown that daily weight gain during their first two grazing seasons is a useful performance parameter to identify animals in need of anthelmintic treatment (Höglund *et al.*, 2009, 2013; O'Shaughnessy *et al.*, 2015b). But there is a critical need to make these treatment decisions practical, accessible, and attractive to US farmers (see Table 9.4). Unless deworming practices are changed, complete treatment failure will become increasingly common (Kaplan, 2020), with huge economic consequences for a national multibillion-dollar industry.

Moreover, studies done in sheep comparing productivity of groups in which both traditional and targeted selective treatment (TST) programs were used demonstrated no significant differences in the growth of lambs (Busin *et al.*, 2013; Kenyon *et al.*, 2013). In the US, one recent study has been completed in cattle in which a TST group that left 10% of the animals untreated was compared over 131 days of grazing with a whole-herd treatment group. No differences were observed in production parameters overall, even when leaving the 10% of animals with the highest FEC untreated (Kipp *et al.*, 2023). However, though this study was a good proof of concept, animals had low levels of infections, which may limit its applicability in situations where cattle are harboring higher levels of infection. Additionally, in this study animals with the highest FEC were left untreated; this would not be a recommended strategy for farmers. Instead, cattle producers should leave untreated only those animals that will not likely benefit from treatment. The use of effective drugs (and preferably combinations of drugs) and management of refugia by leaving some animals untreated are likely to both improve overall herd productivity and sustain the susceptibility of worms on the farm well into the future.

Clearly, there is a great need for new research to address this issue, but waiting for this research to be completed before acting is not advisable. The high cost of performing long-term studies in cattle practically guarantees that the necessary data to prove the effectiveness of these strategies will never be collected in time to be useful. Therefore,

we cannot escape the reality that we must deal with the uncertainty of which approaches will be best for reducing the rate at which anthelmintic resistance evolves in cattle, while not sacrificing significant levels of production. Thus, we must use the data we have, and given the great biological similarities, it is logical to pursue the strategies proven successful for sheep that can be reasonably applied to cattle production systems. Given the substantial evidence that traditional approaches to parasite control in cattle are yielding suboptimal efficacy and economic returns, and that drug resistance is rapidly worsening, to do nothing is both irrational and short-sighted.

Approaches to Control Parasite Resistance Worms in Cattle

As discussed previously, sheep offer some success stories about managing anthelmintic resistance that can provide valuable insights to the cattle community. Some of these successful parasite control programs have included the following approaches: (i) not treating the ewes and only treating the lambs, (ii) leaving a percentage of the flock untreated (e.g. the heaviest 10%), (iii) treating selectively based on some measure of parasitism or growth rate, and (iv) using drug combinations (two or more active compounds from different drug classes administered at the same time) (Leathwick *et al.*, 2008, 2012; Bartram *et al.*, 2012).

In cattle, however, only a few refugia-based strategies have been explored in studies conducted in Europe and Australasia (Höglund *et al.*, 2009, 2013; McAnulty *et al.*, 2011; O'Shaughnessy *et al.*, 2014, 2015a, b), and only one study has been conducted in the US (Kipp *et al.*, 2023). These studies use the following criteria for applying anthelmintic treatments.

- Anthelmintic was administered to individuals that failed to meet predetermined growth rates (McAnulty *et al.*, 2011).
- Weight gain-based anthelmintic treatments were given when individual calf performance was inferior to the average of the poorer 50% of calves in a control group receiving monthly anthelmintic treatments (Höglund *et al.*, 2013).

- Individual calves in the TST groups were treated with anthelmintic when (i) positive for lungworm larvae using the modified Baermann technique or (ii) positive or negative for lungworm larvae using the modified Baermann technique with plasma pepsinogen concentrations (PP) ≥ 2 international units of tyrosine/l (Utyr) and FEC ≥ 200 epg (O'Shaughnessy *et al.*, 2014, 2015a).
- Animals were treated with anthelmintic if thresholds based on a combination of plasma pepsinogen concentrations, FEC, and/or the presence of *Dictyocaulus viviparus* larvae in feces were surpassed (O'Shaughnessy *et al.*, 2015b).
- All calves from the control group were administered a combination treatment, while in the refugia group, the steer with the highest FEC within the paddock was left untreated (Kipp *et al.*, 2023).

Some of these strategies have produced a good initial proof of concept for cattle, but a considerable amount of fine tuning is needed to make them feasible to implement at farm level. Furthermore, only one strategy has been examined under US farming conditions (Kipp *et al.*, 2023). In addition, none of these studies performed a FECRT to determine the farm-level resistance status of the anthelmintics being used, and only two studies used a combination of anthelmintics.

Simulation studies have clearly shown that the success of the TST strategy is strongly linked to the efficacy of treatments (Leathwick, 2012; Leathwick *et al.*, 2012; Bartram *et al.*, 2012). Given what is known about current levels of resistance, if using drugs only from the macrocyclic lactone group (e.g. ivermectin), then it is highly likely that some nematode species are not being adequately controlled. Thus, the methods used in these studies did not provide the full potential benefits of the TST approach. Other limitations of the above studies include the reduced number of animals used, large weighing intervals, and the use of a suppressively treated group as a control. And even more important, none of these strategies is entirely practical or includes the use of tests that could be done pen-side. Animals would have to be gathered on a second opportunity to

be able to treat them selectively. So, even when in some cases anthelmintic use was reduced by over 90%, these strategies become very hard to implement on a commercial cattle farm setting.

Bearing in mind that cattle are not sheep, we can adapt some of the parasite control strategies from sheep into use in cattle farms. Nonetheless, some of these practices may be more difficult to implement and/or be less effective in cattle but we cannot know until more research is available on the matter. For instance, leaving cows untreated can be a very beneficial source of refugia for *Ostertagia*. Cows are predominantly infected with *Ostertagia*, so not treating cows but treating calves is likely to be quite beneficial for slowing the development of resistance in *Ostertagia*. This is an easily implemented strategy that will provide refugia when calves are being treated. However, it is notable that strategies that may work for one parasite species may not work for another. For *Cooperia*, this strategy would not be very effective, since cows develop good immunity to this genus and shed relatively few eggs of *Cooperia*. In contrast, *Cooperia* usually makes up the majority of eggs shed by calves. The high levels of resistance to the macrocyclic lactones that already exist in *Cooperia* make it too late on most farms to implement a refugia-based strategy for this parasite and drug class. However, resistance in *Cooperia* is still relatively low for the other major drug classes, and refugia-based strategies could be implemented to help preserve the efficacy of those other drugs. Such strategies for *Cooperia* would have to involve leaving some calves untreated.

Another easily implemented strategy for cattle that will provide refugia and slow the development of anthelmintic resistance is leaving a proportion of the herd (e.g. 10–30%) untreated. This is sometimes referred to as "selective nontreatment." This strategy differs from TST, where the decision of which animals to treat is based on a measure of infection or productivity. In selective nontreatment, the farmer simply leaves some of the herd untreated when applying anthelmintics to the herd. The nontreated animals can be selected randomly or, preferably, the "best-looking" and/or heaviest (in growing animals) are left untreated. The rationale behind this strategy is that the "best-looking" animals are already performing well compared to the rest of the herd, and therefore are likely to gain minimal benefit from anthelmintic treatment. Hence, little production is lost by not treating these animals, while maintaining a proportion of worms in refugia and slowing down the development of resistance. This strategy could be implemented in growing cattle that will usually harbor a mixed burden of gastrointestinal nematodes. Furthermore, this strategy can be used if cows are treated around calving time. Leaving the "best-looking" cows untreated will provide refugia, while the majority of the herd could benefit by having increased milk yield for feeding the newborn calves (Ploeger *et al.*, 1989; Sanchez *et al.*, 2004).

It is quite relevant and important to appreciate that the evidence in sheep is strong that treating all ewes at lambing will select heavily for resistance, representing a high-risk practice for the rapid development of anthelmintic resistance (Leathwick *et al.*, 1995, 2006; Lawrence *et al.*, 2006). There is no credible reason to believe the same would not be true for cattle. Although selective nontreatment is the most practical means of implementing a refugia-based strategy on cattle farms, and available evidence suggests it is likely to be an effective strategy, definitive evidence is still lacking due to the dearth of research.

Refugia-based parasite control strategies in cattle differ greatly from traditional recommendations provided by veterinarians and pharmaceutical companies. Thus, it can be expected that there will be opposition from farmers to leaving some animals untreated, as this goes against what they have been told for years, and against their common sense of what is best for maximizing productivity. However, the reality is that many cattle producers who continue to treat all cattle in the herd are using anthelmintics that often yield poor efficacy due to resistance without realizing it, as well as using anthelmintics at improper times of the year. So even though they are treating all their cattle, they are getting suboptimal results while simultaneously making the drug resistance worse. Consequently, there is a need to work on improving the understanding of farmers on these issues, so that they will appreciate the importance of managing refugia combined with high-efficacy treatments as pillars of a sound parasite control program. Unless this change occurs at a fairly rapid pace, resistance will continue to worsen

and spread further, decreasing productivity and wasting money by purchasing drugs that do not work.

It is noteworthy that some farms we have tested with FECRT had 0% reduction in FEC, and the cattleman had not suspected resistance at all prior to the test. Studies in sheep have clearly demonstrated that the production cost of subclinical parasitism as a result of using an anthelmintic product that is less than fully effective due to resistance can greatly exceed the cost of routine testing of anthelmintic efficacy (Miller *et al.*, 2012). Cattle farmers would thus be much better off using highly effective anthelmintic treatments and leaving some animals untreated, increasing the sustainability of their production system in the long run.

A Sound Parasite Control Program in Cattle Farms

The goal of any parasite control program should be eliminating clinical presentations of parasitism, minimizing subclinical losses, and preserving the effectiveness of dewormers that still maintain high efficacy for the farm. It is not desirable or advisable to pursue complete "elimination" of gastrointestinal nematodes. This is not possible, and will only accelerate the pace at which resistance to dewormers develops. Therefore, cattle producers and veterinarians need to focus on creating a balance between levels of infection with worms and associated production losses.

Infections with worms are a natural part of being a cow, and in many animals cause little harm. Our goal then is to minimize production losses at the herd level. Whole-herd deworming treatments are not needed to achieve this. Properly timed, highly efficacious deworming treatments given to the majority of the herd (but not all animals) will achieve this, and will be much more effective than frequent whole-herd treatments with a partially effective dewormer. Consequently, the aim is to achieve a result that is both effective and sustainable, and this necessitates following the principles of refugia-based strategies. There are a number of management practices relating to parasite control that should be implemented together with a refugia-based strategy in order to achieve optimal results.

- *Quarantine of all new introductions*, and treatment with a highly efficacious dewormer. This is necessary to prevent the introduction of drug-resistant worms to the herd from newly acquired animals. Since one should always err on the side of caution, one should assume that the new additions carry drug-resistant worms. Therefore, this treatment requires the use of a combination of dewormers from multiple different drug classes (at least two and preferably all three). Failure to perform effective quarantine treatments could result in the introduction of drug-resistant worms that were not previously present on the farm, leading to future problems and challenges in achieving successful control of parasites.

- *Treat animals selectively*, leaving 10–30% of the herd untreated. The number of animals to leave untreated depends on the efficacy of the drugs for a given farm (see Table 9.3). Avoid treating all the animals at one time, especially when pasture refugia are low (e.g. dry summers).

- *Use the appropriate anthelmintic doses* (see Table 9.1). Ideally, weigh the animals prior to treatment or use a weigh tape if a scale is unavailable. Note that several studies have convincingly shown that most cattle producers are not as accurate as they think they are at visual estimation of cattle weights. If treating a group of cattle of a similar age/weight all with the same dose volume, then it is important to treat all the animals at the dose required for the heaviest animal of the group. Note that if one treats a group based on the average weight, half the animals will be underdosed. No matter what dosing strategy is used, it is important to avoid underdosing at all costs!

- *Perform a FECRT on the herd* to test the effectiveness of the various dewormers being used or that are being considered to be used. Anthelmintic (dewormer) resistance is very common, but most cattle producers are unaware that they have resistant worms on their farm. Drug resistance can develop fairly quickly, so the FECRT should be repeated every 2–3 years. Perform the FECRT following the latest guidelines (see Kaplan *et al.*, 2023).

- *Use highly efficacious treatments*; achieve this by measuring the effectiveness of dewormers using a FECRT, and then combining anthelmintics from different drug classes.

- *Avoid "dose and move" strategies*, where cattle are dewormed and immediately moved to a new pasture not recently grazed. Pastures ungrazed for extended periods of time will have a low level of refugia. Treating and moving to such a pasture will allow the resistant worms which survived the treatment to contaminate the "new" pasture with a high proportion of resistant worms (Waghorn *et al.*, 2009). Studies in sheep have demonstrated that the best approach is to move and then dose a few days or more later, or to delay moving cattle for several weeks after dosing.

- *Monitor production parameters* such as weight gains and/or feed conversion ratio year over year to enable detection of subclinical reductions in productivity.

- *Reduce dependance on dewormers* by incorporating other strategies, such as improved pasture management and/or improved overall nutritional management.

- *Identify and mitigate high-risk management practices*. Identifying the high-risk practices for a given farm (e.g. frequent treatments, whole-herd treatments, underdosing, treating with low refugia, not testing the efficacy of dewormers being used, etc.) will provide an opportunity to make changes that will improve the results and sustainability of the parasite control program.

- *Parasite control is dynamic*; strategies being used should be reassessed every season in consultation with a veterinarian or a specialist in parasitology to determine what is working and what is not. Note that things that worked in the past may not continue to work optimally in the future. Plan ahead but stay flexible!

Conclusion

Parasite control programs in cattle should be planned carefully to account for the increasing levels of dewormer resistance occurring in livestock production systems worldwide. Refugia-based strategies have proven highly successful in studies on sheep at delaying the development and/or further increase of anthelmintic resistance. However, in order to gain the full benefits of managing refugia, treatments need to be highly efficacious. Direct evidence of the benefits of this strategy is limited for cattle, and the high cost of doing such studies in cattle means that gaining that evidence will remain a challenge. Consequently, we need to adapt the strategies that have proven successful in the small ruminant sector, and implement them in cattle production systems.

In this chapter, we highlight the importance of such strategies and provide a guide for how to select and implement some of these strategies in cattle production systems. Rapid adoption of refugia-based sustainable strategies for parasite control in cattle will be critical in preventing the further worsening of parasite drug resistance, which threatens cattle production systems worldwide. Implementing these strategies in a practical and flexible fashion will have an immediate impact on the effectiveness and sustainability of parasite control in cattle and will help preserve the efficacy of any new class of anthelmintic introduced for cattle in the future.

References

Armour, J. (1989) The influence of host immunity on the epidemiology of trichostrongyle infections in cattle. *Veterinary Parasitology* 32, 5–19. DOI: 10.1016/0304-4017(89)90152-0.

Barnes, E.H., Dobson, R.J. and Barger, I.A. (1995) Worm control and anthelmintic resistance: Adventures with a model. *Parasitology Today* 11, 56–63. DOI: 10.1016/0169-4758(95)80117-0.

Bartram, D.J., Leathwick, D.M., Taylor, M.A., Geurden, T. and Maeder, S. (2012) The role of combination anthelmintic formulations in the sustainable control of sheep nematodes. *Veterinary Parasitology* 186, 151–158. DOI: 10.1016/j.vetpar.2011.11.030.

Bath, G. and Van Wyk, J. (2009) The Five Point Check© for targeted selective treatment of internal parasites in small ruminants. *Small Ruminant Research* 86, 6–13. DOI: 10.1016/j.smallrumres.2009.09.009.

Bentounsi, B., Meradi, S. and Cabaret, J. (2012) Towards finding effective indicators (diarrhoea and anaemia scores and weight gains) for the implementation of targeted selective treatment against the gastro-intestinal nematodes in lambs in a steppic environment. *Veterinary Parasitology* 187, 275–279. DOI: 10.1016/j.vetpar.2011.12.024.

Busin, V., Kenyon, F., Laing, N., Denwood, M., McBean, D. *et al.* (2013) Addressing sustainable sheep farming: Application of a targeted selective treatment approach for anthelmintic use on a commercial farm. *Small Ruminant Research* 110, 100–103. DOI: 10.1016/j.smallrumres.2012.11.013.

Charlier, J., Höglund, J., Morgan, E.R., Geldhof, P., Vercruysse, J. *et al.* (2020) Biology and epidemiology of gastrointestinal nematodes in cattle. *Veterinary Clinics of North America Food Animal Practice* 36, 1–15. DOI: 10.1016/j.cvfa.2019.11.001.

Corwin, R.M. (1997) Economics of gastrointestinal parasitism of cattle. *Veterinary Parasitology* 72, 451–457. DOI: 10.1016/j.prevetmed.2020.105103.

Cristel, S., Fiel, C., Anziani, O., Descarga, C., Cetra, B. *et al.* (2017) Anthelmintic resistance in grazing beef cattle in central and northeastern areas of Argentina—an update. *Veterinary Parasitology: Regional Studies and Reports* 9, 25–28. DOI: 10.1016/j.vprsr.2017.04.003.

Crook, E.K., O'Brien, D.J., Howell, S.B., Storey, B., Whitley, N. *et al.* (2016) Prevalence of anthelmintic resistance on sheep and goat farms in the mid-Atlantic region and comparison of *in vivo* and *in vitro* detection methods. *Small Ruminant Research* 143, 89–96. DOI: 10.1016/j.smallrumres.2016.09.006.

Dobson, R.J., Barnes, E.H., Tyrrell, K.L., Hosking, B.C., Larsen, J.W. *et al.* (2011) A multi-species model to assess the effect of refugia on worm control and anthelmintic resistance in sheep grazing systems. *Australian Veterinary Journal* 89, 200–208. DOI: 10.1111/j.1751-0813.2011.00719.x.

Edmonds, M.D., Johnson, E.G. and Edmonds, J.D. (2010) Anthelmintic resistance of *Ostertagia ostertagi* and *Cooperia oncophora* to macrocyclic lactones in cattle from the western United States. *Veterinary Parasitology* 170, 224–229. DOI: 10.1016/j.vetpar.2010.02.036.

Eysker, M., Van Der Aar, W.M., Boersema, J.H., Githiori, J. and Kooyman, F. (1998) The effect of repeated moves to clean pasture on the build up of gastrointestinal nematode infections in calves. *Veterinary Parasitology* 76, 81–94. DOI: 10.1016/S0304-4017(97)00211-2.

FDA (2023) Green Book Reports: Active Ingredients. Available at: www.fda.gov/animal-veterinary/produc ts/approved-animal-drug-products-green-book (accessed 15 July 2025).

Fox, M.T. (1993) Pathophysiology of infection with *Ostertagia ostertagi* in cattle. *Veterinary Parasitology* 46, 143–158. DOI: 10.1016/0304-4017(93)90055-R.

Gallidis, E., Papadopoulos, E., Ptochos, S. and Arsenos, G. (2009) The use of targeted selective treatments against gastrointestinal nematodes in milking sheep and goats in Greece based on parasitological and performance criteria. *Veterinary Parasitology* 164, 53–58. DOI: 10.1016/j.vetpar.2009.04.011.

Gasbarre, L.C., Smith, L.L., Hoberg, E. and Pilitt, P. (2009) Further characterization of a cattle nematode population with demonstrated resistance to current anthelmintics. *Veterinary Parasitology* 166, 275–280. DOI: 10.1016/j.vetpar.2009.08.019.

Gasbarre, L.C., Ballweber, L.R., Stromberg, B.E., Dargatz, D., Rodriguez, J. *et al.* (2015) Effectiveness of current anthelmintic treatment programs on reducing fecal egg counts in United States cow-calf operations. *Canadian Journal of Veterinary Research* 79, 296–302.

Geary, T.G., Hosking, B.C., Skuce, P.J., von Samson-Himmelstjerna, G., Maeder, S. *et al.* (2012) World Association for the Advancement of Veterinary Parasitology (WAAVP) Guideline: Anthelmintic combination products targeting nematode infections of ruminants and horses. *Veterinary Parasitology* 190, 306–316. DOI: 10.1016/j.vetpar.2012.09.004.

Gianechini, L.S., Paras, K.L., George, M.M., Howell, S.B., Storey, B. *et al.* (2025) Corrigendum to "Multiple-species resistance to avermectin/milbemycin anthelmintics on beef cattle farms in Georgia, USA [*Vet. Parasitol.* 336 (2025) 110435]. *Vet Parasitol* 337:110494. Epub 2025 May 8. DOI: 10.1016/j.vetpar.2025.110494.

Gibbs, H. (1992) The effects of subclinical disease on bovine gastrointestinal nematodiasis. *Compendium on Continuing Education for the Practicing Veterinarian* 14, 669–677.

Gilleard, J.S. and Beech, R.N. (2007) Population genetics of anthelmintic resistance in parasitic nematodes. *Parasitology* 134, 1133–1147.

Greer, A.W., Van Wyk, J.A., Hamie, J.C., Byaruhanga, C. and Kenyon, F. (2020) Refugia-based strategies for parasite control in livestock. *Veterinary Clinics of North America Food Animal Practice* 36, 31–43. DOI: 10.1016/j.cvfa.2019.11.003.

Hildreth, M.B. and McKenzie, J.B. (2020) Epidemiology and control of gastrointestinal nematodes of cattle in northern climates. *Veterinary Clinics of North America Food Animal Practice* 36, 59–71. DOI: 10.1016/j.cvfa.2019.11.008.

Höglund, J., Morrison, D.A., Charlier, J., Dimander, S. and Larsson, A. (2009) Assessing the feasibility of targeted selective treatments for gastrointestinal nematodes in first-season grazing cattle based on mid-season daily weight gains. *Veterinary Parasitology* 164, 80–88. DOI: 10.1016/j.vetpar.2009.04.016.

Höglund, J., Dahlstrom, F., Sollenberg, S. and Hessle, A. (2013) Weight gain-based targeted selective treatments (TST) of gastrointestinal nematodes in first-season grazing cattle. *Veterinary Parasitology* 196, 358–365. DOI: 10.1016/j.vetpar.2013.03.028.

Kaplan, R.M. (2004) Drug resistance in nematodes of veterinary importance: A status report. *Trends in Parasitology* 20, 477–481. DOI: 10.1016/j.pt.2004.08.001.

Kaplan, R.M. (2020) Biology, epidemiology, diagnosis, and management of anthelmintic resistance in gastrointestinal nematodes of livestock. *Veterinary Clinics of North America Food Animal Practice* 36, 17–30. DOI: 10.1016/j.cvfa.2019.12.001.

Kaplan, R.M. and Vidyashankar, A.N. (2012) An inconvenient truth: Global worming and anthelmintic resistance. *Veterinary Parasitology* 186, 70–78. DOI: 10.1016/j.vetpar.2011.11.048.

Kaplan, R.M., Denwood, M.J., Nielsen, M.K., Thamsborg, S., Torgerson, P. *et al.* (2023) World Association for the Advancement of Veterinary Parasitology (W.A.A.V.P.) guideline for diagnosing anthelmintic resistance using the faecal egg count reduction test in ruminants, horses and swine. *Veterinary Parasitology* 318, 109936. DOI: 10.1016/j.vetpar.2023.109936.

Kenyon, F., Mcbean, D., Greer, A.W., Burgess, C., Morrison, A. *et al.* (2013) A comparative study of the effects of four treatment regimes on ivermectin efficacy, body weight and pasture contamination in lambs naturally infected with gastrointestinal nematodes in Scotland. *International Journal for Parasitology Drugs and Drug Resistance* 3, 77–84. DOI: 10.1016/j.ijpddr.2013.02.001.

Kipp, K., Cummings, D.B., Goehl, D., Wade, H., Davidson, J. *et al.* (2023) Evaluation of a refugia-based strategy for gastrointestinal nematodes on weight gain and fecal egg counts in naturally infected stocker calves administered combination anthelmintics. *Veterinary Parasitology* 319, 109955. DOI: 10.1016/j.vetpar.2023.109955.

Leathwick, D.M. (2007) Refugia – why, how and how much? proceedings of the 38th seminar, society of sheep and beef cattle veterinarians. *New Zealand Veterinary Association* 85–91.

Leathwick, D.M. (2012) Modelling the benefits of a new class of anthelmintic in combination. *Veterinary Parasitology* 186, 93–100. DOI: 10.1016/j.vetpar.2011.11.050.

Lawrence, K.E., Rhodes, A.P., Jackson, R., Leathwick, D., Heuer, C. *et al.* (2006) Farm management practices associated with macrocyclic lactone resistance on sheep farms in New Zealand. *New Zealand Veterinary Journal* 54, 283–288. DOI: 10.1080/00480169.2006.36712.

Leathwick, D.M., Vlassoff, A. and Barlow, N.D. (1995) A model for nematodiasis in New Zealand lambs: The effect of drenching regime and grazing management on the development of anthelmintic resistance. *International Journal for Parasitology* 25, 1479–1490. DOI: 10.1016/0020-7519(95)00059-3.

Leathwick, D.M., Miller, C.M., Atkinson, D.S., Haack, N., Waghorn, T. *et al.* (2008) Managing anthelmintic resistance: Untreated adult ewes as a source of unselected parasites, and their role in reducing parasite populations. *New Zealand Veterinary Journal* 56, 184–195. DOI: 10.1080/00480169.2008.36832.

Leathwick, D.M., Miller, C.M., Atkinson, D.S., Haack, N., Alexander, A. *et al.* (2006) Drenching adult ewes: Implications of anthelmintic treatments pre- and post-lambing on the development of anthelmintic resistance. *New Zealand Veterinary Journal* 54, 297–304. DOI: 10.1080/00480169.2006.36714.

Leathwick, D.M., Waghorn, T.S., Miller, C.M., Candy, P. and Oliver, A. (2012) Managing anthelmintic resistance--use of a combination anthelmintic and leaving some lambs untreated to slow the development of resistance to ivermectin. *Veterinary Parasitology* 187, 285–294. DOI: 10.1016/j.vetpar.2011.12.021.

McAnulty, R.W., Gibbs, S.J. and Greer, A.W. (2011) Liveweight gain of grazing dairy calves in their first season subjected to a targeted selective anthelmintic treatment (TST) regime. In: *Proceedings of the New Zealand Society of Animal Production*. Available at: www.nzsap.org/system/files/proceedings/2011/ab11068.pdf (accessed 15 July 2025).

McArthur, M.J. and Reinemeyer, C.R. (2014) Herding the U.S. cattle industry toward a paradigm shift in parasite control. *Veterinary Parasitology* 204, 34–43. DOI: 10.1016/j.vetpar.2013.12.021.

McBean, D., Nath, M., Lambe, N., Morgan-Davies, C. and Kenyon, F. (2016) Viability of the happy factor™ targeted selective treatment approach on several sheep farms in Scotland. *Veterinary Parasitology* 218, 22–30. DOI: 10.1016/j.vetpar.2016.01.008.

Michel, J.F. (1963) The phenomena of host resistance and the course of infection of *Ostertagia ostertagi* in calves. *Parasitology* 53, 63–84. DOI: 10.1017/S0031182000072541.

Miller, C.M., Waghorn, T.S., Leathwick, D.M., Candy, P., Oliver, A. *et al.* (2012) The production cost of anthelmintic resistance in lambs. *Veterinary Parasitology* 186, 376–381. DOI: 10.1016/j.vetpar.2011.11.063.

Myers, G.H. and Taylor, R.F. (1989) Ostertagiasis in cattle. *Journal of Veterinary Diagnosis Investigation* 1, 195–200. DOI: 10.1177/104063878900100225.

Navarre, C.B. (2020) Epidemiology and control of gastrointestinal nematodes of cattle in southern climates. *Veterinary Clinics of North America Food Animal Practice* 36, 45–57. DOI: 10.1016/j.cvfa.2019.11.006.

Nisbet, A., Meeusen, E., González, J. and Piedrafita, D. (2016) Immunity to *Haemonchus contortus* and vaccine development. *Advances in Parasitology* 93, 353–396. DOI: 10.1016/bs.apar.2016.02.011.

O'Shaughnessy, J., Earley, B., Mee, J.F., Doherty, M., Crosson, P. *et al.* (2014) Nematode control in spring-born suckler beef calves using targeted selective anthelmintic treatments. *Veterinary Parasitology* 205, 150–157. DOI: 10.1016/j.vetpar.2014.07.009.

O'Shaughnessy, J., Earley, B., Mee, J.F., Doherty, M., Crosson, P. *et al.* (2015a) Controlling nematodes in dairy calves using targeted selective treatments. *Veterinary Parasitology* 209, 221–228. DOI: 10.1016/j.vetpar.2015.02.024.

O'Shaughnessy, J., Earley, B., Mee, J.F., Doherty, M., Crosson, P. *et al.* (2015b) Nematode control in suckler beef cattle over their first two grazing seasons using a targeted selective treatment approach. *Irish Veterinary Journal* 68, 13. DOI: 10.1186/s13620-015-0038-1.

O'Sullivan, B.M. and Donald, A.D. (1970) A field study of nematode parasite populations in the lactating ewe. *Parasitology* 61, 301–315. DOI: 10.1017/s0031182000041135.

Ploeger, H.W., Schoenmaker, G.J.W., Kloosterman, A. and Borgsteede, F. (1989) Effect of anthelmintic treatment of dairy cattle on milk production related to some parameters estimating nematode infection. *Veterinary Parasitology* 34, 239–253. DOI: 10.1016/0304-4017(89)90054-X.

Prichard, R.K. (2005) Is anthelmintic resistance a concern for heartworm control? What can we learn from the human filariasis control programs. *Veterinary Parasitology* 133, 243–253. DOI: 10.1016/j.vetpar.2005.04.008.

Ramos, F., Portella, L.P., Rodrigues, F.S., Reginato, C., Potter, L. *et al.* (2016) Anthelmintic resistance in gastrointestinal nematodes of beef cattle in the state of Rio Grande do Sul, Brazil. *International Journal for Parasitology Drugs and Drug Resistance* 6, 93–101. DOI: 10.1016/j.ijpddr.2016.02.002.

Rendell, D.K. (2010) Anthelmintic resistance in cattle nematodes on 13 south-west Victorian properties. *Australian Veterinary Journal* 88, 504–509. DOI: 10.1111/j.1751-0813.2010.00648.x.

Rose Vineer, H., Morgan, E.R., Hertzberg, H., Bartley, D., Bosco, A. *et al.* (2020) Increasing importance of anthelmintic resistance in European livestock: Creation and meta-analysis of an open database. *Parasite* 27, 69. DOI: 10.1051/parasite/2020062.

Sanchez, J., Dohoo, I., Carrier, J. and DesCoteaux, L. (2004) A meta-analysis of the milk-production response after anthelmintic treatment in naturally infected adult dairy cows. *Preventive Veterinary Medicine* 63, 237–256. DOI: 10.1016/j.prevetmed.2004.01.006.

Smith, G. (1990) A mathematical model for the evolutions of anthelmintic resistance in a direct life cycle nematode parasite. *International Journal for Parasitology* 20, 913–921. DOI: 10.1016/0020-7519(90)90030-q.

Soutello, R.G., Seno, M.C. and Amarante, A.F. (2007) Anthelmintic resistance in cattle nematodes in northwestern São Paulo State, Brazil. *Veterinary Parasitology* 148, 360–364. DOI: 10.1016/j.vetpar.2007.06.023.

Stear, M., Bishop, S., Henderson, N. and Scott, I. (2003) A key mechanism of pathogenesis in sheep infected with the nematode *Teladorsagia circumcincta*. *Animal Health Research Review* 4, 45–52. DOI: 10.1079/AHRR200351.

Stromberg, B.E., Gasbarre, L.C., Waite, A., Bechtol, D., Brown, M. *et al.* (2012) *Cooperia punctata*: Effect on cattle productivity. *Veterinary Parasitology* 183, 284–291. DOI: 10.1016/j.vetpar.2011.07.030.

Suarez, V.H. and Cristel, S.L. (2007) Anthelmintic resistance in cattle nematode in the western Pampeana Region of Argentina. *Veterinary Parasitology* 144, 111–117. DOI: 10.1016/j.vetpar.2006.09.016.

Sykes, A.R. (1994) Parasitism and production in farm animals. *Animal Production* 59, 155–172. DOI: 10.1017/S0003356100007649.

Sykes, A.R. and Greer, A.W. (2003) Effects of parasitism on the nutrient economy of sheep: An overview. *Australian Journal of Experimantal Agriculture* 43, 1393–1398. DOI: 10.1071/EA02228.

Taylor, E.L. (1935) Seasonal fluctuation in the number of eggs of trichostrongylid worms in the faeces of ewes. *Journal of Parasitology* 21, 175–179. DOI: 10.2307/3271470.

Toledo, M.G., Porcel, J.O., Peris, J.C. and Munoz, M. (2019) *Atlas of Parasitic Diseases in Ruminants: A Diagnostic Tool for the Identification of Parasites and the Lesions They Cause.* Boehringer Ingelheim Vetmedica, Ingelheim am Rhein, Germany.

USDA (2020) Beef 2017. Beef Cow-calf Management Practices in the United States. Report 1. USDA–APHIS–VS–CEAH–NAHMS, Fort Collins, CO. Available at. Available at: www.aphis.usda.gov/sites/default/files/beef2017_dr_partl.pdf (accessed 15 July 2025).

Van Wyk, J.A. (2001) Refugia-overlooked as perhaps the most potent factor concerning the development of anthelmintic resistance. *Onderstepoort Journal of Veterinary Research* 68(1), 55–67.

Van Wyk, J.A. and Bath, G.F. (2002) The FAMACHA© system for managing haemonchosis in sheep and goats by clinically identifying individual animals for treatment. *Veterinary Research* 33, 509–529. DOI: 10.1051/vetres:2002036.

Veglia, F. (1915) Anatomy and Life-History of the *Haemonchus contortus* (Rud.). Third and Fourth Reports of the Director of Veterinary Research. Available at: https://repository.up.ac.za/items/1b34d373-902f-451d-84c6-891d48ce86ed (accessed 15 July 2025).

Vercruysse, J. and Claerebout, E. (1997) Immunity development against *Ostertagia ostertagi* and other gastrointestinal nematodes in cattle. *Veterinary Parasitology* 72, 309–316. DOI: 10.1016/S0304-4017(97)00103-9.

Waghorn, T., Miller, C., Oliver, A.-M. and Leathwick, D. (2009) Drench-and-shift is a high-risk practice in the absence of refugia. *New Zealand Veterinary Journal* 57, 359–363. DOI: 10.1080/00480169.2009.64723.

Waghorn, T.S., Miller, C.M. and Leathwick, D.M. (2016) Confirmation of ivermectin resistance in *Ostertagia ostertagi* in cattle in New Zealand. *Veterinary Parasitology* 229, 139–143.   DOI: 10.1016/j.vetpar.2016.10.011.

Walker, J.G., Ofithile, M., Tavolaro, F.M., van Wyk, J., Evans, K. *et al.* (2015) Mixed methods evaluation of targeted selective anthelmintic treatment by resource-poor smallholder goat farmers in Botswana. *Veterinary Parasitology* 214, 80–88. DOI: 10.1016/j.vetpar.2015.10.006.

Waghorn, T.S., Leathwick, D.M., Rhodes, A.P., Jackson, R., Pomroy, W. *et al.* (2006) Prevalence of anthelmintic resistance on 62 beef cattle farms in the North Island of New Zealand. *New Zealand Veterinary Journal* 54, 278–282. DOI: 10.1080/00480169.2006.36711.

Waller, P.J., Rudby-Martin, L., Ljungström, B.L. and Rydzik, A. (2004) The epidemiology of abomasal nematodes of sheep in Sweden, with particular reference to over-winter survival strategies. *Veterinary Parasitology* 122, 207–220. DOI: 10.1016/j.vetpar.2004.04.007.

Wang, T., Avramenko, R.W., Redman, E.M., Wit, J., Gilleard, J. *et al.* (2020) High levels of third-stage larvae (L3) overwinter survival for multiple cattle gastrointestinal nematode species on western Canadian pastures as revealed by ITS2 rDNA metabarcoding. *Parasites and Vectors* 13, 458. DOI: 10.1186/s13071-020-04337-2.

10 The Role of Extension in Gastrointestinal Nematode Control and Management

Niki C. Whitley[1]* and Kwame Matthews[2]

[1]*Department of Agricultural Sciences, Cooperative Extension, Fort Valley State University, Fort Valley, Georgia, USA; [2]Department of Agriculture & Natural Resources, Delaware State University, Dover, Delaware, USA*

Abstract

Personnel from Land-Grant University Cooperative Extension programs collaborate with researchers, veterinarians, and other outreach organizations, providing information about client needs for research, conducting applied research and demonstration, and translating results of research into practical recommendations and resources for those clients. For small ruminant producers, the primary needs are related to methods for controlling gastrointestinal nematodes, the worst of which, the blood-sucking *Haemonchus contortus*, exhibits a growing resistance to commercially available deworming drugs. Tools developed from Cooperative Extension collaborations (nationally and internationally) and by other outreach organizations to address this issue include websites with educational materials including training manuals, presentation slide sets, factsheets, infographics, newsletters, blogs, webinars, and videos as well as events such as in-person workshops, field days and seminars, ram and buck performance testing demonstrations, social media platforms, and more.

Introduction

In 1862, the Morrill Act established land-grant colleges and universities which provide teaching, research, and educational outreach to the public. In 1914, the Smith-Lever Act formalized Cooperative Extension (Extension) by establishing a partnership between land-grant colleges and the US Department of Agriculture (USDA NIFA, 2023) to provide a nationwide, informal educational network that brings the research and knowledge of the land-grant university to people in their homes and on their farms. The Extension partnership is facilitated through approximately 2900 county Extension offices and 105 land-grant colleges and universities.

Cooperative Extension serves a more diverse audience and operates with fewer resources than it has in the past, but it still plays a vital role in improving the efficiency of agricultural production. Administered through the state universities and funded through financing by county/parish, state, and federal collaboration, Extension continues to serve the educational needs of the public, including those of small ruminant producers. Recognizing its continued importance, many federal grant programs now require an extension (outreach) component.

*Corresponding author: whitleyn@fvsu.edu

© CAB International 2026. *Management Practices for Controlling Nematode Parasites of Small Ruminants* (eds James E. Miller and Joan M. Burke)
DOI: 10.1079/9781800623767.0010

Need for Extension

Extension programs play a key role in agriculture by providing farmers and other individuals from rural and urban communities with nonformal education and technical assistance to improve farming practices, production, and quality of life. In general, Extension personnel utilize information gained from new developments in research and educational methods to help agricultural and nonagricultural individuals create a positive change in their farming practices, consumption, nutritional understanding, and/or farm business practices. The demand for small ruminant products such as meat, fiber, and milk products, including soap/lotion, and eco-services is still strong in the United States. This demand and the perception of small ruminant enterprises as attractive, affordable, and profitable results in an increased need for individuals with knowledge in small ruminant production to assist those attempting to enter or stay in the small ruminant industry.

Shortages in livestock veterinarians (Weltzein, 2023) and existing large animal/food animal veterinary practices' lack of interest or training related to small ruminants further support the need for well-trained Cooperative Extension personnel and their collaborators to assist small ruminant producers. Though non-veterinarian Extension staff cannot legally diagnose and suggest treatments, especially those that are not labeled for the species or doses in question, they are critical for relaying research-based information from veterinarians that would allow producers to diagnose and treat their own animals. They can also provide small ruminant parasite control resources for producers to share with their veterinarians. Along with shortages in veterinarians, funding issues in some states may also limit Extension personnel, and resources available and competition with social media and other nonresearch-based informational outlets provide challenges to the small ruminant industry. Therefore, collaborations among Extension staff and veterinarians (among others) to help producers combat the issue of gastrointestinal nematode (GIN) infections that have led to major production losses and increased mortality in many herds/flocks are even more imperative.

Parasite Problem

According to a 2015 USDA Animal and Plant Health Inspection Service (USDA APHIS) report, 25% of all nonpredator death losses in goat kids on farms with less than 100 goats was caused by internal parasites and other digestive disorders (USDA APHIS, 2017). Additionally, 15.7% of all nonpredator death losses in sheep and lamb production was caused by internal parasites (USDA APHIS, 2022). The major GINs that affect these small ruminants are *Haemonchus contortus*, *Trichostrongylus* spp., *Teladorsagia circumcincta*, *Oesophagostomum* spp., *Nematodirus* spp., *Trichuris ovis*, *Bunostomum* spp., *Strongyloides papillosus*, and *Cooperia* spp. (Kaplan, 2013). The most problematic of these GINs is the blood-sucking abomasal parasite *Haemonchus contortus* (Zajac, 2006), the barber pole worm, which has developed extensive resistance to anthelmintics (deworming drugs). The size of the issue of dewormer-resistant GINs in small ruminants paired with the lack of qualified local veterinarians willing and/or able to treat these species, and the preponderance of online misinformation, exacerbates the need for collaboration of Cooperative Extension personnel with veterinarians, researchers, and other organizations such as producer groups, industry organizations, and agricultural educational groups to help address the problem.

Recognizing the importance of the widespread emergence of dewormer-resistant worms, the American Consortium for Small Ruminant Parasite Control (Consortium) was established in 2003. This group of veterinarians/veterinary parasitologists, animal and plant scientists, Cooperative Extension personnel, and members of other outreach organizations began a collaboration focused on helping small ruminant producers manage internal parasites on their farms.

Extension Efforts

Extension efforts by the Consortium and many others nationally and internationally related to small ruminant parasite control include developing and maintaining websites or webpages, conducting and/or translating results from practical research and demonstration projects, providing education and training sessions both in person and online, developing train-the-trainer materials in print and electronic/online formats, providing parasite-related factsheets, newsletters, webinars, videos, and in-person workshops, field days and seminars, and establishing ram/buck genetic selection tests with focus areas including parasite resistance, among others.

The work of Extension is often international in scope as livestock production issues, especially those related to small ruminant parasite control, are found worldwide. For example, along with efforts of Consortium members from South Africa who have worked across the African continent, Consortium Extension, outreach and research personnel have exchanged small ruminant education and/or resources with countries including Brazil, Australia, New Zealand, China, Japan, Mexico, Egypt, Hungary, France, El Salvador, Guatemala, Poland, Nepal, Bangladesh, Jordan, Iran, Afghanistan, Russia, Dominican Republic, Costa Rica, Scotland, Austria, Switzerland, Germany, Britain and several Caribbean islands, among many others.

Websites

Disseminating research-based recommendations to get information to small ruminant producers in a timely manner is the goal of many websites supporting the industry. The Consortium developed a website in 2004 to provide up-to-date information to stakeholders. The website (www.wormx.info) was upgraded in 2012 by Consortium member Susan Schoenian, University of Maryland Extension, but moved to Louisiana State University in January of 2025 with Consortium member Dr. Sanjok Poudel at North Carolina A&T State University serving as webmaster. According to the free version of UberSuggest™ (an online service that estimates site views externally), organic/nonpaid traffic for the site was 53,650 for 2024 (up from 44,993 users in 2019). Most of the users were from the US, with 83.8% viewing in English and another 7.9% viewing in Spanish. Non-US countries with the most user numbers included the UK, Australia, and Canada.

The Consortium website includes information in a variety of formats that can be widely accessed by producers, trainers, veterinarians, and others worldwide. Educational articles like 'Timely Topics' provide the latest information on parasite management and research. Factsheets such as the 'Best Management Practices' series provide detailed information developed through collaborative efforts on the part of the Consortium on topics related to alternatives or supplements to effective chemical dewormers (sericea lespedeza, copper oxide wire particles, and nematophagus fungi), proper dewormer use to delay resistance, genetic selection, supportive therapies, and more. The website provides links to recorded webinars, videos, and podcasts created by Extension and research personnel, among others, to lend practical advice for GIN control in an alternative (to text) format. Short infographics offer a simplified presentation format for targeted parasite management topics. A subset of different types of the educational resources on the site have also been translated into Spanish (wormx.info/enespanol).

Backlinks to and from the wormx.info site include those from other websites providing educational outreach for small ruminant GIN control. Australia's paraboss site (paraboss.com.au) is a premier source of internal and external parasite control information (wormboss, flyboss, liceboss, tickboss). Developed through a collaboration of Meat & Livestock Australia (MLA), Australian Wool Innovation (AWI), and the University of New England (UNE), it is managed and implemented by UNE. The site provides an abundance of information, including control programs designed to improve adoption of best management practices for control of internal and external parasites for the Australian sheep, goat, and cattle industries. Designed to decrease losses from productivity, market access, and animal welfare issues, the site provides vital information that is relevant to small ruminant producers in other countries as well.

The website for the Action from the European Cooperation in Science and Technology (COST) organization known as 'combatting anthelmintic resistance in ruminants' (COMBAR; www.combar-ca.eu) highlights its work to research and disseminate results and recommendations related to small ruminant GIN control. The group of parasitologists, social scientists, agricultural economists, and others focuses on research and information dissemination in the area of GIN diagnostics, vaccines, selective treatment stragies, bioactive forages, and decision support tools. A unique aspect of the COMBAR work is the inclusion of the study of socioeconomic/behavioral factors impacting GIN control methodologies. Extension personnel in the US also use surveys, focus groups, and individual interactions with producers to determine producer needs and impacts of programming efforts to meet those needs.

Another program with an associated website (scops.org.uk) is offered through SCOPS (Sustainable Control of Parasites in Sheep) in the UK, a voluntary, industry-led group supporting the sheep industry. New Zealand has Wormwise, a program developed by a farmer-owned organization, Beef + Lamb New Zealand, and available through their website (beeflambnz.com/wormwise). The University of Rhode Island has a webpage entitled 'Northeast Small Ruminant Parasite Control' (web.uri.edu/sheepngoat) that provides information on their research and educational materials. This site hosts the first approved online FAMACHA© integrated parasite control training that results in certification and attainment of a FAMACHA© card, videos for that training as well as for fecal egg counting, and factsheets/other educational tools related to GIN control in small ruminants.

Cornell University's Small Ruminant Parasite Research page provides research and outreach resources for educators and producers for goat and sheep GIN control (https://blogs.cornell.edu/smallruminantparasites/). The Maryland Small Ruminant Page website provides a wide variety of small ruminant educational resources, including those on GIN control, providing links to multiple educational materials on the topic in different formats (www.sheepandgoat.com/). The Appropriate Technology Transfer for Rural Areas (ATTRA)/National Center for Appropriate Technology (NCAT) website provides resources, including printable materials, blogs, videos, and podcasts, on many topics for sustainable agriculture, including over 70 publication search results of 'parasites' with at least 33 related to sheep and goat production (https://attra.ncat.org/about/). Many other sites, including the Consortium's and the Maryland Small Ruminant Page, link to ATTRA publications.

Land-grant university Extension websites with small ruminant programs, including most of the 1890 Historically Black Land-Grants, will provide GIN control-related information, including links to programs and notices of events such as workshops, field days, webinars, and more. Many more university or even local county office Extension sites have general small ruminant or sheep and/or goat pages with resources to download or view along with links to outside materials, some of which are related to parasite management (internal and external).

Along with these traditional websites, social media sites are popular among many small ruminant producers, so several of the organizations previously mentioned also have social media networking accounts through which they provide information. Social media sites/posts from producers and organizations using anecdotal information without a peer-reviewed research foundation should be carefully screened for validity.

Applied research and demonstration projects

Collaborative research and demonstration projects have been conducted by Extension personnel and researchers throughout the US, including members of the Consortium, to find the most effective ways to help producers manage GIN infection. During this process, for *H. contortus* in the US, research found farms with multiple-anthelmintic resistance and even total anthelmintic failure (Mortensen *et al.*, 2003; Howell *et al.*, 2008; Crook *et al.*, 2016; Schoenian *et al.*, 2019).

Prompted by this information, small ruminant Extension specialists, county Extension agents, researchers, and others have worked together to investigate alternative methods for GIN control. Although many possible alternative or natural dewormers, essential oils, and/or plants and plant products have been tested (i.e. herbal dewormers, pumpkin seeds, garlic, ginger, papaya seeds, cranberry vines, cowpea, sainfoin, sulla, sericea lespedeza, and big and birdsfoot trefoil; Burke and Miller, 2009; Burke *et al.*, 2009a, b; Strickland *et al.*, 2009; Matthews *et al.*, 2016; Worku *et al.*, 2018; Barone *et al.*, 2018), the most effective supplemental dewormers presented to farmers by the Consortium are the use of copper oxide wire particles, nematode-trapping fungi, and forages containing condensed tannin (particularly sericea lespedeza) (Burke and Miller, 2009; Terrill *et al.*, 2012). Recommendations to small ruminant producers also arose from on-farm research with producers in collaboration with the National Sheep Improvement Program to develop estimated breeding values (EBV) for specific sheep breeds (and for goats) that can be used for genetic selection to assist in GIN management (reviewed in Burke and Miller, 2009).

Reviews of related research also show that good nutrition, pasture and grazing management such as rotational grazing and multispecies grazing, and use of resistant breeds (Burke and Miller, 2009; Terrill *et al.*, 2012) are additional tools small ruminant producers should use to manage GIN on their farms. Research and demonstration projects at university facilities as well as on producer farms result in research data collection while providing information and resources to farmers. Projects currently under way that combine research and extension efforts for farmers are designed to develop new technologies for use in GIN control using bioelectrical impedance analysis (BIA) and radiofrequency (RF) measurements to determine if they can be used to more quickly determine when animals are parasitized. New mobile applications (apps) are also being researched to determine if mobile devices could be used to determine the need for deworming, which would reduce subjectivity associated with FAMACHA©. In addition, studies in genomics with the goal of eventually being able to conduct a simple DNA test for genetic resistance to parasites also seek to make GIN control easier for farmers.

Collaborative grant writing among universities as well as among diverse personnel from research and extension arms within the land-grant university system has supported both research and outreach/demonstration efforts such as the Western Maryland Pasture-Based Meat Goat Performance Test. This was the first pasture-based meat goat buck performance test to include GIN measures. The test ran from 2006 to 2016 and was incredibly popular, with 639 goats from 84 herds in 20 states being evaluated (www.slideshare.net/schoenian/ 10-years-of-buck-test). As is typically found for livestock peformance tests, the University of

Maryland Extension buck test provided genetic selection opportunities for consigning farms as well as for buyers based on animal resistance to parasite infection, but also provided a demonstration of best management practices for GIN control in small ruminants. In addition, unique to this test for the most part, projects were also included that looked at impacts of combination dewormers and by-product feed supplementation among others. For more information see: www.sheepandgoat.com/goattest.

Eastern Oklahoma State College also had a forage-based goat buck test from 2013 to 2023 and Langston University (OK) ran a buck performance test from 2000 to 2009. The Kerr Center in Oklahoma (2007–2011), and Fort Valley State University in Georgia also hosted buck tests in which fecal egg counts were provided for estimates of parasitism in the animals. Current buck or ram performance tests with a GIN component (typically fecal egg counts measured) include the Virginia Tech/Southwest Agricultural Research and Extension Center pasture-based ram test (since 2012), West Virginia University buck test (since 2016), Mississippi State University/ Southeast Buck Performance Test (since 2023), Pennsylvania Department of Agriculture/Penn State University buck and ram performance tests, and, most recently (started 2023), the University of Florida buck test. The University of Florida forage-based test measured fecal egg counts as well as FAMACHA© eyelid color scores as a measure of parasitism.

Information from research and demonstration efforts as described above is incorporated into educational materials by Cooperative Extension and other outreach organization personnel for training agricultural professionals and veterinarians as well as livestock producers.

Educational materials

Along with the website (2004), early efforts of the Consortium related to extension/outreach included work to consolidate research-based information related to GIN issues and dewormer resistance in small ruminant GIN. Collaborative work funded by the USDA southern region Sustainable Agriculture Research and Education (SARE) program in 2006 (ES06-084) resulted in the development of a research-based train-the-trainer program with a resource manual in print and portable electronic form (also posted to the website). These educational materials focused on the use of integrated parasite management (IPM), including the FAMACHA© eyelid color scoring sytem which was brought to the US in 2003 from South Africa to determine the need for deworming small ruminants. As new research provides information, the FAMACHA©/IPM materials are updated and new materials developed. Recently, in response to a decrease in the number of Extension specialists in most states and fewer researchers working in small ruminants and able to conduct training, a FAMACHA© trainer certification program was developed to expand the number of trainers providing this critical information to producers. The Consortium website hosts the trainer certification program materials as well as a list of certified trainers and opportunities for producer FAMACHA© certification. Access to the FAMACHA© eyelid color scoring cards is strictly regulated through members of the Consortium. For more information, contact famacha@lsu.edu.

Extension personnel at universities and local or regional offices as well as other outreach organizations write grants to conduct research and provide educational resources on many topics, including small ruminant GINs. For example, through USDA NIFA Beginning Farmer Rancher Development Program grant funding, the University of Georgia developed a Journeyman Farmer Program curriculum consisting of PowerPoint presentations and associated webinar type videos, trainer facilitator's guides, and farmer activity manuals for Extension educators. It provides resources for small business training for farmers and a small ruminant production track that includes FAMACHA© integrated training and certification. Regularly scheduled Master Goat, Master Small Ruminant, and similar programs (in-person and/or online formats) are conducted by many Extension or other outreach organizations, including those by University of Georgia, Tuskegee University, University of Tennessee, ATTRA/NCAT, Southern University Ag Center, Oklahoma State University (Goat Boot Camp), and the Kentucky Sheep & Goat Development Office. Many others have hosted individual

programs of this type over the years. Because GINs are the number one health problem for goats and sheep for many producers, any comprehensive small ruminant production program such as Master Goat and Master Small Ruminant will have sessions involving GIN management.

Educational events

Over the years, Extension personnel have spent a significant amount of time planning and executing workshops, short courses, seminars, field days, and webinar series geared towards helping producers control GIN infection on their farm. Several events were mentioned in the previous section because the program is online or the information provided during those events is converted into educational materials. Due to its importance in GIN control, most events include GIN control education, including FAMACHA©.

The FAMACHA© eyelid color scoring system for estimation of anemia is one of the most prominent and successful indicators used to identify small ruminants with *H. contortus* infections (Van Wyk and Bath, 2002; Flay *et al.*, 2022). It is included in the subsequent Five Point Check© decision-making tool (Bath and van Wyk, 2009) along with other indicators of GIN infection such as body condition score, submandibular edema (bottle jaw), fecal soiling, body condition, and more. Extension personnel (and others) use these training events, which are preferentially held in person, to educate farmers on the major GINs that affect small ruminants, the major classes of anthelmintic treatments and parasite resistance to those treatments, the best methods of avoiding GIN infection and treating parasitized animals, nondrug management methods, and the FAMACHA© technique. As of September, 2025, there were 152 certified FAMACHA© instructors in 36 of the 50 states in the US (wormx.info/instructors), with the majority of the instructors having an Extension role. Additionally, because there are still areas in which trainers are not available, online FAMACHA©/IPM training and certification programs were developed and are available at the Consortium website, including a Spanish-translated version developed by the University of Rhode Island.

The FAMACHA©/IPM training is beneficial to producers as it is affordable and effective in limiting the costs (Leask *et al.*, 2013) associated with consistent use of anthelmintics as well as limiting the increase of anthelmintic resistance on farms. In a 2014 publication of the impacts of prior years' FAMACHA© training, 95.1% of the participants responding to a survey agreed that the training made a difference in their ability to control and monitor GIN infection in their herd or flock. Nearly all (96.3%) respondents reported that they employed IPM practices they learned to control GIN, with the most popular being rotational grazing (71.2%), genetic selection (i.e. using a parasite-resistant breed and/or removing susceptible animals from the breeding herd; 52.7%), supplementation with grain to improve nutrition (44.0%), and managing the height of plants grazed (41.8%).

Other relevant Extension work includes events such as the Small Ruminant All Worms All Day Conference which included Extension specialists and county educators from four different states (MD, DE, VA, GA) conducting an in-person 3-year annual workshop starting in 2017. The conference offered presentations on many of the topics covered in FAMACHA©/IPM workshops, plus a presentation on common myths that Extension personnel work hard to dispel related to GIN control that can negatively impact animal health and performance.

Although many Extension programs were using webinars before COVID, the pandemic boosted the popularity of Extension/outreach webinars. Several GIN control-related webinars were conducted during that time (and since), including a collaborative Weekly Worm Webinar series created to address the periparturient egg rise, fecal egg counting parameters, the barber pole worm, the use of BioWorma®, grazing away parasites, deworming, tips for what to do when deworming is not enough, and selection for worm-resistant animals. As is common in Extension programming, the webinars were turned into educational videos (available at sheepandgoat.com/webinars) and many of the topics were also converted into written materials and posted on the wormx.info website for use by Extension and other outreach programs/personnel and producers nationally and internationally. Another example is the 2022 and 2024 University of Wisconsin Extension webinar series videos on YouTube™.

Conclusion

Extension plays a major role in assisting farmers and consumers by translating university-based research into a practical format. Working together with researchers, veterinarians, and other outreach agencies, Cooperative Extension and outreach organizations nationally and internationally are providing integrated parasite control education and support for small ruminant producers nationwide.

References

Barone, C.D., Zajac, A.M., Manzi-Smith, L.A., Howell, A., Reed, J. *et al.* (2018) Anthelmintic efficacy of cranberry vine extracts on ovine *Haemonchus contortus*. *Veterinary Parasitology* 253, 122–129.

Bath, G.F. and van Wyk, J.A. (2009) The Five Point Check© for targeted selective treatment of internal parasites in small ruminants. *Small Ruminant Research* 86, 6–13.

Burke, J.M. and Miller, J.E. (2009) Sustainable approaches to parasite control in ruminant livestock. *Veterinary Clinics of North America: Food Animal Practice* 36, 89–107.

Burke, J.M., Wells, A., Casey, P. and Kaplan, R. (2009a) Herbal dewormer fails to control gastrointestinal nematodes in goats. *Veterinary Parasitology* 160, 168–170.

Burke, J.M., Wells, A., Casey, P. and Miller, J. (2009b) Garlic and papaya lack control over gastrointestinal nematodes in goats and lambs. *Veterinary Parasitology* 159, 171–174.

Crook, E.K., O'Brien, D.J., Howell, S.B., Storey, B., Whitley, N. *et al.* (2016) Prevalence of anthelmintic resistance on sheep and goat farms in the mid-Atlantic region and comparison of *in vivo* and *in vitro* detection methods. *Small Ruminant Research* 143, 89–96.

Flay, K.J., Hill, F.I. and Hernandez Muguiro, D. (2022) A review: *Haemonchus contortus* infection in pasture-based sheep production systems, with a focus on the pathogenesis of anaemia and changes in haematological parameters. *Animals* 12(10), 1238.

Howell, S.B., Burke, J.M., Miller, J.E., Terrill, T., Valencia, E. *et al.* (2008) Prevalence of anthelmintic resistance on sheep and goat farms in the southeastern United States. *Journal of the American Veterinary Medicine Association* 233, 1913–1919.

Kaplan, R.M. (2013) Recommendations for control of gastrointestinal nematode parasites in small ruminants: These ain't your father's parasites. *Bovine Practitioner* 47, 97–109.

Leask, R., van Wyk, J.A., Thompson, P.N. and Bath, G. (2013) The effect of application of the FAMACHA© system on selected production parameters in sheep. *Small Ruminant Research* 110, 1–8.

Matthews, K.K., O'Brien, D.J., Whitley, N.C., Burke, J., Miller, J. *et al.* (2016) Investigation of possible pumpkin seeds and ginger effects on gastrointestinal nematode infection indicators in meat goat kids and lambs. *Small Ruminant Research* 136, 1–6.

Mortensen, L.L., Williamson, L.H., Terrill, T.H., Kircher, R., Larsen, M. *et al.* (2003) Evaluation of prevalence and clinical implications of anthelmintic resistance in gastrointestinal nematodes of goats. *Journal of the American Veterinary Medicine Association* 23, 495–500.

Schoenian, S., O'Brien, D. and Whitley, N. (2019) Determining anthelmintic resistance on sheep farms in the southeastern US. *Journal of the National Association of County Agricultural Agents*. Available at: www.nacaa.com/journal/06066564-af4f-416f-9a5a-41f69f09cc5f (accessed 16 July 2025).

Strickland, V.J., Krebs, G.L. and Potts, W. (2009) Pumpkin kernel and garlic as alternative treatments for the control of *Haemonchus contortus* in sheep. *Animal Production Science* 49, 139–144.

Terrill, T.H., Miller, J.E. and Burke, J.M. (2012) Experiences with integrated concepts for the control of *Haemonchus contortus* in sheep and goats in the United States. *Veterinary Parasitology* 186, 28–37.

USDA APHIS (2017) Goat and kid predator and nonpredator death loss in the United States, 2015. Available at: www.aphis.usda.gov/sites/default/files/goat_kid_deathloss_2015.pdf (accessed 16 July 2025).

USDA APHIS (2022) Death loss trends in the U.S. sheep industry: 1994–2019 sheep death loss study 2020. Available at: www.aphis.usda.gov/sites/default/files/sheep-death-loss-trends-us-2020.pdf (accessed 16 July 2025).

USDA NIFA (2023) History. Available at: www.nifa.usda.gov/about-nifa/who-we-are/history (accessed 16 July 2025).

Van Wyk, J.A. and Bath, G.F. (2002) The FAMACHA© system for managing haemonchosis in sheep and goats by clinically identifying individual animals for treatment. *Veterinary Research* 33, 509–529.

Weltzein, L.M. (2023) The livestock veterinarian shortage. Implications for food safety and security. Available at: https://clf.jhsph.edu/sites/default/files/2023-06/the-livestock-veterinarian-shortage.pdf (accessed 16 July 2025).

Worku, M., Adjei-Fremah, S., Whitley, N. and Jackai, L. (2018) Effect of cowpea (*Vigna unguiculata*) pasture grazing on growth, gastrointestinal parasite infection and immune response biomarkers of goats. *Journal of Agricultural Science* 10, 27–37.

Zajac, A.M. (2006) Gastrointestinal nematodes of small ruminants: Life cycle, anthelmintics, and diagnosis. *Veterinary Clinics of North America: Food Animal Practice* 22, 529–541.

Index